Water-soluble Vitamin Assays in Human Nutrition

Water-soluble Vitamin Assays in Human Nutrition

G.F.M. Ball

SPRINGER-SCIENCE+BUSINESS MEDIA, B.V.

First edition 1994

Typeset in Palatino 10/12 pt by Cambrian Typesetters, Frimley, Surrey

ISBN 978-0-412-58370-4 ISBN 978-1-4615-2061-0 (eBook)
DOI 10.1007/978-1-4615-2061-0

A catalogue record for this book is available from the British Library

Printed on permanent acid-free text paper, manufactured in accordance with ANSI/NISO Z39.48-1992 and ANSI/NISO Z39.48-1984 (Permanence of Paper).

Contents

Preface

The demand for rapid, accurate and reproducible analytical methods for the quantitative determination of vitamins in foods is growing, due to an increased consumption of processed and convenience foods for which nutritional data are lacking. Such methods are also needed for the quality control of manufacturing processes and to investigate rates of vitamin loss during handling, processing and storage. Existing food compositional data for natural products are unreliable for certain vitamins (notably B_6 and folate), owing to recently discovered problems with the assay methodology. In addition, new varieties of traditional food plants, including the cereal grains, have been introduced since the early analyses.

There are a number of factors which complicate the assessment of a food commodity or diet in terms of its value in providing vitamins in a form that can be assimilated and utilized by the consumer. All natural foods are derived from animal or plant products and are therefore subject to biological variation in vitamin content. The variation is further compounded by losses incurred during processing, storage and cooking, especially for the more labile vitamins. Many of the B-group vitamins are present in coenzyme and other bound forms, often at extremely low levels, in animal and plant tissues, and these bound forms are absorbed and utilized by the body to varying extents. The dietary significance of a food or diet is complicated by interaction of the vitamins with other nutrients, and especially by alcohol, during intestinal absorption. Physiological factors such as age and state of health further complicate the evaluation.

In the past, *in vitro* analytical methods have been developed to determine the total (potential) vitamin content of a food using the most rigorous extraction method commensurate with the stability of the vitamin. The data obtained have been used to compile food composition tables, which provide information about typical amounts of vitamin for raw and processed foods as measured by microbiological or physicochemical assay, but they do not evaluate the nutritional value of the food in terms of biological vitamin activity. The determination of total vitamin content is useful when animal growth assays are being carried out on the same test material, as it allows the bioavailability of a nutrient to be determined as a ratio of standardized biological activity to the total nutrient content. On its own, however, the total vitamin content can sometimes grossly overestimate the biologically active vitamin content. There is an increasing trend nowadays toward the estimation of biologically active vitamin, rather than total vitamin content, using *in vitro* methods with selective extraction techniques.

The purpose of this book is to survey current methodologies of determining the water-soluble vitamins in foods, with the theme of human nutrition very much in mind. This book has been published as a companion volume to an earlier book entitled *Fat-Soluble Vitamin Assays in Food Analysis. A Comprehensive Review*, G.F.M. Ball, Elsevier Applied Science, London and New York, 1988.

As to the scope of this book, the introductory chapter establishes the nutritional theme and introduces the concepts of biological activity and bioavailability. A detailed discussion of animal bioassays is beyond the scope of this book, since such assays are the province of specialized laboratories equipped with the personnel and facilities for their evaluation. Chapter 2 sets out to acquaint the reader with a brief account of the chemical and biological properties of thiamin, riboflavin, niacin, vitamin B_6, pantothenic acid, biotin, folate, vitamin B_{12} and vitamin C. Emphasis is placed upon the vitamins' chemical structures, including the various bound forms, their stabilities and their occurrence in natural materials. Chapter 3 sets the stage for the subsequent analytical chapters by defining the analytical objectives and summarizing the scope of current analytical techniques in determining the vitamins and related vitamers. Chapter 4 is entirely devoted to the extraction of the vitamins from the food matrix. The chemistry of the extraction process and the quantitative efficiency have a great influence upon the accuracy of an assay method, yet extraction methods are the least studied and least characterized component of vitamin assays. Chapters 5–8 present the basic principles of the various physicochemical, microbiological and biospecific techniques encountered in vitamin analysis and discuss the applications of these techniques by reference to representative published methods. In the concluding chapter the various techniques are appraised by reference to comparative studies.

Absorption and fluorescence spectra were kindly provided by A.C. Cowling.

For the preparation of the manuscript, I am indebted to Ruth Harrisson, proprietor of Action Desk.

G.F.M. Ball

Introduction 1

1.1 DEFINITION AND CLASSIFICATION OF VITAMINS

The vitamins comprise a diverse group of organic compounds required by animals in small amounts to ensure normal growth and maintenance of health. It is often stated that vitamins cannot be produced in the body and must, therefore, be supplied in the diet. However, this is not strictly true for certain vitamins: niacin can be synthesized *in vivo* from an amino acid precursor, tryptophan, and variable amounts of B-group vitamins may be produced by the microflora in the gut, although it is difficult to ascertain to what extent, if any, this endogenous source is available to the host. Generally speaking, vitamins are essential micronutrients because the animal cannot synthesize such compounds in amounts adequate for its daily needs. Plants have the ability to synthesize most of the vitamins and serve as primary sources of these dietary essentials. An insufficiency of a vitamin in the animal's diet, or its poor absorption from the digestive tract, frequently induces a disease with characteristic symptoms. More recently, marginal (subclinical) deficiency states have been reported, especially for vitamin B_6, folate and vitamin B_{12} (Counsell, 1988).

Vitamins may be classified, according to their solubility, into two groups: the fat-soluble vitamins (A, D, E and K) and the water-soluble vitamins (B group and C). This simple classification reflects to some extent the function of the vitamins, as the solubility affects their natural distribution in tissues and their physiological role therein.

The water-soluble vitamins discussed in this book are vitamin C and the members of the vitamin B group, namely thiamin (vitamin B_1), riboflavin (vitamin B_2), niacin, vitamin B_6, pantothenic acid, biotin, folate and vitamin B_{12}. For some of these vitamins, biological activity is attributed to a number of structurally related compounds known as vitamers, which exhibit varying degrees of biological activity or potency.

1.2 BIOCHEMICAL ROLE OF THE B-GROUP VITAMINS

Several of the B-group vitamins serve as precursors for enzyme cofactors that function in the catabolism of foodstuffs to produce energy for the organism. The dietary macronutrients – carbohydrates, lipids and proteins – are degraded in a three-stage process to liberate energy (Figure 1.1). The first step is digestion, during which the macronutrients are hydrolysed into their component substituents: carbohydrates to glucose and other monosaccharides, lipids to glycerol and fatty acids, and proteins to amino acids. In the second stage the monosaccharides,

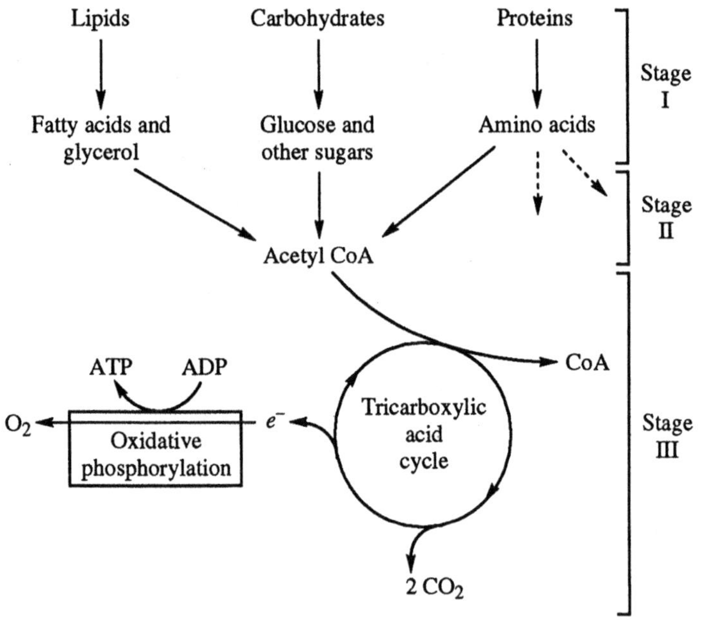

Figure 1.1 Catabolism of macronutrients in foods.

glycerol and fatty acids, and some of the amino acids are further degraded intracellularly to the key metabolite acetyl coenzyme A (acetyl-CoA) by processes that generate small amounts of energy-rich adenosine tri-phosphate (ATP). In the third stage acetyl-CoA is oxidized in the tricarboxylic acid cycle, during which ATP is produced in large amounts by oxidative phosphorylation. Many enzymatic reactions involved in the catabolism of foodstuffs depend upon the presence of specific vitamins, and hence deficiencies of these vitamins lead to metabolic disorders, sometimes with fatal consequences. The biochemical roles of specific vitamins in food catabolism and other essential metabolic processes are briefly discussed in Chapter 2.

1.3 DIETARY CONSIDERATIONS

The water-soluble vitamins are widely distributed in unprocessed foods of both animal and vegetable origin, except for vitamin B_{12}, which is found almost exclusively in animal-derived foods. In foods derived from animal and plant tissues, the B-group vitamins occur as their coenzyme derivatives, usually associated with their protein apoenzyme. In addition, niacin in cereals and vitamin B_6 in certain fruits and vegetables occur largely as bound storage forms. In milk and eggs, which are derived from animal secretions, the B-group vitamins occur, at least to some extent, in the underivatized form, a proportion of which is associated with specific binding proteins. Vitamin C usually occurs as free ascorbic acid, and underivatized B-group vitamins will be found in fortified foods. Representative food sources of water-soluble vitamins are presented in Table 1.1.

Food composition tables must be interpreted in terms of Reference Nutrient Intakes (Table 1.2), concentration of vitamin in the food commodity, and the amount of that commodity consumed. Thus a staple food that may have only a modest content of a certain vitamin may nevertheless constitute an important source of that vitamin. Tryptophan is an additional and variable dietary source of niacin, the contribution depending upon the amino acid balance of the whole diet and the hormonal status of the recipient. Another important factor which affects the dietary significance of a food is the bioavailability of a particular vitamin, which has been defined as the proportion of that vitamin in the food sample of interest that undergoes intestinal absorption and metabolic conversion to functional coenzymic forms (utilization) (Gregory, 1989). Certain foodstuffs exhibit very low bioavailabilities for a particular vitamin. For example, in mature cereal grains up to 90% of the total niacin content exists in a chemically bound form of nicotinic acid (Ghosh, Sarkar and Guha, 1963) and this is nutritionally unavailable unless released by prior treatment with alkali.

Table 1.1 Water-soluble vitamin contents per 100 g of selected foods (from Holland *et al.*, 1991)

	Thiamin (mg)	Riboflavin (mg)	Niacin (mg)	Tryptophan/60 (mg)	Vitamin B_6 (mg)	Pantothenic acid (mg)	Biotin (μg)	Folic acid (μg)	Vitamin B_{12} (μg)	Vitamin C (mg)
Wheat flour, wholemeal	0.47[a]	0.09	5.7[a]	2.5	0.50	0.8	7	57	0	0
Brown rice, raw	0.59	0.07	5.3	1.5	N	N	N	49	0	0
Cow's milk, whole, pasteurized	0.04	0.17	0.1	0.7	0.06	0.35	1.9	6	0.4	1
Eggs, chicken, whole, raw	0.09	0.47	0.1	3.7	0.12	1.77	20.0	50	2.5	0
Beef, lean only, raw	0.07	0.24	5.2	4.3	0.32	0.70	Tr	10	2	0
Lamb, lean only, raw	0.14	0.28	6.0	4.4	0.25	0.70	2	5	2	0
Pork, lean only, raw	0.89	0.25	6.2	3.8	0.45	1.10	3	5	3	0
Chicken, meat only, raw	0.10	0.16	7.8	3.8	0.42	1.20	2	12	Tr	0

Liver, ox, raw	0.23	3.10	13.4	4.5	0.83	8.10	33	330	110.0	23
Cod, raw, fillet	0.08	0.07	1.7	3.2	0.33	(0.20)	(3)	12	2	Tr
Potato, main crop, old, raw, flesh only	0.21	0.02	0.6	0.5	0.44	0.37	0.3	35	0	11
Soya beans, dried, raw	0.61	0.27	2.2	5.7	0.38	0.79	65.0	370	0	Tr
Peas, raw	0.74	0.02	2.5	1.1	0.12	(0.15)	0.5	62	0	24
Brussels sprouts, raw	0.15	0.11	0.2	0.7	0.37	1.00	0.4	135	0	115
Oranges, flesh only	0.11	0.04	0.4	0.1	0.10	0.37	1.0	31	0	54
Peanuts, plain	1.14	0.10	13.8	5.5	0.59	2.66	72.0	110	0	0
Yeast extract (Marmite)	3.10	11.00	58.0	9.0	1.30	N	N	1010	0.5	0

Values in parentheses are estimated.
Tr, Trace; N, the nutrient is present in significant quantities but there is no reliable information on the amount.
[a]These levels are for fortified flour.

Table 1.2 Reference Nutrient Intakes for vitamins (from Department of Health, 1991)

Age	Thiamin (mg/day)	Riboflavin (mg/day)	Niacin (nicotinic acid equivalent) (mg/day)	Vitamin B_6 (mg/day)[a]	Vitamin B_{12} (µg/day)	Folate (µg/day)	Vitamin C (mg/day)
0–3 months	0.2	0.4	3	0.2	0.3	50	25
4–6 months	0.2	0.4	3	0.2	0.3	50	25
7–9 months	0.2	0.4	4	0.3	0.4	50	25
10–12 months	0.3	0.4	5	0.4	0.4	50	25
1–3 years	0.5	0.6	8	0.7	0.5	70	30
4–6 years	0.7	0.8	11	0.9	0.8	100	30
7–10 years	0.7	1.0	12	1.0	1.0	150	30
Males							
11–14 years	0.9	1.2	15	1.2	1.2	200	35
15–18 years	1.1	1.3	18	1.5	1.5	200	40
19–50 years	1.0	1.3	17	1.4	1.5	200	40
50+ years	0.9	1.3	16	1.4	1.5	200	40
Females							
11–14 years	0.7	1.1	12	1.0	1.2	200	35
15–18 years	0.8	1.1	14	1.2	1.5	200	40
19–50 years	0.8	1.1	13	1.2	1.5	200	40
50+ years	0.8	1.1	12	1.2	1.5	200	40
Pregnancy	+0.1[b]	+0.3	[c]	[c]	[c]	+100	+10
Lactation							
0–4 months	+0.2	+0.5	+2	[c]	+0.5	+60	+30
4+ months	+0.2	+0.5	+2	[c]	+0.5	+60	+30

[a] Based on protein providing 14.7% of estimated average requirement for energy.
[b] For last trimester only.
[c] No increment.

Vitamin stability is another important issue when considering the nutritional value of a food. Processing and storage losses depend upon conditions such as pH, temperature and moisture content. Niacin and biotin are relatively stable, but the other water-soluble vitamins are labile to varying extents and under different conditions. Riboflavin is notoriously susceptible to decomposition by light, and as much as 85% of the riboflavin content of milk in glass bottles may be destroyed after only 2 h exposure to bright sunlight (Horwitt, 1972). During domestic cooking, the vitamins are easily leached out into the cooking water or exuded from meat, but are not lost if the cooking fluids are consumed. In the case of vitamin C, rapid heat treatment, such as the blanching of fruits and vegetables or the pasteurization of fruit juices, actually serves to prevent vitamin loss during post-processing storage by inactivating enzymes that promote the direct oxidation of ascorbic acid.

The milling of cereals to produce white flour removes most of the B-group vitamins with the bran, and hence wheat flour is fortified with thiamin, riboflavin and niacin to compensate for the loss of these vitamins. Processed cereal foods such as breakfast cereals, bread, macaroni and spaghetti are frequently enriched with vitamins at concentrations much higher than those occurring in the natural raw materials to make a product more marketable.

In summary, the assessment of a food commodity or a diet as a good nutritional source of a vitamin is based on the amount of vitamin contained in the original commodity or diet, the amount remaining following processing and cooking, the amount actually eaten by the consumer, and the amount digested and absorbed (Kies, Kan and Fox, 1984).

1.4 BIOLOGICAL ACTIVITY AND BIOAVAILABILITY

Vitamins are regarded in the nutritional context as physiological substances, rather than as chemical entities. The ideal assay procedure should therefore reflect the biological activity or potency of the vitamin analyte in a food sample by measuring the combined response of all vitamers in relation to their biological activity. Biological activity refers to the vitamin's ability to fulfil a specific metabolic requirement, and should be distinguished from bioavailability, which (as defined earlier) refers to the extent of absorption and metabolic utilization of the vitamin (Gregory, 1988a). The direct determination of biological vitamin activity of foods is performed by means of animal bioassays, using rats or chicks, which serve as models for human assays. It would be more practicable to use an *in vitro* (microbiological or physicochemical) assay as a substitute for a bioassay but, unless a statistical correlation (r = >0.95) can be demonstrated between the results of *in vitro* assay and bioassay for a particular food sample, there is no alternative to the use of bioassays for the evaluation of biological activity. To determine bioavailability, it is necessary to measure the total amount of the vitamin present in the food, using a microbiological or physicochemical assay performed after an extraction procedure designed to liberate all bound forms of the vitamin. Bioavailability is then calculated by dividing the concentration of biologically active forms of the vitamin (as determined by animal bioassay) by the total concentration of the vitamin (Gregory, 1988a).

Growth assays are based on comparison of responses of rats fed test diets to those of rats fed standard diets fortified with the vitamin in question. When the rat is used to determine biological activity there is a possible bias due to coprophagy or direct absorption of vitamins synthesized by intestinal microflora (Gregory and Litherland, 1986). Absorption can be assessed independently using intralumenal perfusions of intestinal segments. Measurements of plasma levels of vitamins, urinary levels of vitamin metabolites and (for some vitamins) specific enzyme activity provide information about utilization in animals and humans (Gregory, 1988b).

To summarize, *in vitro* assays permit the quantification of the substances that are responsible for the biological activity but, because of the extreme difficulty of devising sample extraction procedures which would adequately model mammalian (or avian) digestion and absorption processes, they do not reflect the actual biological activity of the vitamin. Hence, *in vitro* assays may provide a poor and sometimes highly inaccurate estimate of the sample's nutritional value.

REFERENCES

Counsell, J.N. (1988) Vitamin fortification of foods. *Fd Technol. Int. Europe*, 211–8.

Department of Health (1991) *Dietary Reference Values for Food Energy and Nutrients for the United Kingdom*. Report on Health and Social Subjects No. 41. HM Stationery Office, London.

Ghosh, H.P., Sarkar, P.K. and Guha, B.C. (1963) Distribution of the bound form of nicotinic acid in natural materials. *J. Nutr.*, **79**, 451–3.

Gregory, J.F. (1988a) Methodology for nutrient analysis. In *Nutritional Evaluation of Food Processing* (eds E. Karmas and R.S. Harris), Van Nostrand Reinhold Company Inc., New York, pp. 719–43.

Gregory, J.F. (1988b) Recent developments in methods for the assessment of vitamin bioavailability. *Fd Technol.*, **42**(10) 230, 233, 235, 237–8.

Gregory, J.F. (1989) Bioavailability of vitamin B_6 from plant foods. *Am. J. Clin. Nutr.*, **49**, 717.

Gregory, J.F. and Litherland, S.A. (1986) Efficacy of the rat bioassay for the determination of biologically available vitamin B_6. *J. Nutr.*, **116**, 87–97.

Holland, B., Welch, A.A., Unwin, I.D. *et al.* (1991) *McCance and Widdowson's The*

Composition of Foods, 5th edn, Royal Society of Chemistry and Ministry of Agriculture, Fisheries and Food.

Horwitt, M.K. (1972) Riboflavin. V. Occurrence in food. In *The Vitamins. Chemistry, Physiology, Pathology, Methods*, 2nd edn, Vol. V, (ed. W.H. Sebrell Jr and R.S. Harris), Academic Press, New York, pp. 46–9.

Kies, C., Kan, S. and Fox, H.M. (1984) Vitamin B_6 availability from wheat, rice and corn brans for humans. *Nutr. Rep. Int.*, **30**, 483–91.

Chemical and biological nature of the water-soluble vitamins 2

2.1 THIAMIN

2.1.1 HISTORY

Eijkman, between 1890 and 1897, discovered that feeding chickens on polished rice induced a polyneuritis resembling beriberi, which could be prevented by addition of rice polishings (bran) to the avian diet. A few years later Grijns extracted a water-soluble heat-labile 'polyneuritis protective factor' from rice polishings and correctly concluded that beriberi is the result of a dietary lack of an essential nutrient. By 1926, Jansen and Donath had succeeded in isolating the factor in crystalline form from rice bran extracts. Ten years later R.R. Williams elucidated the structure of thiamin and accomplished its synthesis.

2.1.2 STRUCTURE

The thiamin molecule (Figure 2.1) comprises substituted pyrimidine and thiazole moieties linked by a methylene bridge and systematically named as 3-(2′-methyl-4′-amino-5′-pyrimidylmethyl)-4-methyl-5-(ß-hydroxyethyl)-thiazole. In living tissues thiamin, in the form of the diphosphate ester, thiamin pyrophosphate (TPP) (Figure 2.1), functions as the prosthetic group of several enzymes in which it has a tight but noncovalent binding affinity for the apoenzyme (enzyme protein). Small amounts of the monophosphate (TMP) and triphosphate (TTP) esters of thiamin occur in animal tissues. For food supplementation purposes thiamin is chiefly used in the form of its chloride hydrochloride double salt (known commercially as thiamin hydrochloride), $C_{12}H_{17}N_4OSCl$. HCl, of molecular weight (MW) 337.28.

2.1.3 PHYSICAL AND CHEMICAL PROPERTIES

Thiamin hydrochloride is a colourless crystalline substance with a yeast-like odour and a salty nut-like taste. It is readily soluble in water (100 g/100 ml), less soluble in glycerol (5 g/100 ml), sparingly soluble in 95% ethanol (1 g/100 ml) and absolute ethanol (0.3 g/100 ml) and insoluble in fat solvents such as diethyl ether, chloroform, benzene and hexane. Since the thiamin molecule contains a quaternary nitrogen, it is a strong base and will be completely ionized over the entire range of pH normally encountered in foods. The pH of a 1% solution of thiamin hydrochloride in water is 3.13 and that of a 0.1% solution is 3.58. The hydrochloride salt is hygroscopic and usually exists as the hemihydrate containing the

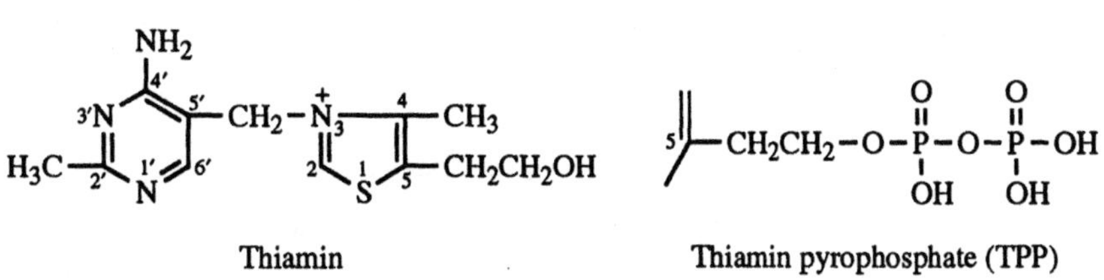

Figure 2.1 Structures of thiamin and thiamin pyrophosphate.

equivalent of about 4% water. The melting point (m.p.) is about 207 °C, with decomposition. Another commercial form of the vitamin, thiamin mononitrate, is practically nonhygroscopic and is especially recommended for the enrichment of flour mixes.

2.1.4 STABILITY

The phosphorylated and protein-bound thiamin present in most foods is quite stable when food samples in a medium of 0.1 N HCl are heated to 95–100 °C or autoclaved at 121–123 °C for 30 min, but higher concentrations of acid are likely to decompose thiamin. The nonphosphorylated thiamin that occurs in cereal grain products is partly destroyed when autoclaved under the above conditions, but it can resist autoclaving at 108–109 °C for 20 min (McRoberts, 1954). As the pH of the medium is increased, the vitamin becomes increasingly susceptible to deactivation by heat and chemical reaction. Mild oxidation produces thiamin disulphide without loss of thiamin activity; more vigorous oxidation with alkaline potassium hexacyanoferrate(III) (potassium ferricyanide) produces the biologically inactive thiochrome (Figure 2.2). Thiamin phosphate esters are oxidized to thiochrome compounds in a similar manner without splitting the phosphate bonds. Thiamin is deactivated by sulphite ion even at room temperature, owing to methylene bridge cleavage. Solutions of thiamin are degraded by ultraviolet (UV) irradiation (Dwivedi and Arnold, 1973). The thiamin content of foods is protected to some extent by the matrix and further stabilized through protein binding.

2.1.5 SPECTROSCOPIC PROPERTIES

Absorption

The absorption spectrum of thiamin hydrochloride is pH-dependent as shown in Figure 2.3. At pH 2.9 a single maximum at 246 nm occurs. At pH 5.5 two maxima occur at 234 nm and 264 nm which correspond to the substituted pyrimidine and thiazole moieties, respectively. The $A_{1\,\mathrm{cm}}^{1\%}$ values corresponding to the maxima at 246, 234 and 264 nm are, respectively, *c.* 425, 345 and 255 (Hashmi, 1973).

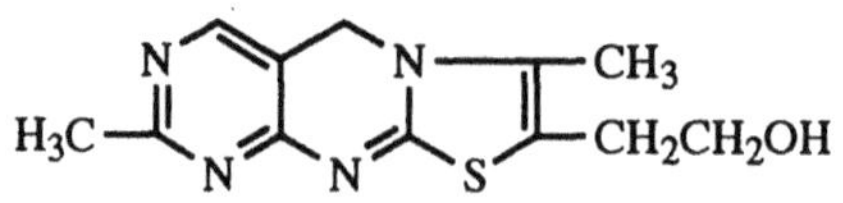

Figure 2.2 Structure of thiochrome.

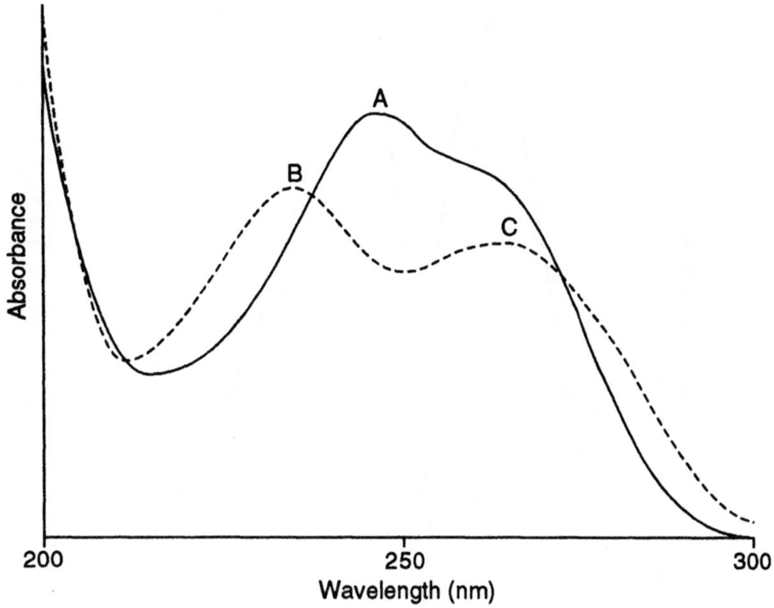

Figure 2.3 Absorption spectra of thiamin hydrochloride in 0.1 M phosphate buffer at pH 2.9 (solid line) and 5.5 (broken line) (λ_{max} of peak A = 246 nm; B = 234 nm; C = 264 nm).

Fluorescence

Thiamin does not exhibit native fluorescence, but the vitamin and its phosphate esters react *in vitro* with chemical oxidizing agents at an alkaline pH to form the corresponding thiochrome compound, which displays a strong blue fluorescence (Figure 2.4). Equimolar amounts of the thiochrome derivatives of thiamin, TMP, TPP and TTP produce different fluorescent intensities (Ishii *et al.*, 1979a).

2.1.6 DIETARY SOURCES

All plant and animal tissues contain thiamin and it is therefore present in all natural unprocessed foods. Rich sources of thiamin include yeast and yeast extract, wheat bran, oatmeal, whole-grain cereals, pulses, nuts, lean pork, heart, kidney and liver. Beef, lamb, chicken, eggs, vegetables and fruits contain intermediate amounts, while milk contains a relatively low amount (see Table 1.1). In cereal grains the thiamin is very unevenly distributed, being relatively low in the starchy endosperm and high in the germ. The milling of cereals removes most of the

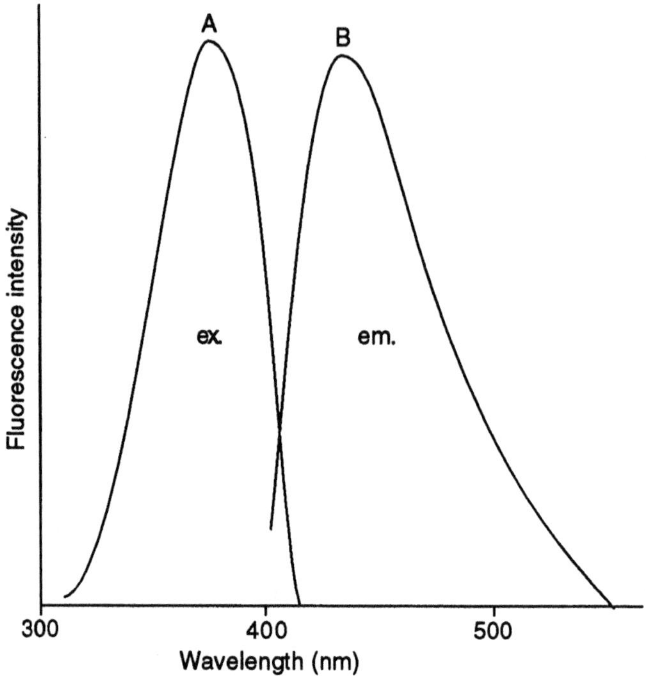

Figure 2.4 Fluorescence excitation and emission spectra of thiochrome (λ_{max} of peak A = 375 nm; B = 432–435 nm).

thiamin, so white flour, breakfast cereals and, in certain countries, polished rice are enriched by addition of the vitamin. Other frequently enriched foodstuffs are breads, macaroni, spaghetti and milk modifiers (chocolate, malt, etc.).

The major form of thiamin in meat products is TPP, which exists as a protein complex. Small amounts of the TMP, TTP and non-phosphorylated thiamin have been detected in the liver, heart, kidney and brain of the rat (Ishii *et al.*, 1979b). Of the total thiamin present in milk, 50–70% is free thiamin, 5–17% is protein-bound thiamin, and 18–45% is TMP, which has no thiamin activity (Hartman and Dryden, 1974). The natural thiamin content of most cereals and cereal products, including white flour made from wheat, is present almost entirely in the form of nonphosphorylated thiamin; exceptions are wheat germ and bran which contain TPP (Andrews and Nordgren, 1941; Hoffer, Alcock and Gedders, 1943). There is evidence that the absence of phosphorylated thiamin in plant material is caused by phosphatase activity when the material is extracted for assay (Obermeyer, Fulmer and Young, 1944). White bread contains TPP due to the phosphorylation of thiamin added for enrichment during the yeast fermentation of the dough as well as the contribution from the yeast itself (McRoberts, 1957).

2.1.7 EFFECTS OF FOOD PROCESSING AND STORAGE

Storage losses of thiamin in foods depend upon conditions such as pH, temperature and moisture content. Frozen foods and dehydrated foods incur little loss of thiamin during storage. An alkaline environment during processing or cooking will promote loss of thiamin; for instance, the use of baking powder in cake making can destroy over 50% of the original thiamin content of the flour. In the baking of bread with yeasts the medium is slightly acidic and the loss is reduced to 15–30%, mostly in the crust. The addition of sulphiting agents to fruit and minced meat to inhibit enzymatic and nonenzymatic browning can cause total destruction of thiamin, but these foods are not important sources of the vitamin. In the processing of milk the following losses have been reported: pasteurization, 9–20%; sterilization, 30–50%; spray-drying, 10%; roller drying, 15%; and condensing (canning), 40% (Gubler, 1984).

2.1.8 BIOCHEMICAL AND PHYSIOLOGICAL FUNCTIONS

Thiamin, in the form of TPP, participates in carbohydrate metabolism by functioning as a cofactor in a number of reactions involving the tricarboxylic acid cycle (Figure 2.5) and the pentose phosphate pathway.

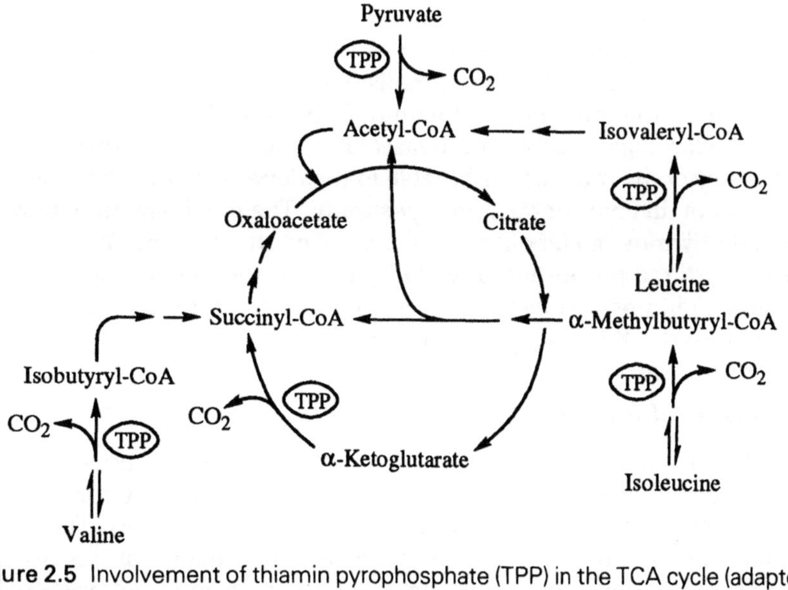

Figure 2.5 Involvement of thiamin pyrophosphate (TPP) in the TCA cycle (adapted from McCormick, 1988a). From M.E. Shils and V.R. Young, *Modern Nutrition in Health and Disease*, 7th edn, Philadelphia, Lea & Febiger, 1988. Used with permission.

Pyruvate undergoes a TPP-dependent oxidative decarboxylation to form the important energy-rich thioester acetyl-CoA, and α-ketoglutarate undergoes a similar decarboxylation to form the analogous succinyl-CoA. TPP participates in transketolase reactions in the pentose phosphate pathway, the principal function of which is to provide a source of ribose for nucleotide and nucleic acid synthesis, and reduced nicotinamide adenine dinucleotide phosphate (NADPH) for the synthesis of fatty acids. Furthermore, TPP is required for the oxidative decarboxylation of the branched-chain keto acids formed after deamination of the amino acids leucine, isoleucine and valine (Gubler, 1984). There is also evidence that thiamin is involved directly in nerve transmission.

Deficiency signs

The classic pathological condition resulting from a gross deficiency of thiamin in humans is beriberi, which is prevalent in Far Eastern populations where unfortified polished rice is the staple diet. The symptoms of beriberi vary according to circumstances. Wet beriberi, which is manifested as a generalized oedema and cardiac malfunction, results from severe physical exertion and high carbohydrate intake. Dry beriberi is characterized by a pronounced muscle wasting accompanied by a variety of neurological disorders; it results from relative inactivity with caloric restriction during the chronic deficiency. Subclinical deficiencies are more common and are characterized by mental disturbances, fatigue and loss of weight resulting from reduced appetite and digestive problems. Chronic alcoholism leads to a deficiency syndrome arising from the inhibition of thiamin absorption (Gubler, 1984).

The neurological and cardiovascular disorders that arise from a deficiency of thiamin are attributable to the dependence of the brain and heart upon thiamin for their energy supply. The involvement of thiamin in carbohydrate metabolism explains why the thiamin requirement varies with the proportion of carbohydrate in the diet and is increased under conditions that elevate the metabolic rate. Both dietary lipid and protein exert a thiamin-sparing action.

Expression of dietary value

The international unit (IU) of vitamin B_1 activity is defined as the activity of 3 μg of crystalline thiamin hydrochloride, i.e. 1 g corresponds to 333 000 IU (Association of Vitamin Chemists, Inc., 1966). The IU for thiamin is no longer used in practice, and analytical results are expressed in terms of weight (mg) of pure thiamin hydrochloride. Thiamin activity can be determined either by the curative growth test or the brachycardia test in rats.

Toxicity

Thiamin is of extremely low toxicity when administered orally to humans, excess amounts being excreted in the urine. Large parenteral doses administered over a long period of time have been reported to produce clinical manifestations and, in some cases, even death (Cumming, Briggs and Briggs, 1981).

2.1.9 METABOLISM

Thiamin is absorbed in the small intestine by an active transport process and is rapidly deposited in the muscle, liver and other organs, where it is phosphorylated to the biologically active form, TPP. Approximately 80% of the total thiamin deposited exists as TPP, with 10% as TTP and the remainder as unesterified thiamin and TMP. Of the three phosphate esters, TPP possesses full thiamin activity, TMP is completely inactive, and any activity previously attributed to TTP results from partial conversion to TPP by *in vivo* enzymatic hydrolysis of the terminal ester bond (Gubler, 1984).

2.1.10 BIOAVAILABILITY

Thiamin appears to be well utilized, whether supplied by diets containing wheat or animal protein (Edwards *et al.*, 1971). Certain shellfish and freshwater fish contain thiaminases whose action can cause symptoms of beriberi in those Southeast Asian populations that consume fermented raw fish (Vimokesant *et al.*, 1982). The tannins and other polyphenol compounds present in tea and coffee have marked anti-thiamin activity (Hilker and Somogyi, 1982).

2.2 RIBOFLAVIN

2.2.1 HISTORY

The existence of a heat-stable growth factor in yeast extracts was first discovered by Emmett and Luros in 1920. In 1932, Warburg and Christian isolated from yeast a yellow enzyme which contained a non-protein component subsequently shown to be a phosphate ester of an alloxazine derivative. The structure of riboflavin was determined by Kuhn's group in 1933 and the vitamin was first synthesized by Karrer's group in 1935.

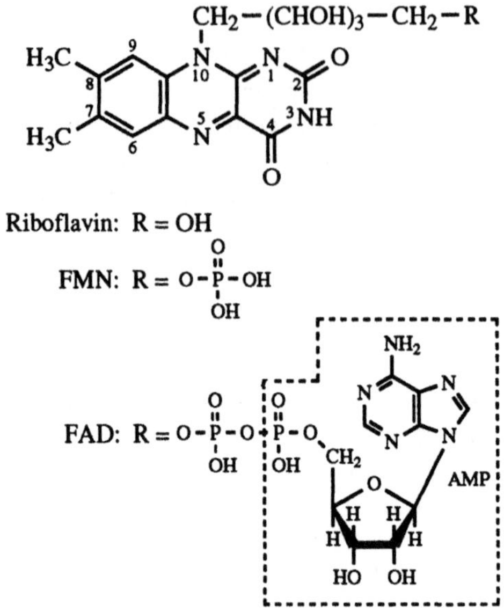

Figure 2.6 Structures of riboflavin, FMN and FAD.

2.2.2 STRUCTURE

The structures of the riboflavin compounds that occur in nature are depicted in Figure 2.6. The parent riboflavin molecule comprises a substituted isoalloxazine moiety with a ribitol side chain and is systematically named as 7,8-dimethyl-10-(1′-D-ribityl)-isoalloxazine ($C_{17}H_{20}O_6N_4$, MW = 376.36). The principal forms of riboflavin found in nature are riboflavin-5′-phosphate (= flavin mononucleotide, FMN) and riboflavin-5′-adenosyldiphosphate (= flavin adenine dinucleotide, FAD). FMN is actually not a nucleotide, as the compound attached to the flavin moiety is the sugar alcohol ribitol and not the aldose sugar ribose, and the isoalloxazine ring is not a purine or a pyrimidine. FAD is composed of a nucleotide (adenosine monophosphate, AMP) and the so-called flavin pseudonucleotide. In biological tissues, FAD and, to a lesser extent, FMN occur almost entirely as prosthetic groups for a variety of flavin enzymes (flavoproteins) concerned with oxidoreductive processes. In most flavoproteins the flavins are bound tightly but noncovalently to the apoenzyme. In mammalian tissues less than 10% of the FAD is covalently attached to specific amino acid residues of four important apoenzymes. These are found within succinate and sarcosine dehydrogenases, monoamine oxidase and L-gluconolactone oxidase, in which FAD is peptide-linked to an *N*-histidyl or *S*-cysteinyl residue via the 8-methyl group (McCormick, 1988b).

2.2.3 PHYSICAL AND CHEMICAL PROPERTIES

Riboflavin crystallizes in the form of yellow to orange–yellow needles with a melting point of about 280 °C. The compound is odourless and has an unpleasant bitter taste. In neutral aqueous solution riboflavin exhibits a strong yellow–green fluorescence which reaches a maximum at pH 6.7–6.8. Riboflavin is only sparingly soluble in water (10–13 mg/100 ml at 25–27.5 °C; 19 mg/100 ml at 40 °C; 230 mg/100 ml at 100 °C) and even less soluble in absolute ethanol (4.5 mg/100 ml at 27 °C). The vitamin is readily soluble, but unstable, in dilute alkali. There is no solubility in acetone, diethyl ether, chloroform or benzene. A saturated aqueous solution of riboflavin has a pH of 5.5–7.2; pK_a values are 1.9 and 10.2 (20 °C). The solubility of riboflavin in water is increased in the presence of aromatic compounds such as nicotinamide, and practical use of this property is made in pharmaceutical preparations. The sodium salt of FMN is very soluble in water, and FAD is freely soluble in water (Yagi, 1962).

2.2.4 STABILITY

Crystalline riboflavin is stable in dry form under normal lighting. In solution, vitamin activity is destroyed by exposure to both UV radiation and visible light, the rate of destruction increasing with an increase in temperature and pH. If protected from light, aqueous solutions of riboflavin in the pH range between 2 and 5 are heat stable up to 120 °C; above pH 7 the isoalloxazine ring is rapidly destroyed at elevated temperatures. Optimal stability is obtained at pH 3.5–4.0. The principal photodegradation produce under neutral and acidic conditions is lumichrome (7,8-dimethylalloxazine) while, under alkaline conditions, the major product is lumiflavin (7,8,10-trimethylisoalloxazine) (Figure 2.7). The latter degradation product exhibits a strong blue fluorescence, which has been used as a means of detection in many assay procedures. Riboflavin is stable towards oxygen and many oxidizing agents in the absence of light.

The flavin cofactors naturally present in biological tissues are stabilized through protein binding, and riboflavin added to foods is protected to some extent by the food matrix. FMN is partially hydrolysed to riboflavin when food samples are heated to 95–100 °C or autoclaved at 121–123 °C with 0.1 N HCl for 30 min. A substantial fraction of the FMN is converted to the biologically active isomeric 2′-, 3′- and 4′-phosphates (Nielsen, Rauschenbach and Bacher, 1986). FAD is totally hydrolysed to FMN when food samples are heated with 0.1 N HCl under the above conditions or incubated with 10% (w/v) trichloro-acetic acid (TCA) at 38 °C overnight; no destruction of FAD occurs at

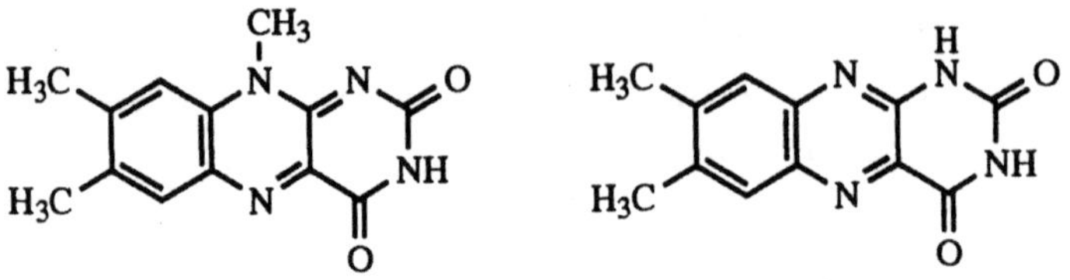

Figure 2.7 Photodegradation products from riboflavin.

0 °C for 30 min in 10% TCA (Koziol, 1971). Flavins, in their role as enzyme cofactors for hydrogen transport, undergo reversible reduction with active hydrogen to 1,5-dihydro forms known as leuco bases.

2.2.5 SPECTROSCOPIC PROPERTIES

Absorption

Riboflavin in aqueous solution exhibits a UV–visible spectrum containing four major bands centred around 223, 266, 373 and 445 nm (Figure 2.8). The positions of the maxima and their absorbance coefficients vary somewhat according to the nature of the solvent in which the compound is dissolved. The 373-nm band is the most affected by solvents, generally shifting to shorter wavelengths with decreasing solvent polarity. The position of the visible 445-nm band is not greatly affected. The spectra of riboflavin and FMN are almost identical to one another under similar conditions, but that of FAD is slightly different. All three flavins lose their absorbance in the visible region when they are reduced to their colourless leuco bases. Molar absorptivity (ε) values of flavins dissolved in 0.1 M phosphate buffer, pH 7.0, are given in Table 2.1.

Fluorescence

Riboflavin, FMN and FAD all show fluorescence emission at around 530 nm when excited at 440–500 nm. Neutral aqueous solutions of riboflavin display an intense yellowish-green fluorescence with an emission maximum at 521 nm (Figure 2.9). The fluorescence is quenched by strong alkali or strong acid (Yagi, 1962). The emission of flavins is a characteristic of uncharged neutral forms of isoalloxazines; anions and cations do not fluoresce. Riboflavin shows a maximum and equal fluorescence intensity in the pH range between 3.5 and 7.5. The same is true for FMN and lumiflavin, whereas FAD displays maximal intensity

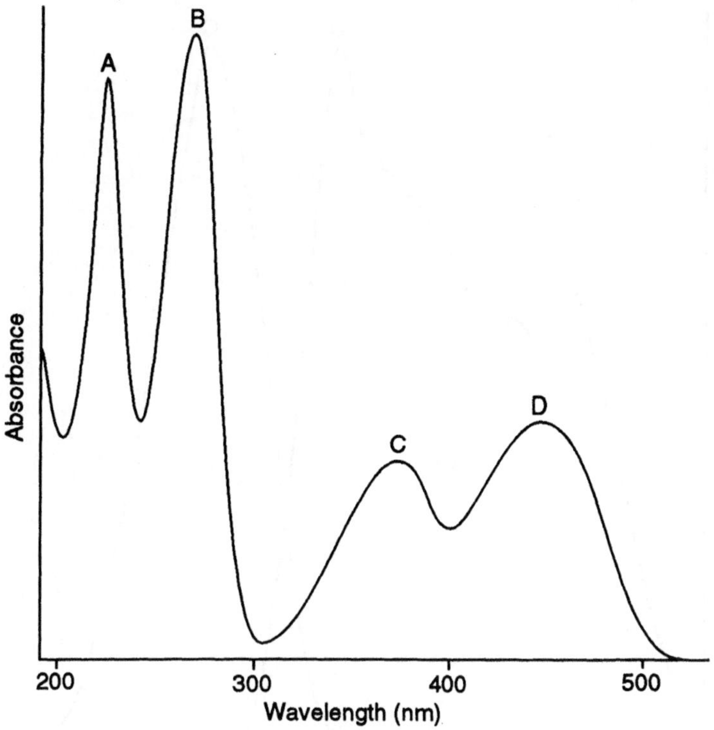

Figure 2.8 Absorption spectrum of riboflavin dissolved in water (pH 7.4) (λ_{max} of peak A = 223 nm; B = 266 nm; C = 373 nm; D = 444 nm).

Table 2.1 The molar absorptivity (ε) values of flavins dissolved in 0.1 M phosphate buffer, pH 7.0

	Wavelength (nm)		
	260	375	450
Riboflavin	27 700	10 600	12 200
FMN	27 100	10 400	12 200
FAD	37 000	9 300	11 300

From Yagi, K. (1962) *Methods of Biochemical Analysis*, Vol. 10 (ed. D. Glick), Copyright © 1962, by John Wiley & Sons, Inc. Reprinted by permission of John Wiley & Sons, Inc.

at pH 2.7–3.1. In equimolar neutral aqueous solutions, riboflavin and FMN exhibit practically the same fluorescence intensity, whereas that of FAD is only about 15% of that of riboflavin. The binding of flavins to proteins generally results in a dramatic quenching of fluorescence. Reduced forms of flavins do not fluoresce (Koziol, 1971).

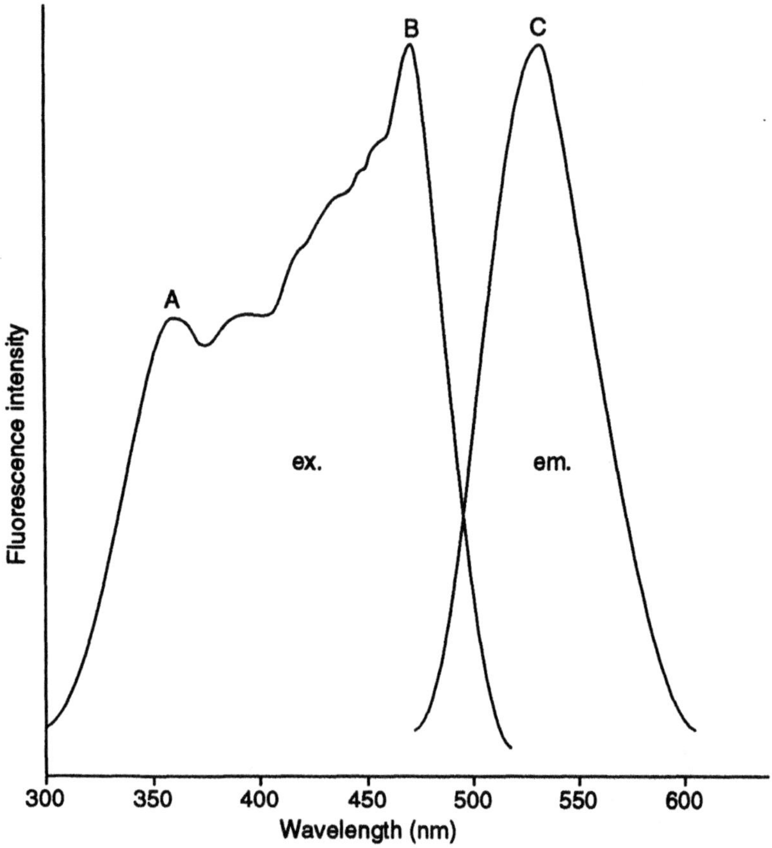

Figure 2.9 Fluorescence excitation and emission spectra of riboflavin dissolved in water (pH 7.4) (λ_{max} of peak A = 360 nm; B = 465 nm; C = 521 nm).

2.2.6 DIETARY SOURCES

Living cells require FMN and FAD as the prosthetic groups of a variety of enzymes, and hence the flavins are found at least in small amounts in all natural unprocessed foods. Yeast extract is exceptionally rich in riboflavin, and liver and kidney are also rich sources. Wheat bran, eggs, meat, milk and cheese are imported sources in diets containing these foods (see Table 1.1). Cereal grains contain relatively low concentrations of riboflavin, but are imported sources in those parts of the world where cereals constitute the staple diet. The milling of cereals results in considerable loss of riboflavin, so white flour is enriched by addition of the vitamin. The enrichment of bread and breakfast cereals contributes significantly to the dietary supply of riboflavin. Polished rice is not usually enriched, since the yellow colour of the vitamin would present problems. However, most of the riboflavin content of the whole brown rice is retained if the rice is steamed prior to milling. This process drives the water-soluble vitamins in the germ and aleurone layers into the endosperm (Cooperman and Lopez, 1984).

In most foods the riboflavin is present in the form of protein-bound flavins, predominantly as FAD. Several investigators have reported that from 54% to 95% of the total riboflavin in bovine milk is present as free (underivatized) riboflavin; the rest is present as FMN and FAD (Hartman and Dryden, 1974). In milk a small proportion (14% in whole milk) of the flavins is bound noncovalently to specific proteins (Kanno *et al.*, 1991). Egg white and egg yolk contain specialized riboflavin-binding proteins that are required for storage of free riboflavin in the egg for use by the developing embryo (Merrill *et al.*, 1981).

2.2.7 EFFECTS OF FOOD PROCESSING

Significant losses of riboflavin are caused in milk by photodegradation. As much as 85% of the vitamin content of milk in glass bottles may be destroyed after only 2 h exposure to bright sunlight (Horwitt, 1972). Wavelengths between 400 and 550 nm were shown to be responsible for the destruction (Dunkley, Franklin and Pangborn, 1962). The breakdown product, lumichrome, is a much stronger oxidizing agent than is riboflavin and catalyses massive destruction of the ascorbic acid content. The formation of highly reactive singlet oxygen during the photodegradation of riboflavin promotes the rapid autoxidation of unsaturated fatty acids in the milk fat, resulting in an unpleasant 'off' flavour (Coultate, 1989). The pasteurization, evaporation and condensing of milk has little effect on riboflavin content. Riboflavin is stable during the heat processing and normal cooking of foods if light is excluded.

2.2.8 BIOCHEMICAL AND PHYSIOLOGICAL FUNCTIONS

The flavin enzymes play a vital role in carbohydrate and lipid catabolism by catalysing: (1) the reoxidation of reduced nicotinamide adenine dinucleotide (NADH); (2) the oxidation of the tricarboxylic acid cycle intermediary, succinate, to fumarate; and (3) the oxidation of saturated fatty acid acyl-CoA to α,β-unsaturated fatty acyl-CoA in the β-oxidation of fatty acids. In all of these reactions the reduced flavin ($FADH_2$ or $FMNH_2$) is reoxidized by the cytochrome electron-transport chain with the eventual transfer of the hydrogen to molecular oxygen to form water (Figure 2.10). The flavin enzymes are also involved in the biosynthesis of long-chain saturated fatty acids and in the catabolism of biogenic amines and purine bases arising from the degradation of nucleic acids. In addition, they are necessary for the conversion of

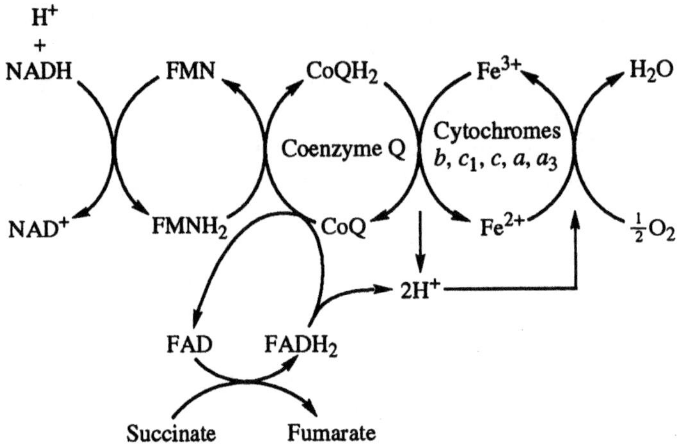

Figure 2.10 Simplified representation of the cytochrome electron-transport chain showing the interrelationship between FMN and NADH and the reoxidation of reduced flavins ($FADH_2$ and $FMNH_2$). The specific entry of $FADH_2$ from succinic dehydrogenase is also shown.

vitamin B_6 and folic acid to their coenzyme forms and in the conversion of tryptophan to NAD^+.

Deficiency signs

Unlike the case with gross thiamin deficiency, no pathologically severe signs attributed to riboflavin deficiency have been observed in humans. Signs of riboflavin deficiency have been induced experimentally in volunteers whose diets were lacking only in riboflavin or who were fed riboflavin antagonists. Deficiency signs in man usually include lesions of the lips (cheilosis) and angles of the mouth (angular stomatitis), a fissured and magenta-coloured tongue (glossitis), seborrhoeic follicular keratosis of the nose and forehead, and dermatitis of the anogenital region. Ophthalmic symptoms are a superficial vascularization of the cornea accompanied by intense photophobia.

Expression of dietary value

Riboflavin, FMN and FAD are equally active as vitamins in nutrition (Yagi, 1962). No IU of vitamin B_2 activity has been defined, and analytical results are expressed in terms of weight (mg) of chemically pure riboflavin. The biological activity of preparations containing riboflavin can be examined in the curative rat growth test using crystalline riboflavin as the reference standard.

Toxicity

The low solubility of riboflavin and the limited capacity of intestinal absorption mechanisms probably account for the lack of toxicity following oral doses of up to 20 mg daily (Cumming, Briggs and Briggs, 1981).

2.2.9 METABOLISM

The FAD and FMN present in the ingested food are released from their mainly noncovalent association with proteins by gastric acidification and are enzymatically dephosphorylated in the upper gut. The free riboflavin is absorbed in the small intestine by an active transport process and is phosphorylated in the mucosal cells to FMN. FMN then enters the portal system, where it becomes loosely associated with plasma albumin, and is transported to the liver. Conversion of FMN to FAD and binding to specific flavoproteins occurs in most tissues, but particularly in the small intestine, liver, heart and kidney. The liver is the major storage site of the vitamin and contains about one-third of the total body flavins, 70–90% of which is in the form of FAD. Free riboflavin constitutes less than 5% of the stored flavins (Cooperman and Lopez, 1984). Other storage sites are the spleen, kidney and cardiac muscle. These depots maintain significant amounts of the vitamin even in severe deficiency states.

2.2.10 BIOAVAILABILITY

Riboflavin is obtained directly from foods naturally rich in the underivatized vitamin, such as bovine milk and eggs, and from foodstuffs to which riboflavin has been added during manufacture; the flavoprotein content of food containing noncovalently bound flavins provides an indirect source of riboflavin. Experimental evidence using rats suggests that the fraction (<10%) consisting of covalently bound flavins is largely unavailable as a source of riboflavin (Chia, Addison and McCormick, 1978).

2.3 NIACIN

2.3.1 HISTORY

The human disease of pellagra was first described in Spain by Casal in 1735 after the introduction of maize into Europe from the Americas. In the 1920s, Goldberger (USA) reported that pellagra and black tongue in dogs responded to treatment with animal protein and also to boiled protein-free extracts of yeast. In 1937, Elvehjem found that the active component in liver extracts used to successfully treat canine black tongue was nicotinamide, and reports that nicotinic acid cured pellagra soon followed. Because nicotinic acid has been known chemically since 1897, it has never been assigned a letter, but it is included among the vitamins of the B group.

Nicotinic acid and nicotinamide had been isolated from the coenzymes now known as NADP and NAD by 1934–1935; hence knowledge of their biochemical roles in electron-transfer reactions preceded the discovery of their nutritional significance. By 1946, the metabolism of dietary tryptophan to an active form of the vitamin had been demonstrated.

2.3.2 STRUCTURE

Niacin is the generic descriptor for two vitamers, nicotinic acid and nicotinamide, which are systematically named as pyridine-3-carboxylic acid ($C_6H_5O_2N$, MW = 123.11) and pyridine-3-carboxamide ($C_6H_6ON_2$, MW = 122.12), respectively (Figure 2.11). This nomenclature is not to be confused with American usage of the term niacin to denote specifically nicotinic acid, and niacinamide to denote the amide. In living tissues nicotinamide is the reactive moiety of the coenzymes NAD and NADP. The coenzymes are composed of a nucleotide (AMP) and a pseudo-nucleotide containing the nicotinamide moiety (Figure 2.11). The oxidized forms of the coenzymes carry a positive charge (NAD^+ and $NADP^+$); reduced forms carrying two electrons and one proton (and associated with an additional proton) are represented as NADH and NADPH. Although the coenzymes are only loosely associated with the apoenzyme during catalysis, most cellular NAD and NADP is stored in the cytoplasm bound to protein (Weiner and van Eys, 1983).

2.3.3 PHYSICAL AND CHEMICAL PROPERTIES

Nicotinic acid crystallizes into colourless needles (m.p. 235 °C) which are odourless and have a tart taste; the crystals of nicotinamide (m.p. 129 °C) are similar but have a bitter taste. Nicotinic acid is sparingly soluble in water (1.67 g/100 ml at 25 °C) and ethanol (0.73 g/100 ml) and insoluble in acetone and diethyl ether. It is, however, freely soluble in boiling water. The pH of a saturated aqueous solution is 3 and the pK_a is 4.8 (25 °C). The sodium salt of nicotinic acid is readily soluble in water (71 g/100 ml) and yields a solution of about pH 7. Nicotinamide is readily soluble in water (100 g/100 ml) and ethanol (67 g/100 ml); there is solubility in acetone and very slight solubility in diethyl ether and chloroform. An aqueous solution of nicotinamide yields a pH of 6 and

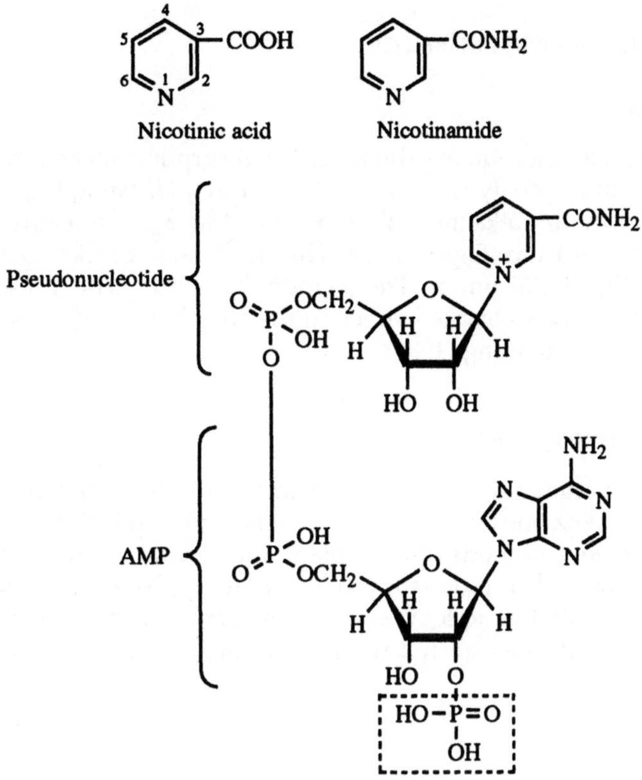

NAD$^+$ and NADP$^+$ (phosphate group within dotted area is absent in NAD$^+$)

Figure 2.11 Structures of niacin compounds and the nicotinamide nucleotides.

the pK_a is 3.3 (20 °C). Both nicotinic acid and nicotinamide have the properties of bases and form quaternary ammonium salts when in acid solution. Nicotinic acid, being amphoteric, forms carboxylic acid salts when in a basic solution, but nicotinamide possesses no acidic properties.

2.3.4 STABILITY

Both nicotinic acid and nicotinamide are unaffected by atmospheric oxygen, light and heat in the dry state and in neutral aqueous solution. Nicotinamide is hydrolysed quantitatively to nicotinic acid when autoclaved with 1 N mineral acid or alkaline solutions, the nicotinic acid being resistant to these conditions. The oxidized coenzymes (NAD$^+$ and NADP$^+$) are labile to alkali (Guilbert and Johnson, 1977), whereas the reduced coenzymes (NADH and NADPH) are labile to acid (Chaykin, 1967).

2.3.5 SPECTROSCOPIC PROPERTIES

Absorption

Nicotinic acid and its amide exhibit similar absorption spectra in the UV region. The absorptivity is strongly affected by pH, being higher in an acidic than in an alkaline solution, but the λ_{max} remains almost unchanged at 261 nm (Figure 2.12). The $A_{1\,cm}^{1\%}$ value of nicotinamide in 0.1 N H_2SO_4 at 261 nm is 478 (Windholz, 1983). The presence of electrolytes also has a marked effect on the absorbances of the solutions (Strohecker and Henning, 1966).

2.3.6 DIETARY SOURCES

All plant and animal tissues require niacin in the form of nicotinamide nucleotide coenzymes for normal metabolism, and the vitamin is therefore present in foods of both plant and animal origin. Because of the contribution of tryptophan, foods containing balanced protein are important contributors to total niacin equivalent intake. Food composition tables should itemize the niacin equivalent content of foods and

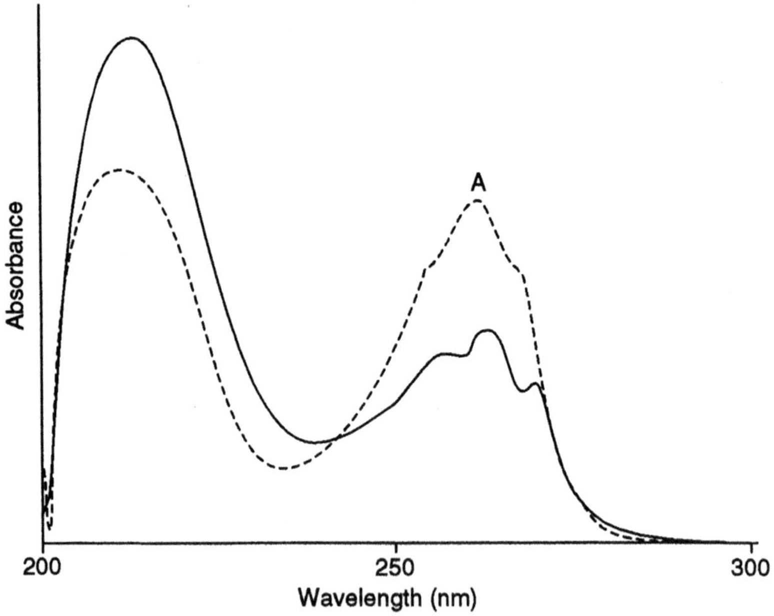

Figure 2.12 Absorption spectra of nicotinic acid in 0.1 M phosphate buffer at pH 7.0 (solid line) and 2.0 (broken line) (λ_{max} of peak A = 261 nm).

ideally provide data for both preformed niacin and tryptophan. Yeast extract is exceptionally rich in niacin, while wheat bran, liver, heart, kidney, lean meat, fish, whole-grain cereals, peanuts and pulses constitute other rich sources. Fruits and vegetables provide useful amounts, depending upon the dietary intake. Cheese and eggs are relatively poor sources of preformed niacin, but these high-protein foods contain ample amounts of tryptophan and therefore have a high niacin equivalent (see Table 1.1).

In mature cereal grains (including maize, wheat, rice and barley) 85–90% of the total niacin content exists in a chemically bound form of nicotinic acid (Ghosh, Sarkar and Guha, 1963) and this is nutritionally unavailable (to the pig) unless released by prior treatment with alkali (Kodicek *et al.*, 1956). In the preparation of Mexican tortillas the vitamin is made available by soaking the maize with limewater before cooking (Kodicek *et al.*, 1959), and the use of baking powder liberates much of the bound vitamin from cereal flours (Bender and Bender, 1986). The niacin is concentrated in the aleurone and germ portions of the grain (Wall and Carpenter, 1988), and hence milling to produce white flour removes most of the vitamin with the bran. The steaming of rice prior to milling does not significantly increase the niacin content of polished rice as, unlike other B-group vitamins, the nicotinic acid in its bound form does not diffuse into the endosperm (Koetz and Newkom, 1977). About 70% of the niacin in commercial flour is present in the bound form (Koetz and Neukom, 1977). In many countries nicotinamide is added to white flour and to maize meal for enrichment. In wheat bran the nicotinic acid is bound within a number of macromolecules that are both polysaccharide and glycopeptide in character (Mason, Gibson and Kodicek, 1973). Chemical analysis of bound nicotinic acid preparations from wheat bran yielded nicotinoyl glucose as a subunit, the nicotinic acid moiety being ester-linked through the 3-position of a single glucose molecule (Koetz, Amadò and Neukom, 1979). Nicotinic acid is also bound to lipid material in wheat bran, presumably esterified to long-chain fatty alcohols or to sterols (Koetz, Amadò and Neukom, 1979). The binding of nicotinic acid to proteins through amide linkages is also possible. Pulses do not contain any bound nicotinic acid (Ghosh, Sarkar and Guha, 1963). The niacin of immature sweetcorn occurs as NAD and NADP for seed metabolism, as opposed to the bound storage forms in mature cereal grains (Wall and Carpenter, 1988), and is nutritionally available. Nicotinic acid is formed during the roasting of coffee beans, owing to the thermal decomposition of the alkaloid trigonelline (Viani and Horman, 1974). The amount formed is generally 10 mg per 100 g of raw beans but can rise to 40 mg in a dark roast (Bender and Bender, 1986). In animal tissues the nicotinamide nucleotides are rapidly hydrolysed *post mortem* and hence most of the niacin content of meat exists as free nicotinamide (Bender and Bender, 1986). Almost all of the niacin content of milk is present as nicotinamide (Krehl *et al.*, 1946).

2.3.7 EFFECTS OF FOOD PROCESSING AND STORAGE

Niacin is generally stable during the commercial processing, storage and domestic cooking of foods. Losses of 25–30% occur during the maturation of meat (i.e. the first days *post mortem*) due to biochemical changes (Belitz and Grosch, 1987), but no further loss occurs during subsequent storage at −18 °C for at least 1 year (Hankes, 1984). There is no significant loss of niacin during milk processing (Tannenbaum, Young and Archer, 1985).

Tryptophan (a precursor of NAD) is also very stable to the usual treatment encountered in food processing, storage and cooking (FAO/WHO, 1967).

2.3.8 BIOCHEMICAL AND PHYSIOLOGICAL FUNCTIONS

The nicotinamide nucleotide coenzymes, NAD and NADP, function as proton and electron carriers in a wide variety of oxidation–reduction reactions. Examples are reactions concerned with the release of energy from carbohydrates, fatty acids and amino acids, and with the synthesis of amino acids, fatty acids and pentoses for nucleotide and nucleic acid production.

Carbohydrate catabolism involves the conversion of glucose to pyruvate by anaerobic glycolysis and, under aerobic conditions, the oxidative decarboxylation of pyruvate to acetyl-CoA, which is further metabolized in the tricarboxylic acid cycle. A number of NAD^+-linked substrate dehydrogenations occur during this process (Figure 2.13) and the NADH so formed is itself dehydrogenated by the flavin enzymes. Under anaerobic conditions the NADH generated during glycolysis is oxidized by transferring its hydrogen to pyruvate to form lactate.

The reducing equivalents (NADPH) for fatty acid biosynthesis are produced by the pentose phosphate pathway. NADH required for gluconeogenesis is generated via the oxidation of fatty acids and deamination of amino acids.

Deficiency signs

A deficiency in niacin results in pellagra, which is a nutritional disease endemic among poor communities who subsist chiefly on maize. The prognosis is complicated by signs of protein–energy malnutrition and by

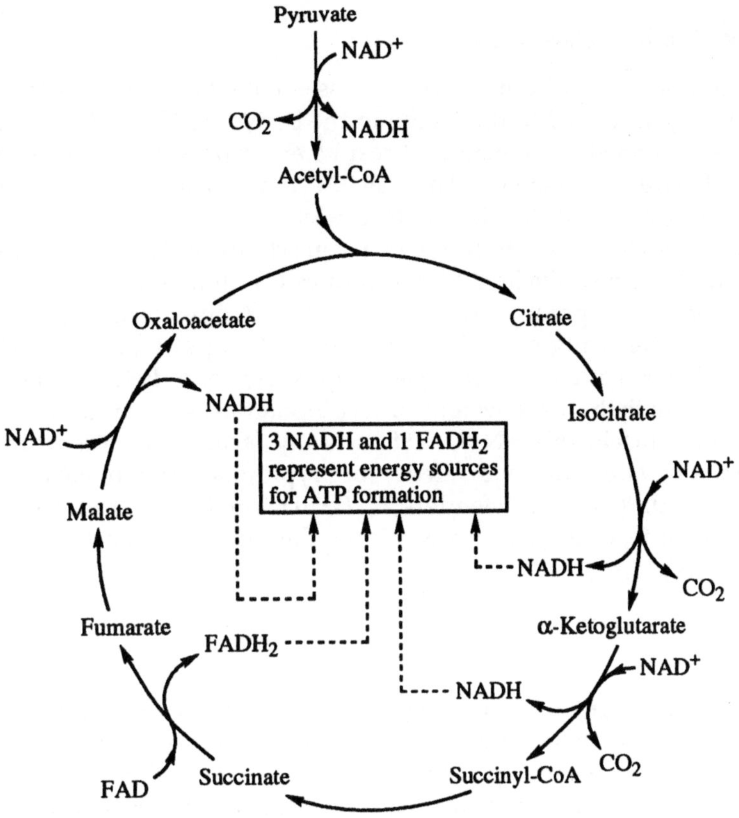

Figure 2.13 Involvement of NAD^+ in the TCA cycle.

an imbalance of amino acid intake, particularly low levels of tryptophan and high levels of leucine. The disease is diagnosed in the early stages by a sunburn-like dermatitis affecting skin areas exposed to light. The dermatitis may progress to a scaled and cracked condition, and in chronic cases the skin becomes rough and thickened with a brown pigmentation. Gastrointestinal disturbances (abdominal pain, diarrhoea and loss of appetite) may also appear, accompanied by oral lesions similar to those described for riboflavin. Early neurological symptoms include tremor, irritability, anxiety and depression, with delirium and dementia sometimes occurring in severe and chronic cases. The response to nicotinamide therapy is rapid and dramatic: untreated pellagra results eventually in death. Because of the widespread occurrence of niacin in its coenzyme forms, primary deficiencies are rare (at least in industrialized countries), but secondary deficiencies may arise from gastrointestinal disorders or alcoholism.

Expression of dietary value

Nicotinic acid and nicotinamide possess equal vitamin activity, the free acid being converted to the amide in the body. No IU of niacin activity has been defined, and analytical results are expressed in weight units (mg) of pure nicotinamide. The niacin activity of food samples can be assayed by a growth test in rats or chicks.

To account for the contribution to niacin activity by dietary tryptophan, the term 'niacin equivalent' was introduced. In humans, approximately 60 mg of L-tryptophan yield 1 mg of niacin, so one niacin equivalent is equal to either 1 mg of available niacin or 60 mg of tryptophan (FAO/WHO, 1967). To calculate the niacin equivalent of a diet, one therefore adds one-sixtieth of the weight of tryptophan present to the weight of preformed niacin (NAS/NRC, 1989). Many factors, such as hormonal status, can affect the equivalence of tryptophan and dietary niacin. Horwitt, Harper and Henderson (1981) predicted that 89 mg of tryptophan to 1 mg of niacin would be the ratio to cover 97.5% of the population.

Toxicity

Nicotinic acid administered orally at doses as low as 100 mg/day causes peripheral vasodilatation with the appearance of skin flushing. In high doses, nicotinic acid competes with uric acid for excretion, leading to an increase in the incidence of acute gouty arthritis. Of greatest concern is possible liver damage, and in one report severe jaundice occurred at doses of 750 mg/day for only 3 months. Nicotinamide does not cause vasodilatation, but is otherwise two to three times as toxic as the acid (Miller and Hayes, 1982; Alhadeff, Gualtieri and Lipton, 1984).

2.3.9 METABOLISM

Ingested nicotinamide nucleotides are hydrolysed in the small intestine, and the liberated nicotinamide, along with nicotonic acid and tryptophan, is absorbed and transported to the liver. In the liver, tryptophan and the niacin vitamers are converted via a common intermediary (nicotonic acid ribonucleotide) into NAD, some of which is utilized by the liver itself. Vitamin B_6 is a required coenzyme for at least four steps in the tryptophan–niacin pathway. The surplus NAD is hydrolysed in the liver to free nicotinamide, which is then released into the general circulation accompanied by the nicotinic acid that was not metabolized. On reaching the tissues, the niacin vitamers are used for the intracellular synthesis of NAD and NADP. There is a continuous turnover of these nucleotides in the body and very little storage. Excess niacin is converted in the liver to methyl derivatives, which are excreted in the urine (McCormick, 1988c).

2.3.10 BIOAVAILABILITY

The *in vivo* conversion of tryptophan to NAD is inadequate to meet the total coenzyme requirement in humans, and niacin must be included in the diet. The utilization of tryptophan as a precursor of NAD depends upon the dietary supply of other essential amino acids. If the supply falls, less tryptophan is utilized in protein synthesis and more becomes available for conversion to NAD. A high dietary intake of leucine interferes with tryptophan metabolism and increases the requirement for niacin. This essential amino acid is found in high concentration in sorghum. In parts of India, where sorghum is the staple cereal, niacin deficiency is likely to occur because of the excess leucine intake (Passmore and Eastwood, 1986). The unavailability of niacin in alkali-untreated maize, coupled with a very low proportion of tryptophan in zein (the major protein in maize), almost certainly explains the high incidence of pellagra in those communities which rely on maize for their staple diet.

It has been suggested (Mason and Kodicek, 1973; Mason, Gibson and Kodicek, 1973) that the nutritional unavailability of bound nicotinic acid in cereals is due to its association with indigestible hemicelluloses, which prevents access of the gastrointestinal esterases to the nicotinoyl ester bonds. Alternatively, esterase activity may be poor: the methyl ester of nicotinic acid was only 15% as effective as the free acid in supporting the growth of rats (Wall and Carpenter, 1988). A small fraction of bound nicotinic acid appears to be biologically available as a result of hydrolysis by gastric acid. About 10% of the total niacin was released as free nicotinic acid after extraction of sorghum meal with 0.1 N HCl (Bender and Bender, 1986), and bioavailability studies in humans and rats (Carter and Carpenter, 1982a,b) have shown that bound nicotinic acid can be partially utilized. Several authors have suggested that the measurement of free (0.1 N HCl extractable) niacin in foods would provide an accurate estimate of the content of available niacin but, in view of the apparent partial utilization of bound nicotinic acid, this may underestimate the niacin value.

Feeding tests have shown that the oxidized form of NAD (NAD^+) is biologically available as a source of niacin and supports rat growth in proportion to its content of nicotinamide. Reduced NAD (NADH) is not available, probably because it is labile in acid and breaks down in the gastric juice (Wall and Carpenter, 1988).

2.4 VITAMIN B_6

2.4.1 HISTORY

In 1934 György observed the appearance of a scaly dermatitis (acrodynia) in rats fed on diets free from the whole vitamin B complex and supplemented with thiamin and riboflavin. This observation led to the establishment of a 'rat acrodynia-preventative factor' and its designation as vitamin B_6. The isolation of the pure crystalline vitamin was first reported by Lepkovsky in 1938, and the synthesis of pyridoxine was accomplished by Harris and Folkers in the following year. The existence of pyridoxal and pyridoxamine and the recognition of their phosphorylated forms as coenzymes is largely credited to Snell during 1944–1948.

2.4.2 STRUCTURE

Vitamin B_6 is the generic descriptor for all 3-hydroxy-2-methylpyridine derivatives which exhibit qualitatively in rats the biological activity of pyridoxine (Snell, 1986). Six B_6 vitamers are known, namely pyridoxine or pyridoxol (PN), pyridoxal (PL) and pyridoxamine (PM), which possess, respectively, alcohol, aldehyde and amine groups in the 4-position (Figure 2.14); their 5′-phosphate esters are designated as PNP, PLP and PMP. Pyridoxine is systematically named as 3-hydroxy-4,5-bis(hydroxy-methyl)-2-methylpyridine and is available commercially as its hydrochloride salt ($C_8H_{11}O_3N.HCl$, MW = 205.65).

In aqueous solutions the vitamin B_6 compounds exist in a variety of equilibrium forms, depending upon the pH (Snell, 1958). The structures of some of these forms are shown in Figure 2.14. PN exists as the cation in acidic solutions, as the anion in alkaline solutions, and primarily as the electrically neutral dipolar ion (IV) at neutral pH. PM also exists as the cation in acidic solutions and the anion in alkaline solutions, but at neutral pH the predominant form is the tripolar ion (VI). The situation is more complicated with PL owing to the posssibility of hemiacetal formation or hydration. At neutral pH the predominant form of PL is the hemiacetal dipolar ion (V).

In its role as a coenzyme, PMP binds to the apoenzyme through salt linkage to the coenzyme phosphate group, whereas PLP is bound more tightly to the apoenzyme by a Schiff base (aldimine) linkage formed through condensation of the 4-carbonyl group with the ε-amino group of specific lysine residues (Morino and Nagashima, 1986). The resultant Schiff base compounds may be subject to nucleophilic attack by a neighbouring amino, sulphydryl or imidazole group to form a substituted aldamine (Figure 2.15) (Gregory and Kirk, 1977). All of these forms of

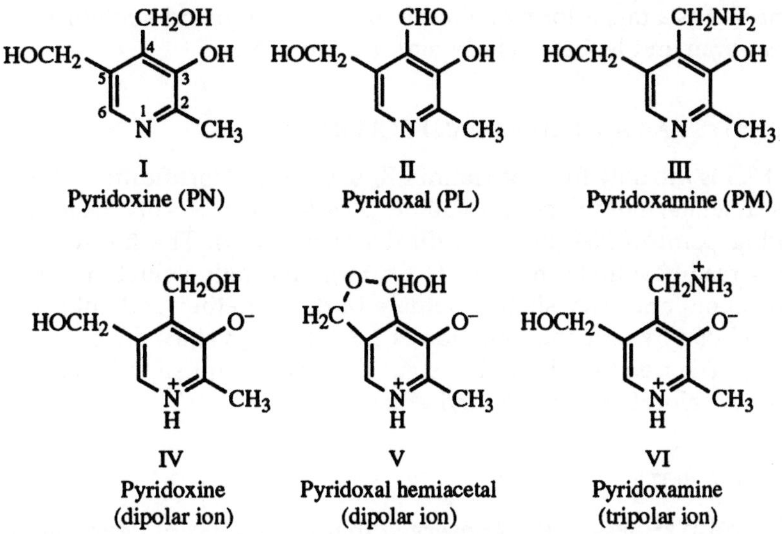

Figure 2.14 Structures of vitamin B_6 compounds. Uncharged neutral forms are I–III; ionic forms as the compounds exist in aqueous solution at neutral pH (IV–VI).

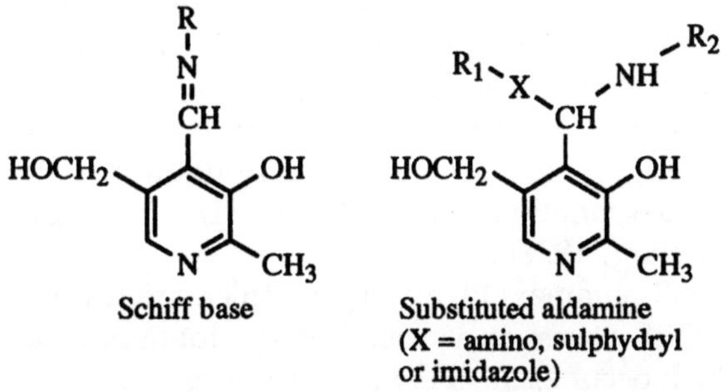

Figure 2.15 Potential interactions involving pyridoxal and amino groups of food proteins. Analogous reactions would occur with pyridoxal phosphate and proteins.

vitamin B_6 are reversibly bound and easily dissociated from the apoenzymes.

A ubiquitous bound form of PN that occurs in plant tissues is a glucoside conjugate, 5′-*O*-(β-D-glucopyranosyl)-pyridoxine, designated in this text as PN-glucoside (Gregory, 1988). Two minor derivatives in which an organic acid is esterified to the C-6 position of the glucosyl moiety of PN-glucoside have been identified in legume seedlings (Gregory, 1988). A more complex derivative of PN-glucoside containing cellobiose and 5-hydroxydioxindole-3-acetic acid moieties has been identified as a major form of vitamin B_6 in rice bran and a minor form in wheat bran and legumes (Tadera and Orite, 1991).

2.4.3 PHYSICAL AND CHEMICAL PROPERTIES

PN.HCl is the only form of vitamin B_6 used in the fortification of foods. It is a white, odourless, crystalline powder with a salty taste and a melting point of 204–206 °C (with decomposition). The hydrochloride salt is readily soluble in water (1 g/5 ml), sparingly soluble in ethanol (1 g/100 ml) and very slightly soluble in diethyl ether and chloroform. The pH of a 5% aqueous solution is 2.3–3.5; pK_a values are 5.0 and 9.0 (25 °C). The free base is readily soluble in water and slightly soluble in acetone, chloroform and diethyl ether.

2.4.4. STABILITY

Saidi and Warthesen (1983) observed that no significant degradation of PN.HCl took place when aqueous solutions protected from light were held at 40 °C and 60 °C for up to 140 days at pH levels from 4 to 7. Under the same conditions, PM.2HCl showed a trend of increasing loss with increasing pH, while PL.HCl showed a marked loss at pH 5, but only a moderate loss above and below that pH. Ang (1979) showed that PN.HCl was the most stable and PM.2HCl the least stable of the three vitamers after exposure of aqueous solutions to normal laboratory light at different pH values. Low-actinic amber glassware or yellow or gold fluorescent lighting protected the vitamers from photodegradation. The principal photodegradation product of PLP is 4-pyridoxic acid 5′-phosphate (Reiber, 1972).

The aldehydic B_6 vitamers PL and PLP, which are reversibly bound to proteins as Schiff bases and substituted aldamines, and the PN-glucosides, which occur exclusively in plant tissues, are readily liberated by acid extraction with autoclaving (Vanderslice *et al.*, 1985). The conjugated form of vitamin B_6 identified in brans and legumes (Tadera and Orite, 1991) released the free vitamin only when hydrolysed with alkali and then with ß-glucosidase (Tadera, Kaneko and Yagi, 1986).

2.4.5 SPECTROSCOPIC PROPERTIES

Absorption

The absorption spectrum of PN.HCl is strongly dependent upon the pH of the solution (Figure 2.16). At pH 1.8 there is a single maximum at 290 nm which diminishes in intensity at pH 4.5 with the appearance of a new maximum at 324 nm. At pH 7.0 the 324-nm maximum increases in intensity, the 290-nm maximum disappears and a new maximum appears at 253 nm. The spectra of PL.HCl at corresponding pH values are similar to those of PN.HCl, the only obvious difference being at pH 7.0, where the maximum occurs at 316 nm. The $A_{1\,cm}^{1\%}$ values of acidified solutions (pH about 2) of PN.HCl and PL.HCl are, respectively, *c.* 430 at λ_{max} 290.5 nm and 440 at λ_{max} 286.5 nm (Strohecker and Henning, 1966). The absorbance maxima of various molecular species of vitamin B_6 compounds are presented in Table 2.2

Fluorescence

PN, PL (hemiacetal) and PM all display native fluorescence whose intensity is pH-dependent (Table 2.2). PM is the most highly fluorescent compound of the three. The phosphorylated forms are only weakly fluorescent, as shown by the relatively low intensity displayed by PLP.

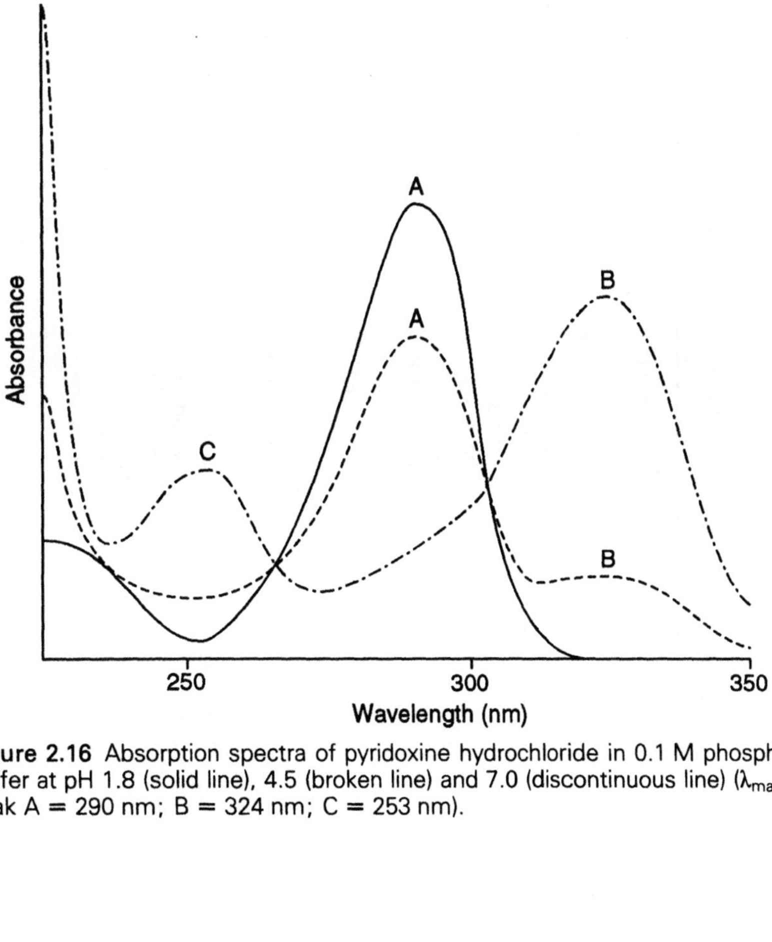

Figure 2.16 Absorption spectra of pyridoxine hydrochloride in 0.1 M phosphate buffer at pH 1.8 (solid line), 4.5 (broken line) and 7.0 (discontinuous line) (λ_{max} of peak A = 290 nm; B = 324 nm; C = 253 nm).

Table 2.2 Absorption and fluorescence properties of vitamin B_6 compounds (Bridges, Davies and Williams, 1966)

Compound	Molecular species	Wavelength (nm)			Intensity of max. fluorescence (corrected)	pH range of max. fluorescence
		Of max. absorption	Of max. excitation	Of max. fluorescence		
Pyridoxine	Cation	291	302	345	10	Highly acidic
	Cation (ex.)[a]	–	302	400	150	2.5
	Dipolar ion	324	332	400	165	6.5–7.5
	Anion	310	320	380	144	12–14
	Neutral form	286	296	335	–	(in ethanol)
Pyridoxal hemiacetal	Cation	288	300	350	13	Highly acidic
	Cation (ex.)[a]	–	300	382	145	0
	Dipolar ion	317	330	382	150	6
	Anion	302	310	356	270	12
	Neutral form	280 (dioxan)	291	330	–	(in ethanol)
Pyridoxamine	Dication	292	306	350	95	Highly acidic
	Dication (ex.)[a]	–	302	400	365	Highly acidic
	Tripolar ion	326	337	400	245	4.9–5.5
	Dipolar ion	–	–	None	0	–
	Anion	310	320	370	345	15
	Neutral form	287 (dioxan)	309	361	–	(in ethanol)

Pyridoxal-5′-phosphate (aldehyde hydrate form)	Cation	291	302	385	<1.0	Highly acidic
	Cation (ex.)[a]	–	302	400	13	1
	Cation-phosphate monoanion	291	302	400	–	–
	Cation-phosphate monoanion (ex.)[a]	–	302	410	–	–
	Dipolar ion–phosphate monoanion	324	330	410	8	6
	Dipolar ion-phosphate dianion	324	330	400	–	7.5–8.5
	Trianion	305	315	370	20.5	12–14
	Trianion aldehyde form?	388	400	525	About 2	12–14

The concentration of each compound was 5 μg/ml.

[a] ex. refers to the excited state ionization as opposed to normal ionization.

The fluorescence spectra of PN.HCl in 0.1 M phosphate buffer, pH 7.0, are shown in Figure 2.17.

2.4.6 DIETARY SOURCES

Vitamin B_6 is present in all natural unprocessed foods, with yeast extract, wheat bran and liver containing particularly high concentrations. Other important sources include whole-grain cereals, nuts, pulses, lean meat, fish, kidney, potatoes and other vegetables. Milk, eggs and fruits contain relatively low concentrations of the vitamin (see Table 1.1).

In raw animal and fish tissue the major form of vitamin B_6 is PLP, which is reversibly bound to proteins as Schiff bases and substituted aldamines. PN and PNP are virtually absent in animal tissues, one exception being liver tissue, in which they are detectable at very low levels. Using a nonhydrolytic extraction procedure and HPLC, the vitamin B_6 content of whole pasteurized homogenized milk was found to comprise the following vitamers: PL (53%), PLP (23%), PMP (12%) and PM (12%); PN was not detected (Gregory and Feldstein, 1985).

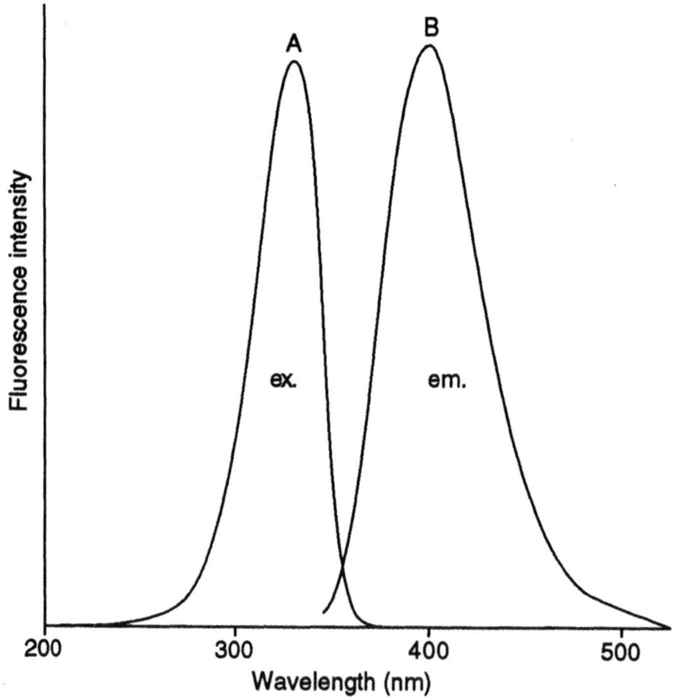

Figure 2.17 Fluorescence excitation and emission spectra of pyridoxine hydrochloride in 0.1 M phosphate buffer at pH 7.0 (λ_{max} of peak A = 327 nm; B = 393 nm).

Siegel, Melnick and Oser (1943) estimated the free and total vitamin B_6 content of milk by assaying aliquots before and after acid hydrolysis; the difference indicated the amount of bound vitamin, which was found to be 14% of the total. PNP does not occur to any measurable extent in natural products. Plant tissue contains mostly PN, a proportion of which may be present as PN-glucoside and/or other conjugates (Kabir, Leklem and Miller, 1983). Typical sources of PN-glucoside (expressed as a percentage of the total vitamin B_6 present) are bananas (5.5%), raw broccoli (35.1%), raw green beans (58.5%), raw carrots (70.1%) and orange juice (69.1%) (Gregory and Ink, 1987). In cereal grains over 90% of the vitamin B_6 is found in the bran and germ (Polansky and Toepfer, 1969a), and 75–90% of the vitamin content of the whole grain is lost in the milling of wheat to low-extraction flour (Sauberlich, 1985).

2.4.7 EFFECTS OF FOOD PROCESSING AND STORAGE

Both the quantity and form of vitamin B_6 are affected by the processes of heating, concentration and dehydration (Sauberlich, 1985; Tannenbaum Young and Archer, 1985). In particular, the retorting process used to sterilize canned foods induces marked losses of vitamin B_6. Most of the research into the effects of heat sterilization has been applied to autoclaved milk products, including canned evaporated milk. The sterilization of milk and nonfortified infant formula induced losses of 36–67% of naturally occurring vitamin B_6 using *Saccharomyces carlsbergensis* as the assay organism; the losses appeared progressively during the first 10 days after processing (Hassinen, Durbin and Bernhart, 1954). The reduction of vitamin activity was due mainly to the loss of PL (the predominant B_6 vitamer in raw milk), although a significant proportion of this vitamer was converted to PM (Gregory, 1959). Only about 50% of the total vitamin B_6 found in sterilized nonfortified milk products by microbiological assay (*S. carlsbergensis*) was biologically available as determined by rat growth assay, whereas the bioassay and the microbiological assay agreed for the analysis of sterilized milk products fortified with PN.HCl (Tomarelli, Spence and Bernhart, 1955). PN.HCl is stable during retort processing, while PM.2HCl and PL.HCl are 2.5- to 3.5-fold less stable (Gregory and Hiner, 1983). The research effort has led to the general conclusion that the thermal processing of milk products and other animal-derived foods promotes the chemical reduction of protein-bound Schiff base forms of PL and PLP to peptide-linked ε-pyridoxyllysine (Figure 2.18) or its 5′-phosphate derivative, which possess low vitamin B_6 availability and are highly stable. This reaction has been demonstrated to take place in evaporated milk, chicken liver and muscle that were autoclaved to simulate retort processing (Gregory, Ink and Sartain, 1986) and in a dehydrated model food system that was stored at 37 °C and 0.6 water activity (a_w) for 128 days (Gregory and Kirk, 1978).

The formation of bis-4-pyridoxyl disulphide has been demonstrated in heat-sterilized milk through reaction between PL added at high concentration before heat treatment and sulphydryl groups liberated through denaturation of the milk proteins (Bernhart, D'amato and Tomarelli, 1960; Wendt and Bernhart, 1960). This thermal reaction product has a low vitamin B_6 activity and it has been proposed that its formation may account for the reported loss of vitamin availability. However, Gregory, Ink and Sartain (1986), using PL and PLP levels comparable to those occurring naturally, did not detect bis-4-pyridoxyl disulphide, which suggested that this compound is not quantitatively important as a form of vitamin B_6 in thermally processed foods.

Vitamin B_6 losses are not as great when processing spray-dried milk products and condensed milk as they are when heat sterilization is employed (Hassinen, Durbin and Bernhart, 1954). High-temperature short-time (HTST) pasteurization (2–3 s at 92 °C) and boiling of milk for 2–3 min gave only 3% loss, while ultra-HTST sterilization (injection of steam at 143 °C into preheated milk for 3–4 s) caused negligible loss of the vitamin (Tannenbaum, Young and Archer, 1985).

Interconversions between the aldehyde (PL and PLP) and amine (PM and PMP) B_6 vitamers via reversible interaction with proteins or carbonyl compounds occur during the processing or storage of meat and dairy products (Gregory, Ink and Sartain, 1986). For example, in hydrolysed extracts of raw pork loin the predominant vitamer is PL, whereas in fully cooked ham it is PM (Polansky and Toepfer, 1969b).

Thermal processing had little effect on the concentration of PN-glucoside in alfalfa sprouts, demonstrating the stability of the glycosidic bond as well as the stability of the PN moiety of the conjugate (Ink, Gregory and Sartain, 1986).

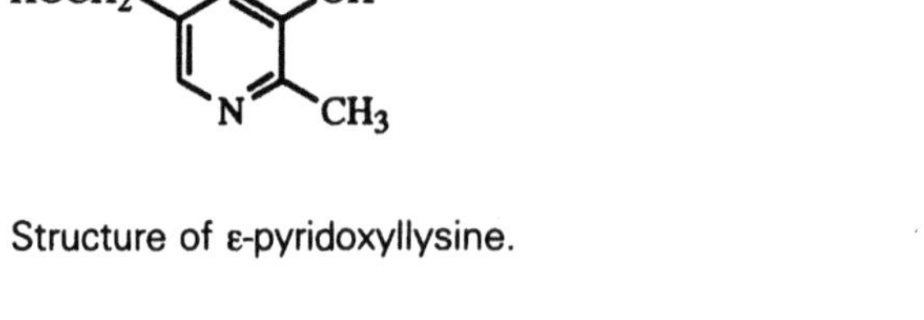

Figure 2.18 Structure of ε-pyridoxyllysine.

2.4.8 BIOCHEMICAL AND PHYSIOLOGICAL FUNCTIONS

Vitamin B_6 in the form of PLP functions as a coenzyme in amino acid metabolism, but in certain transaminases the coenzyme is PMP. Aminotransferases facilitate the transfer of amino groups between amino acids and keto acids, and thus represent an important link between amino acid, carbohydrate and fat metabolism (Figure 2.19). Biogenic amines such as dopamine, serotonin, histamine and gamma-aminobutyric acid (GABA), which are implicated as neurotransmitters, are either synthesized or metabolized with the aid of PLP-dependent enzyme reactions. PLP is also involved in the synthesis of sphingosine, and a deficiency of vitamin B_6 leads to impaired development of brain lipids and incomplete myelination of nerve fibres in the central nervous system (Dakshinamurti, Paulose and Siow, 1985). Hence vitamin B_6 plays a critical role in the structural and functional integrity of the central and peripheral nervous systems. Vitamin B_6 is also involved in the metabolism of folic acid and vitamin B_{12}, and in the synthesis of many hormones.

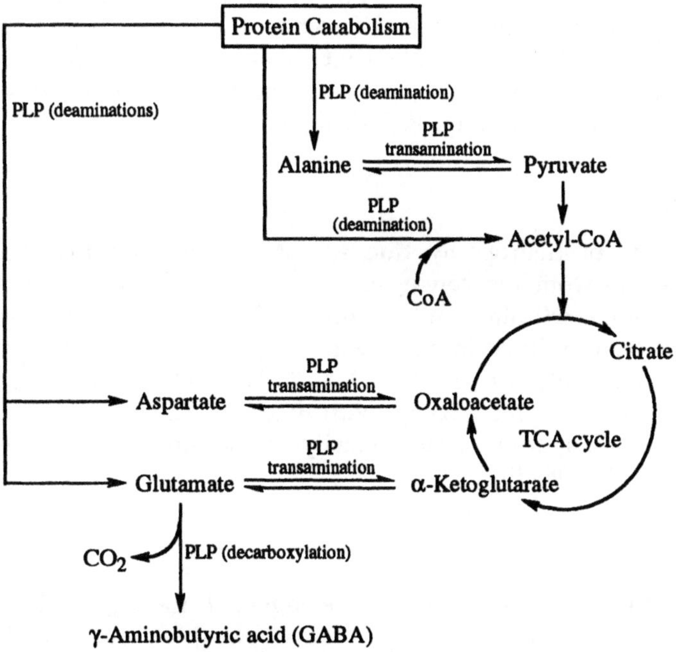

Figure 2.19 Some important reactions involving vitamin B_6 in amino acid metabolism. PLP = pyridoxal 5′-phosphate; CoA = coenzyme A.

Deficiency signs

Vitamin B_6 is widely distributed in foods, and any diet so poor as to be insufficent in this vitamin would most likely lack adequate amounts of other B-group vitamins. For this reason, a primary clinical deficiency of B_6 in the adult human is rarely encountered. In the 1950s, an occurrence of convulsions in infants was traced to a nonfortified liquid milk-based canned formula that had undergone autoclaving in manufacture (Coursin, 1954). There is considerable evidence that the convulsions were caused by an insufficient production of GABA, the major inhibitory neurotransmitter in the brain (Ebadi, 1978). The administration of the antagonist deoxypyridoxine to adult volunteers receiving diets low in vitamin B_6 resulted in lesions of the skin and mouth that resembled those of riboflavin and niacin deficiency. These symptoms responded to B_6 therapy, but did not respond to thiamin, riboflavin or niacin (NAS/NRC, 1980).

Expression of dietary value

No IU of vitamin B_6 activity has been defined, and analytical results are expressed in weight units (mg) of pure PN.HCl. Using plasma PLP concentration as an index of vitamin B_6 status in a rat bioassay, Nguyen *et al.* (1983) found little or no difference in apparent biological activity between PN, PL and PM. All six vitamers have equal biological activity in humans (on a molar basis) as a result of their enzymatic conversion to the major coenzyme form, PLP (Brin, 1978).

Toxicity

Symptoms of neuropathy due to vitamin B_6 overdose have been observed in women receiving upwards of 50 mg of B_6 per day for 6 months or more (Dalton and Dalton, 1987). A B_6 dependency syndrome has also been induced in healthy adults given a 200-mg supplement of the vitamin daily for 33 days (NAS/NRC, 1980). These observations suggest that chronic dosing with vitamin B_6 above 50 mg/day is potentially dangerous. Acute toxicity of the vitamin is, however, low (McCormick, 1988d).

2.4.9 METABOLISM

The various B_6 vitamers which are ingested are absorbed by passive diffusion in the small intestine after dephosphorylation of the phosphorylated compounds in the gastrointestinal tract. The vitamers are transported to the liver, where they are phosphorylated, and where

PNP and PMP are converted to the major active form, PLP. A proportion of the PLP is utilized directly in the liver, and a regulated amount is released and circulated tightly bound to serum albumin. Prior to tissue uptake, the PLP is dissociated from the albumin and dephosphorylated; it is then rephosphorylated after cell entry. Interconversion between PLP and PMP occurs within the tissues. The major body pool of vitamin B_6 is skeletal muscle, in which 90% or more of the vitamin in the form of PLP is bound to the enzyme glycogen phosphorylase. The major end-product of vitamin B_6 metabolism is 4-pyridoxic acid, which is excreted in the urine.

2.4.10 BIOAVAILABILITY

The availability of vitamin B_6 in foods is highly variable, owing to a number of factors, including the presence of PN-glucoside in plant tissues and the formation of reaction products during food processing. In general, vitamin B_6 has a lower availability from plant-derived foods than from animal tissues (Nguyen and Gregory, 1983). Based on plasma PLP levels in male human subjects, the availability of the vitamin in an average American diet ranged from 61% to 81%, with a mean of 71% (Tarr, Tamura and Stokstad, 1981).

Gregory *et al.* (1991) determined the bioavailability of PN-glucoside in humans through the use of a stable-isotope method. The utilization of orally administered deuterated PN-glucoside was 58 ± 13% (mean ± SEM) relative to that of deuterated PN. Intravenously administered PN-glucoside underwent approximately half the metabolic utilization of oral PN-glucoside, which suggested a role of ß-glucosidase(s) of the intestinal mucosa, microflora, or both, in the release of free PN from dietary PN-glucoside. In contrast, the bioavailability of PN-glucoside in the rat is approximately 20–30% relative to PN (Ink, Gregory and Sartain, 1986; Trumbo, Gregory and Sartain, 1988). PN-glucoside accounted for 10–15% of the total vitamin B_6 in the typical mixed diets used in the human study, but would be proportionally higher in vegetarian diets. No significant difference was found in the vitamin B_6 status of vegetarian women compared with nonvegetarians receiving similar vitamin B_6 intakes (Schultz and Leklem, 1987).

Kies, Kan and Fox (1984) obtained experimental data indicating that vitamin B_6 provided by the bran fractions of wheat, rice and corn (maize) is unavailable to humans. However, the presence of fibre in plant foods appears to have only a minor effect on vitamin B_6 availability. A wide variety of dietary fibre material (polysaccharides, lignin and wheat bran) did not bind or entrap B_6 vitamers *in vitro* (Nguyen *et al.*, 1981), and cellulose, pectin and bran had little or no effect on the availability of vitamin B_6 in a chick bioassay (Nguyen, Gregory and Damron, 1981). In humans, the availability of vitamin B_6 from whole wheat bread was only 5–10% less than that from white bread supplemented with vitamin B_6 (Leklem *et al.*, 1980), and the addition of wheat bran (15 g/day) to human diets resulted in only a minor decrease (maximum of 17%) in availability of the vitamin (Lindberg, Leklem and Miller, 1983).

The Schiff base and substituted aldamine forms of vitamin B_6 that occur naturally in foods of animal origin are presumed to be totally available, as these complexes readily dissociate under gastric acid conditions (Gregory and Kirk, 1977). The Schiff base reduction product, ε-pyridoxyllysine, which is formed during the thermal processing of animal-derived foods, is extremely resistant to acid hydrolysis and, in the rat, exhibits approximately 50% availability relative to the molar utilization of free PN (Gregory, 1980a). The effect of ε-pyridoxyllysine on the availability of vitamin B_6 in foods appears to depend upon the total vitamin B_6 content of the diet and the ratio of the protein-bound vitamin to free B_6 vitamers. When fed to rats at low levels in vitamin B_6-deficient diets, ε-pyridoxyllysine demonstrated anti-vitamin B_6 activity, which could be counteracted by dietary supplementation with PN (Gregory, 1980a). This anti-vitamin B_6 activity is attributable, at least in part, to the competitive inhibition of pyridoxal kinase, which is the enzyme that catalyses the 5′-phosphorylation of PL (Gregory, 1980b). This antagonistic effect may have been responsible for the severe deficiency developed in infants fed nonfortified, heat-sterilized, canned infant formulas (Coursin, 1954). The effect does not occur if the diet is adequate in vitamin B_6 content (Gregory and Kirk, 1981).

2.5 PANTOTHENIC ACID

2.5.1 HISTORY

In 1933 R.J. Williams and his associates isolated from a variety of biological materials an acidic substance that acted as a growth factor for yeast. Williams named the substance pantothenic acid because of its apparently widespread occurrence (Greek *pantos*, everywhere). Pantothenic acid was recognized as a vitamin for animals in 1939, when Jukes and Wooley independently reported that pantothenic acid isolated in pure form from liver by R.J. Williams in 1938 was identical to a chick antidermatitis factor first described by Norris and Ringrose in 1930. The biochemical role of pantothenic acid as a constituent of coenzyme A was identified by Lipmann in 1947.

2.5.2 STRUCTURE

Pantothenic acid comprises a derivative of butyric acid (pantoic acid) joined by a peptide linkage to the amino acid ß-alanine, and is systematically named as *d*(+)-*N*-(2,4-dihydroxy-3,3-dimethyl-1-oxobutyl)-ß-alanine ($C_9H_{17}O_5N$, MW = 219.23). The molecule is optically active but only the *d*(+)-enantiomorph occurs in nature. Synthetic pantothenic acid is a racemic mixture and, since only the *d* isomer is biologically active, this fact must be considered if the *dl* mixture is to be used therapeutically. Free pantothenic acid exists as a pale yellow extremely hygroscopic viscous oil which, consequently, is unsuitable for commercial application. For human food supplements, calcium *d*-pantothenate $(C_9H_{16}O_5N)_2Ca$ (MW = 476.53) is used. In nature, pantothenic acid occurs only rarely in the free state, but it is very widely distributed as an integral part of the structures of coenzyme A and 4-phosphopantetheine. The latter serves as a covalently attached prosthetic group of acyl carrier protein (ACP) (Figure 2.20). The term coenzyme A may be abbreviated to CoA-SH to show the functional sulphydryl group, or simply to CoA.

The corresponding alcohol of pantothenic acid, pantothenol (referred to commercially as pathenol), is widely used as a source of pantothenate activity for pharmaceutical vitamin products, because it is more stable than the pantothenate salts, especially in liquid multivitamin products that must be slightly acid to preserve the thiamin content. Pantothenol does not occur naturally and itself has no pantothenate activity, but it is converted quantitatively to pantothenic acid *in vivo* and is equivalent to pantothenic acid in man (Bird and Thompson, 1967).

2.5.3 PHYSICAL AND CHEMICAL PROPERTIES

Calcium pantothenate is a colourless, odourless, bitter-tasting, moderately hygroscopic microcrystalline powder which decomposed at *c.* 200 °C. The pH of an aqueous (1 in 20) solution of calcium pantothenate is 7.2–8.0; the pK_a value is 4.4 (Kutsky, 1973). Pantothenic acid is readily soluble in water and ethyl acetate and slightly soluble in diethyl ether; the calcium salt is more soluble in water (40 g/100 ml), only slightly soluble in ethyl acetate and insoluble in diethyl ether.

2.5.4 STABILITY

The stability of pantothenic acid and its calcium salt in aqueous solution is highly dependent on the pH. In contrast to other B-vitamins, pantothenic acid becomes more stable as the pH of the solution increases. Solutions of calcium pantothenate are most stable between pH 5 and 7 but, even so, are not stable to autoclaving, and therefore sterilization by ultrafiltration is necessary (McCormick, 1988e). Below and above these pH values, solutions of calcium pantothenate are

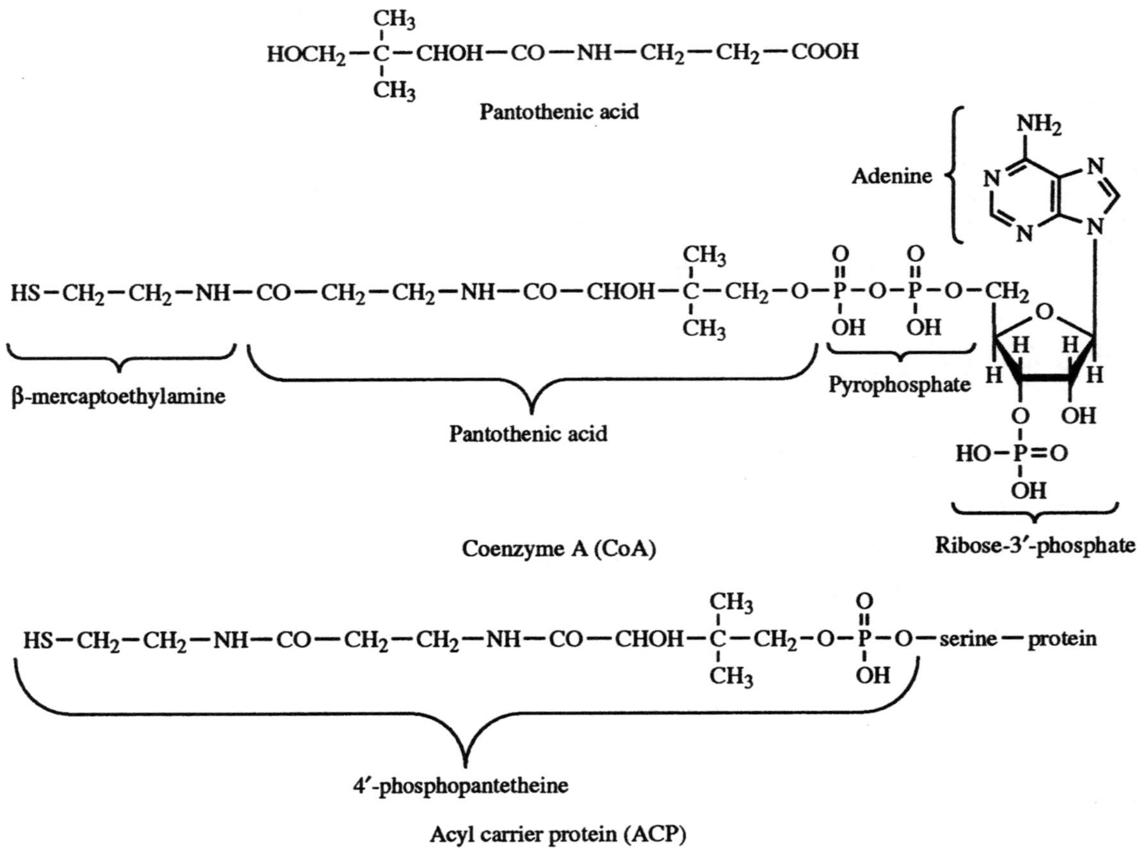

Figure 2.20 Structures of pantothenic acid and compounds containing a pantothenate moiety.

thermolabile. Alkaline hydrolysis yields pantoic acid and β-alanine, whereas acid hydrolysis yields the gamma-lactone of pantoic acid (Tannenbaum, Young and Archer, 1985). Pantothenic acid is unaffected by atmospheric oxygen and light.

2.5.5 SPECTROSCOPIC PROPERTIES

Absorption

The pantothenic acid molecule does not contain a characteristic chromophore, and hence it exhibits only very weak absorbance at 204 nm, owing to the presence of the carbonyl groups.

2.5.6 DIETARY SOURCES

Pantothenic acid is widely distributed in foods of animal and plant origin. Coenzyme A is the major pantothenic acid-containing compound present in animal tissues, but small amounts of other bound forms (phosphopantothenic acid, pantetheine and phosphopantetheine), in addition to free pantothenic acid, have also been detected (Brown, 1959). Significant amounts of bound pantothenic acid other than coenzyme A have been found in milk (Voigt and Eitenmiller, 1978). High concentrations of the vitamin are found in yeast, liver, heart, kidney, eggs, whole-grain cereals and nuts. Lean meat, milk, potatoes and green leafy vegetables contain lesser amounts (see Table 1.1), but are important food sources because of the quantities consumed. Relatively low amounts of the vitamin are found in many highly processed foods (Walsh, Wyse and Hansen, 1981).

2.5.7 EFFECTS OF FOOD PROCESSING

Pantothenic acid is fairly stable during the domestic cooking of natural unprocessed foods. The canning and freezing of foods has been reported by Schroeder (1971) to cause large losses of pantothenic acid. In canned foods of animal origin, losses ranged from 20% to 35%, and in vegetable foods from 46% to 78%. Freezing losses in animal foods ranged from 21% to 70%, and in vegetable foods from 37% to 57%. Grains lost 37%–74% of the original pantothenic acid during conversion to various cereal products, and meats lost 50–75% during conversion to comminuted products. These processing losses were calculated from data on corresponding raw materials rather than on identical materials before and after processing, and have been strongly criticized (Orr and Watt, 1972). However, later studies have also indicated large losses of pantothenic acid in many highly processed foods, including products made from refined grains, fruit products and fat- or cereal-extended meats and fish (Walsh, Wyse and Hansen, 1981). Losses of pantothenic acid during milk pasteurization, sterilization and drying are usually less than 10% (Archer and Tannenbaum, 1979).

2.5.8 BIOCHEMICAL AND PHYSIOLOGICAL FUNCTIONS

The vitamin activity of pantothenic acid is attributable to its incorporation into the molecular structures of CoA and ACP. Though the functional sulphydryl group of these compounds is not part of the pantothenate moiety, the steric configuration of the pantothenate structure is important for enzymatic recognition.

CoA forms energy-rich thioesters with weakly reactive carboxylic acids, so that the acyl (R—CO—) groups can participate in a variety of metabolic processes. In carbohydrate catabolism, the pyruvate produced by glycolysis must undergo an oxidative decarboxylation reaction with CoA to form acetyl-CoA 'active acetate' (CH_3—CO—S—CoA) before the acetyl moiety can react with oxaloacetate to produce citrate in the tricarboxylic acid cycle. Ketogenic amino acids undergo a similar metabolic fate through the formation of acetyl-CoA. The tricarboxylic acid cycle intermediary, α-ketoglutarate, undergoes an oxidative decarboxylation with CoA to form succinyl-CoA, which is a precursor for porphyrin and hence for haemoglobin and cytochromes. Acetyl-CoA is required for the acetylation of amino sugars, which are constituents of various mucopolysaccharides of connective tissues, and also of choline to form the neurotransmitter acetylcholine.

In the biosynthesis of fatty acids (Figure 2.21) the acyl groups of acetyl-CoA and malonyl-CoA are transferred to the —SH group of ACP. The resultant acetyl-ACP and malonyl-ACP molecules react together with the release of CO_2 to form acetoacetyl-ACP, which undergoes further reduction and dehydration reactions to yield butyryl-ACP. This, in turn, reacts with malonyl-ACP, with a repetition of the same sequence of events, to yield a six-carbon fatty acyl-ACP derivative, and so the process is repeated until the palmityl derivative with 16 carbon atoms is formed. The ACP moiety then splits off and the palmitic acid is released. Cholesterol is synthesized from acetyl-CoA via mevalonic acid and squalene.

Deficiency signs

A dietary deficiency of pantothenic acid is virtually impossible apart from circumstances of severe malnutrition. Deficiency symptoms have,

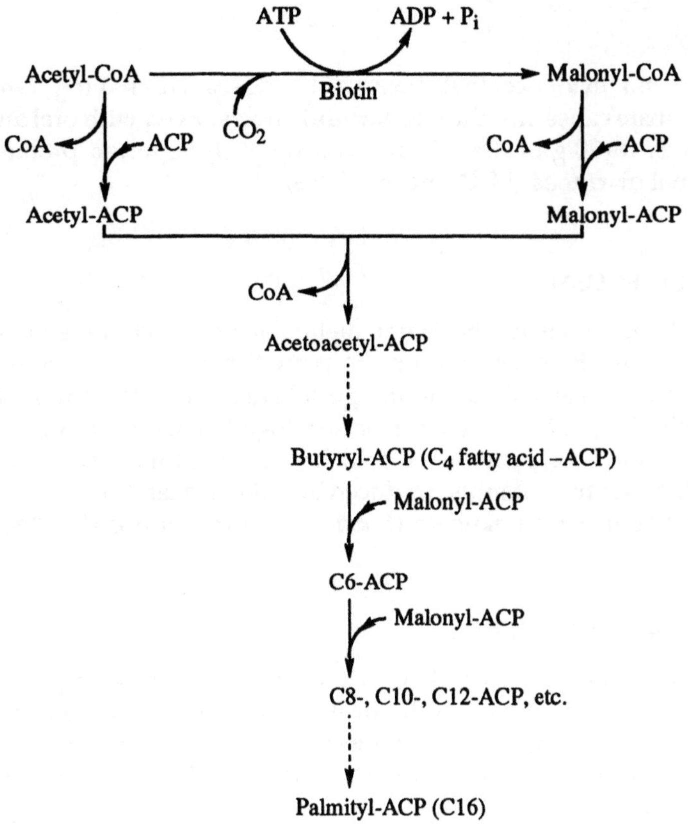

Figure 2.21 The role of acetyl-CoA and ACP in the biosynthesis of fatty acids.

however, been induced by administering a metabolic antagonist omega-methylpantothenic acid, or by providing volunteers with a pantothenate-free semisynthetic diet. The subjects experienced a variety of disorders that included irritability, numbness and tingling of the hands and feet ('burning feet' syndrome), impaired motor co-ordination and gastro-intestinal disturbances (McCormick, 1988e).

Expression of dietary value

No IU of pantothenic acid activity has been defined. Analytical results are generally expressed in weight units (mg) of pantothenic acid, using calcium pantothenate as the standard material: 1 mg of pantothenic acid is equivalent to 1.087 mg of calcium pantothenate. Pantothenate can be assayed biologically in the curative chick growth test.

Toxicity

There is no evidence that therapeutic doses (10–100 mg range) of pantothenate cause any chronic harmful effects. Even with oral amounts as high as 10–20 g of the calcium salt, the only reported problem was occasional diarrhoea (McCormick, 1988e).

2.5.9 METABOLISM

Ingested coenzyme A, the major dietary form of pantothenic acid, is hydrolysed in the small intestine to pantetheine which, together with pantothenate, is absorbed into the portal circulation. Within the tissues the biosynthesis of coenzyme A occurs together with the formation of ACP. Synthesis of pantothenic acid by intestinal microflora has been suspected, but the amounts produced and the availability of the vitamin from this source are unknown (Food and Nutrition Board, 1989).

2.5.10 BIOAVAILABILITY

Little information is at hand regarding the availability of pantothenic acid in food items. Based on the urinary excretion of pantothenic acid, the availability for male human subjects ingesting the 'average American diet' ranged from 40% to 61% with a mean of 50% (Tarr, Tamura and Stokstad, 1981).

2.6 BIOTIN

2.6.1 HISTORY

Biotin was discovered as a result of several independent lines of investigation. In 1916 Bateman reported that the inclusion of large proportions of raw egg white in experimental diets produced a characteristic 'spectacle-eye' hair loss and dermatitis in rats. The causative factor later proved to be avidin, a glycoprotein component of egg white, which binds biotin and renders it unavailable to the rat. Boas in 1927 and later György in 1931 found a curative factor in liver against the egg white injury. In 1936 Kögl and Tönnis isolated from egg yolk a crystalline substance which acted as a growth factor for yeast, and which they named biotin. Independent research conducted by György and du Vigneaud led to the conclusion in 1940 that the above curative and growth factors were chemically identical to each other. The structure of biotin was established in 1942 by du Vigneaud's group.

2.6.2 STRUCTURE

The biotin molecule is a fusion of an imidazolidone ring with a tetrahydrothiophene ring bearing a pentanoic (valeric) acid side chain and systematically named 2′-keto-3,4-imidazolido-2-tetrahydrothiophene-n-valeric acid ($C_{10}H_{16}O_3N_2S$, MW = 244.31). The molecule contains three asymmetric carbon atoms, and hence eight stereoisomers are possible. Of these only the dextrorotatory *d*-biotin occurs in nature and possesses vitamin activity. Biotin synthesized industrially by the Hoffman–La Roche process is also in the *d*-form (Achuta Murthy and Mistry, 1977). The stereochemical structure of *d*-biotin (Figure 2.22) reveals that the two rings are fused in the *cis* configuration and the aliphatic side chain is *cis* with respect to the imidazolidone ring. In animal and plant tissues only a small proportion of the biotin present occurs in the free state. The majority is covalently bound to the protein structure (apoenzyme) of biotin-dependent enzymes via a peptide bond between the carboxyl group of biotin and the ε-amino group of a lysine residue (Zapsalis and Beck, 1985). Proteolysis of the enzyme liberates a natural water-soluble fragment called biocytin (ε-*N*-biotinyl-L-lysine) (Figure 2.23), which is biologically active.

2.6.3 PHYSICAL AND CHEMICAL PROPERTIES

Synthetic *d*-biotin crystallizes as fine colourless needles which melt at 232 °C with decomposition. Biotin in its free acid form is only very sparingly soluble in water at 25 °C (20 mg/100 ml) and in 95% ethanol (80 mg/100 ml) but is more soluble in hot water. It is soluble in dilute alkali, sparingly soluble in dilute acid, and practically insoluble in fat solvents, including chloroform, diethyl ether and petroleum ether. The pH of a 0.01% aqueous solution of biotin is 4.5; the pK_a value is 4.51 (McCormick, 1988f). Biotin salts are significantly more water-soluble than the acid form of biotin.

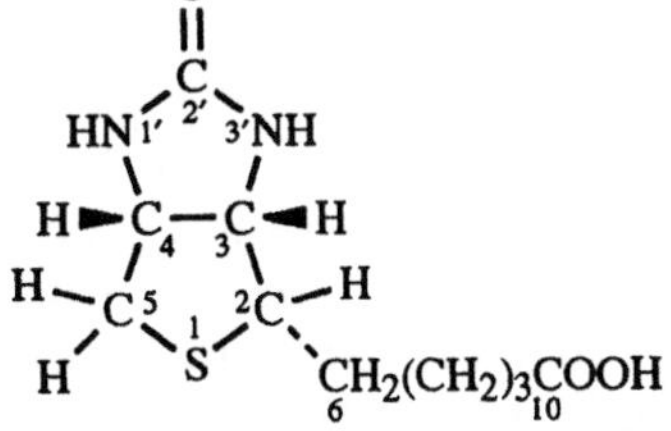

Figure 2.22 The absolute stereochemistry of *d*-biotin.

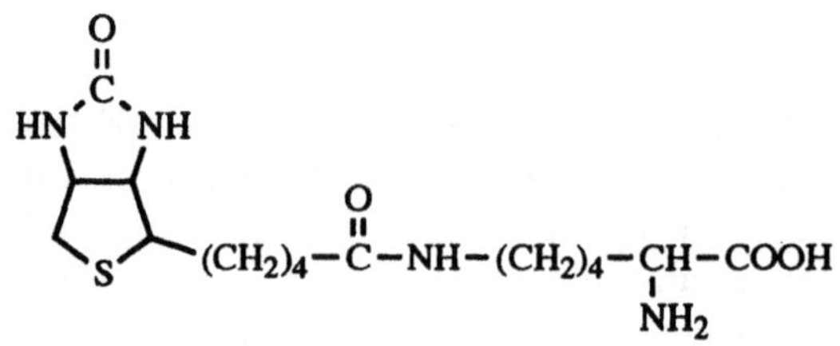

Figure 2.23 Structure of biocytin.

2.6.4 STABILITY

Dry crystalline biotin is stable to heat and atmospheric oxygen but is gradually destroyed by UV radiation. The vitamin shows stability towards strong acids but is unstable to alkali. Aqueous solutions within the pH range 4–9 are stable up to 100 °C, but strongly acid or alkaline solutions are unstable to heating. The sulphur atom can be readily oxidized with various reagents to yield a mixture of isomeric *d*- and *l*-biotin sulphoxides; stronger oxidants form biotin sulphone. These oxidation products are essentially inactive for humans, although the *d*-sulphoxide can be metabolically slowly reduced to biotin (McCormick, 1988f). Bound forms of biotin may be freed by strong acid hydrolysis at elevated temperature or with a proteolytic enzyme (Lampen, Bahler and Peterson, 1942). Aqueous solutions of biotin are very susceptible to mould growth.

2.6.5 SPECTROSCOPIC PROPERTIES

Absorption

The biotin molecule does not contain a characteristic chromophore, apart from the carbonyl groups; hence it exhibits only very weak absorbance at 204 nm.

2.6.6 DIETARY SOURCES

Biotin is present at very low concentration in all natural foodstuffs. Most of the biotin content of animal products, nuts, seeds and yeast is in a protein-bound form. A higher percentage of free water-extractable biotin occurs in vegetables, green plants, fruit, milk and rice bran (Lampen, Bahler and Peterson, 1942). Rich sources of biotin include yeast, wheat bran, oatmeal, nuts, liver, kidney and eggs. Muscle meats, fish, dairy products and cereals contain smaller amounts (see Table 1.1), but are important contributors to the dietary intake.

2.6.7 EFFECTS OF FOOD PROCESSING AND STORAGE

Biotin is quite stable during the commercial processing and storage of foodstuffs. In canned infant foods an approximately 15% reduction in biotin content after a 6-month storage period has been observed (Bonjour, 1984). Biotin is stable towards the sterilization and drying of milk (Benterud, 1977). The cooking of foods can convert a significant portion of biotin to the sulphoxide and sulphone oxidation products, with consequent loss of vitamin activity (Zapsalis and Beck, 1985).

2.6.8 BIOCHEMICAL AND PHYSIOLOGICAL FUNCTIONS

Biotin functions as the prosthetic group in carboxylase enzymes, which are capable of taking up bicarbonate ions as the carboxyl donor and transferring them to specific substrates. The regeneration of glucose (gluconeogenesis) from lactate produced during exercise takes place in the liver and requires means of bypassing several energy barriers in the glycolytic pathway. The bypassing of the phosphoenolpyruvate to pyruvate reaction is achieved by the actions of two enzymes that are unique to gluconeogenesis. The biotin-dependent pyruvate carboxylase catalyses the formation of oxaloacetate from pyruvate, and phosphoenolpyruvate carboxykinase, which is not biotin-dependent, converts oxaloacetate to phosphoenolpyruvate (Figure 2.24). Pyruvate carboxylase is allosterically activated by acetyl-CoA, which will be abundant when energy intake exceeds demand. The glucose thus produced in the liver is then returned to the muscle for energy storage in

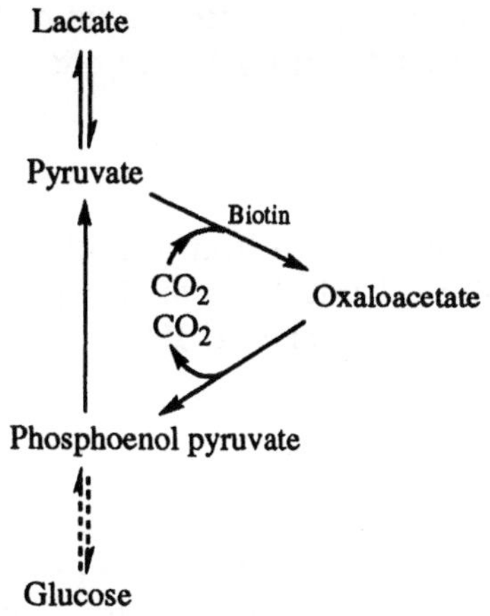

Figure 2.24 The role of biotin in gluconeogenesis.

the form of glycogen. The formation of oxaloacetate is also important in lipid biosynthesis through its role in transporting acetyl-CoA from within the mitochondrion to the cytosol. This involves the continuous removal of oxaloacetate from the mitochondrion, and its replacement by the action of pyruvate carboxylase is necessary to maintain normal tricarboxylic acid cycle activity (Achuta Murthy and Mistry, 1977). Malonyl-CoA, which is required for fatty acid biosynthesis, is formed by the biotin-dependent carboxylation of acetyl-CoA (Figure 2.21).

Deficiency signs

The human requirements for biotin are normally met through the combined dietary supply and endogenous microbial synthesis in the gut. A primary biotin deficiency state is therefore extremely rare, especially where a well-balanced diet prevails. Deficiency states have been induced in adult volunteers by feeding low-biotin diets containing a high proportion of raw egg white. An initial scaly dermatitis was followed by nonspecific symptoms that included extreme lassitude, anorexia, muscular pains, hyperaesthesia and localized paraesthesia. All of these signs and symptoms responded to injections of 150–300 μg of biotin per day. Seborrhoeic dermatitis of the scalp and a more generalized dermatitis known as Leiner's disease have been reported in breast-fed infants when the mother is malnourished. These symptoms are relieved when biotin is administered to the mothers.

Expression of dietary value

No IU of biotin activity has been defined and analytical results are expressed in weight units (μg) of pure *d*-biotin. Biotin can be assayed biologically by the egg white injury test in rats.

Toxicity

Biotin toxicity in humans has not been reported. It is presumably low, since infants have tolerated injections of 10 mg daily for 6 months with no adverse effects (Miller and Hayes, 1982).

2.6.9 METABOLISM

Most of the biotin in foods is incorporated in the biotin-dependent enzymes, although some free biotin may be present. The peptide bond linking the biotin moiety to the lysine residue of the enzyme is resistant to hydrolysis by proteolytic enzymes in the intestinal tract, so the main digestion product is biocytin. Biocytin is readily absorbed, and then enzymatically hydrolysed to free biotin. In the tissues, biotin is covalently bound to the apoenzymes of biotin-dependent enzymes to form the active holoenzyme. Biotin is conserved very efficiently in the body owing to resorption by the kidney and the protein binding of plasma biotin, which reduces filtration at the glomerulus. On catabolism of the biotin-dependent enzymes, the biocytin is hydrolysed by a specific peptidase, permitting reutilization of the vitamin. There is a low, but significant, activity of biotin absorption in the colon, suggesting that biotin synthesized by, and released from, intestinal bacteria can be absorbed (Bowman and Rosenberg, 1987).

2.6.10 BIOAVAILABILITY

Chick growth assays have revealed wide differences in the availability of biotin in cereals. For example, the biotin of maize is completely available, compared with oats and barley (20–30% available) and wheat (almost completely unavailable) (Bonjour, 1984).

Avidin, the glycoprotein in egg white, uniquely binds biotin, both in the free form and as the prosthetic group of enzymes. The complex is stable over a wide pH range and is not dissociated in the gastrointestinal tract. When the eggs are cooked, the avidin is denatured and the biotin is liberated.

2.7 FOLATE

2.7.1 HISTORY

In 1931, Lucy Wills and associates showed that an autolysed yeast preparation (Marmite), which was therapeutically ineffective against the pernicious anaemia caused by vitamin B_{12} deficiency, was effective against nutritional megaloblastic anaemia in pregnant women. These researchers induced a similar anaemia in monkeys which then responded to crude liver extracts. Other factors that cured specific deficiency anaemias in monkeys and chicks were isolated from yeast by different workers and assigned the names 'vitamin M' and 'vitamin B_c'. Another factor isolated from liver was shown to be essential to the growth of *Lactobacillus casei* and therefore called the '*L. casei* factor'. In 1941, Mitchell and co-workers processed 4 tons of spinach to obtain a purified substance with acidic properties which was an active growth factor for rats and *L. casei*. They named the factor 'folic acid' (from *folium*, the Latin word for leaf). Eventually, all of the above factors proved to be the same substance when Angier and co-workers in 1946 accomplished the synthesis and determination of the chemical structure of folic acid.

2.7.2 STRUCTURE

The term folate (or folacin in American usage) is used as the generic descriptor for all derivatives of pteroic acid that demonstrate vitamin activity in humans. The structure (I) depicted in Figure 2.25 is known by the trivial name of folic acid, but is more precisely designated as pteroylmonoglutamic acid. This compound is frequently abbreviated to PteGlu (named after the pteroic acid and glutamate moieties) but in this text it will be referred to in most cases simply as PGA. The fundamental unit of PGA comprises a bicyclic pterin moiety linked by a methylene bridge to *p*-aminobenzoic acid, which is joined by peptide linkage to a single molecule of L-glutamic acid. The latter moiety is essential for vitamin activity. PGA can be systematically named as *N*-(*p*-([2-amino-4-hydrozxy-6-pteridinyl)-methyl]-amino)-benzoyl)glutamic acid ($C_{19}H_{19}N_7O_6$, MW = 441.42). The conformation and absolute configuration of the folates have been described by Temple and Montgomery (1984).

PGA is not a natural physiological form of the vitamin; the pteridine ring of natural folates is reduced to give either the 7,8-dihydrofolate (DHF) or 5,6,7,8-tetrahydrofolate (THF) (Figure 2.25). These reduced forms can be substituted with a covalently bonded one-carbon adduct attached to nitrogen positions 5 or 10 or bridged across both positions. The following substituted forms of THF are important intermediates in folate metabolism: 5-formyl-, 10-formyl-, 5-methyl-, 5-formimino-, 5,10-methylene- and 5,10-methenyl-THF (Figure 2.25). All folate compounds exist predominantly as polyglutamates containing typically from five to seven glutamate residues in gamma-peptide linkage (Gregory, 1989). These conjugates are abbreviated to $PteGlu_n$ derivatives, where *n* is the number of glutamate residues; for example, $5\text{-}CH_3\text{-}H_4PteGlu_3$ refers to triglutamyl-5-methyl-tetrahydrofolic acid. Assuming that the polyglutamyl side chain extends to no more than seven residues, the theoretical number of folates approaches 150 (Baugh and Krumdieck, 1971). An important structural aspect of the 5,6,7,8-tetrahydrofolates is the stereochemical orientation at the C-6 asymmetric carbon of the pteridine ring (Gregory, 1989). Of the two 6*S* and 6*R* stereoisomers (formerly called 6*l* and 6*d*), only the 6*S* isomer is biologically active and occurs in nature. Methods of chemical synthesis of tetrahydrofolates, whether by catalytic hydrogenation or chemical reduction, yield a racemic product (i.e. a mixture of both stereoisomers).

2.7.3 PHYSICAL AND CHEMICAL PROPERTIES

PGA is synthesized commercially for use in food fortification either as the free acid or the disodium salt. Synthetic PGA is an orange–yellow

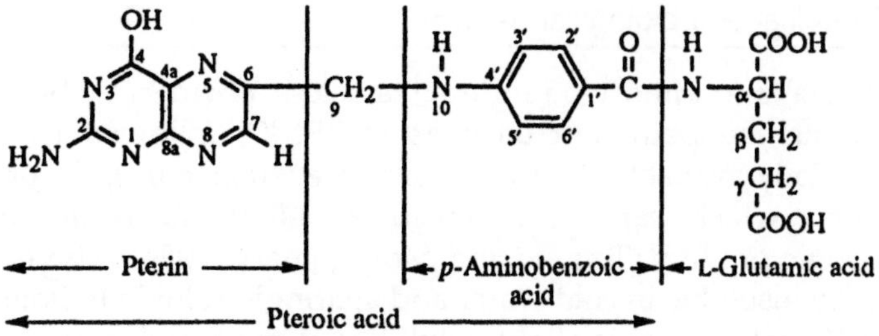

I
Pteroylmonoglutamic acid (PGA)

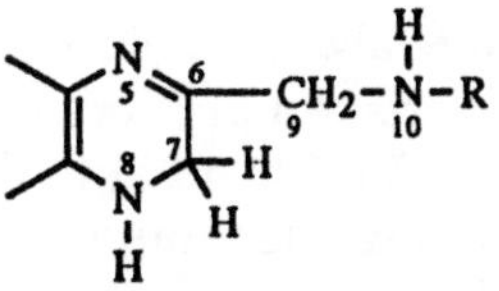

II
7,8-Dihydropteroylmonoglutamic acid (DHF)

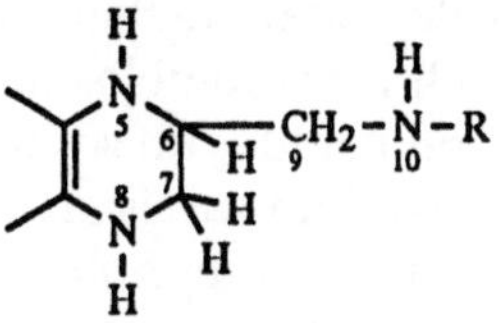

III
5,6,7,8-Tetrahydropteroylmonoglutamic acid (THF)

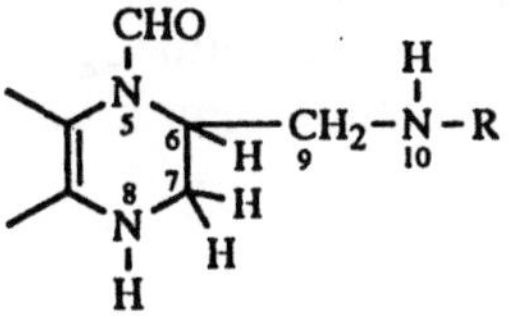

IV
5-Formyl-THF (5-CHO-THF)

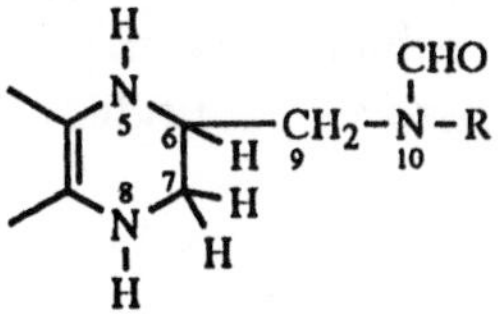

V
10-Formyl-THF (10-CHO-THF)

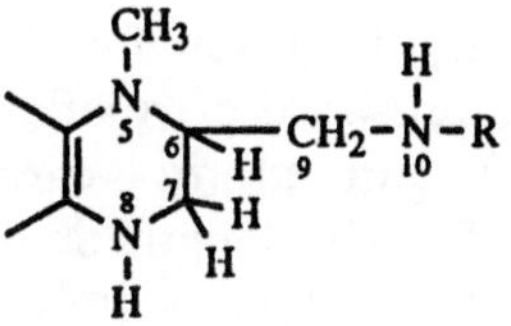

VI
5-Methyl-THF (5-CH_3-THF)

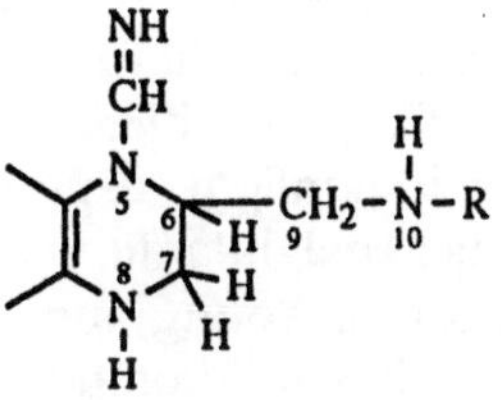

VII
5-Formimino-THF (5-CH=NH-THF)

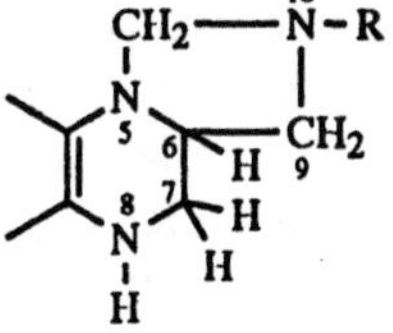

VIII
5,10-Methylene-THF (5,10-CH_2-THF)

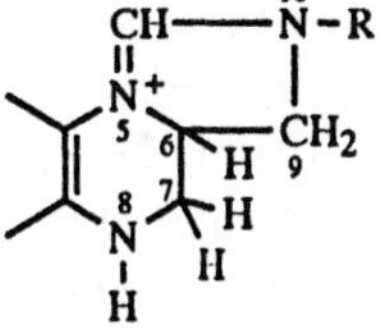

IX
5,10-Methenyl-THF (5,10 =CH-THF)

Figure 2.25 Structures of folate compounds.

microcrystalline, almost odourless, tasteless powder. It has no well-defined melting point but darkens at 250 °C, followed by charring. Commercially available PGA contains on average 8.0–8.5% of water of hydration, which can be removed at 140 °C *in vacuo* to give a hygroscopic product (Temple and Montgomery, 1984). The free acid is practically insoluble in cold water and sparingly soluble in boiling water (20 mg/100 ml). There is slight solubility in methanol, appreciably less solubility in ethanol, and no solubility in acetone, diethyl ether, chloroform or benzene. PGA dissolves in warm dilute hydrochloric acid, but with degradation that increases with increasing temperature and acid strength. It is soluble and stable in dilute alkaline solution; aqueous solutions prepared with sodium bicarbonate have a pH between 6.5 and 6.8. The disodium salt is soluble in water (1.5 g/100 ml at 0 °C). Folates are ionogenic and amphoteric molecules. Ionogenic groups of particular significance in the range of pH values relevant to foods and biological systems are the N-5 positions of THF ($pK_a = 4.8$) and the glutamate carboxyl groups ($\gamma\ pK_a = 4.8$; $\alpha\ pK_a = 3.5$). Polyglutamyl folates, because of the free α-carboxyl groups situated on each glutamate residue, exhibit greater ionic character than the monoglutamyl forms when dissociated under neutral to alkaline conditions (Gregory, 1989).

2.7.4 STABILITY

The folates differ widely with respect to their susceptibility to oxidative degradation, their thermal stability, and the pH dependence of their stability (Gregory, 1985). Folate activity is gradually destroyed by exposure to sunlight, especially in the presence of riboflavin, to yield *p*-aminobenzoylglutamic acid (PABG) and pterin-6-carboxaldehyde (Tannenbaum, Young and Archer, 1985). The length of the glutamyl side chain has little or no influence on the stability properties of the folate compounds (Gregory, 1985).

The most stable of the various folates at ambient and elevated temperatures is PGA (Gregory, 1985). In aqueous solution PGA is stable at 100 °C for 10 h in a pH range 5.0–12.0 when protected from light, but becomes increasingly unstable as the pH decreases below 5.0 (Paine-Wilson and Chen, 1979). Alkaline hydrolysis under aerobic conditions promotes oxidative cleavage of the PGA molecule to yield PABG and pterin-6-carboxylic acid, whereas acid hydrolysis under aerobic conditions yields 6-methylpterin (Tannenbaum, Young and Archer, 1985). The stability of PGA (and indeed all folates) is greatly enhanced in the presence of an antioxidant such as ascorbic acid. Polyglutamyl derivatives of PGA can be hydrolysed by alkali in the absence of air to yield folic and glutamic acids (Tannenbaum, Young and Archer, 1985).

The unsubstituted reduced structure THF is extremely susceptible to oxidative cleavage. DHF is included with the PABG and pterin breakdown products at pH 10 but not at pH 4 or 7 (Reed and Archer, 1980). Trace metals, particularly iron (III) and copper (II) ions, catalyse the oxidation of THF (Hawkes and Villota, 1989). The presence of substituent groups in the N-5 position greatly increases the oxidative stability of the reduced folates relative to that of THF (Gregory, 1985). 5-Methyl-THF exhibited a half-life of 21 min at 100 °C in aqueous solution compared with 2 min for THF (Chen and Cooper, 1979). Maximum thermal stability of 5-methyl-THF was observed at pH 7, while similar rates of decreasing stability occurred with increasing acidity and alkalinity (Paine-Wilson and Chen, 1979). Oxidation of 5-methyl-THF at or near neutral pH yields 5-methyl-5,6-DHF, which exhibits 80% biological activity relative to PGA as measured by a chick bioassay (Gregory *et al.*, 1984). Because of the rapid reduction of 5-methyl-5,6-DHF to 5-methyl-THF by ascorbate and mercaptoethanol, which are common antioxidants in folate analysis, the specific presence of 5-methyl-5,6-DHF would not be detected in most chromatographic methods of folate analysis. In acid media 5-methyl-5,6-DHF undergoes either C-9–N-10 bond cleavage or rearrangement of the pteridine ring system with a consequent loss of folate activity (Gregory, 1985). 10-Formyl-THF is readily oxidized by air to 10-formylfolic acid, which exhibits 100% biological activity relative to PGA as measured by chick bioassay (Gregory *et al.*, 1984), and stability comparable to that of PGA (Gregory, 1985). Under anaerobic conditions, 10-formyl-THF undergoes isomerization to 5-formyl-THF at neutral pH after prolonged standing and especially at elevated temperature (Robinson, 1971). 5-Formyl-THF exhibits equal thermal stability to PGA at neutral pH; under acidic conditions, and especially at high temperatures, 5-formyl-THF loses a molecule of water to form 5,10-methenyl-THF (Paine-Wilson and Chen, 1979). This compound is stable to air oxidation in acid solution and is hydrolysed to 10-formyl-THF in neutral and slightly alkaline solutions (Stokstad and Koch, 1967).

Sulphurous acid and nitrite, two chemicals that are used in food processing, cause a loss of folate activity in aqueous systems. Reactions between folates and sulphurous acid promotes C-9–N-10 bond cleavage (Tannenbaum, Young, and Archer, 1985). Nitrite ions react with PGA to yield exclusively 10-nitrosofolic acid and with 5-formyl-THF to yield the 10-nitroso derivative; interaction with THF and 5-methyl-THF yields PABG and several pterin products (Reed and Archer, 1979).

2.7.5 SPECTROSCOPIC PROPERTIES

Absorption

The absorption spectrum of PGA in phosphate buffer at pH 7.1 exhibits two maxima at wavelengths above 220 nm, namely at 282 and 347 nm. At pH 13, three maxima above 220 nm are observed, namely at 255, 283 and 364 nm. THF in phosphate buffer at pH 7.1 shows a single maximum at 286 nm (Figure 2.26). Additional spectral data relating to PGA and reduced folate derivatives are presented in Table 2.3.

Fluorescence

The naturally occurring folates and several pterin derivatives exhibit native fluorescence, as shown by Uyeda and Rabinowitz (1963) (see Table 2.4). DHF and all the THF derivatives tested, with the exception of 5,10-methenyl-THF, show maximum fluorescence when irradiated at wavelengths between 300 and 320 nm. The fluorescence emission has a maximum at 360–425 nm. The general similarity of the fluorescence properties of these reduced folate derivatives and their similarity to the fluorescence properties of PABG suggest that the fluorescence results from the PABG residue common to all these molecules. This conclusion is further supported by the observations that reduced pterins which lack

Table 2.3 Absorption spectral properties of folates

Compound	pH[a]	λ_{max} (nm)	Molar extinction coefficient (ε)
Folic acid	7	282, 350	27 000, 7000
	13	254, 282, 363	25 000, 23 800, 8700
THF	7	297	27 000
10-Formyl-THF	7	288	18 200
5-Formyl-THF	7	287	31 500
	13	282	32 600
5-Methyl-THF	7	290	32 000
	13	290	31 600
5-Formimino-THF	7	285	35 400
5,10-Methenyl-THF	7	352	25 000
5,10-Methylene-THF	7.2	294	32 000

From Temple, C., Jr and Montgomery, J.A. (1984) *Folates and Pterins*, Vol. 1, *Chemistry and Biochemistry of Folates* (ed. R. Blakley and S.J. Benkovic). Copyright © 1984, by John Wiley & Sons, Inc. Reprinted by permission of John Wiley & Sons, Inc.

[a] pH 7, usually phosphate buffer; pH 13, 0.1 M NaOH.

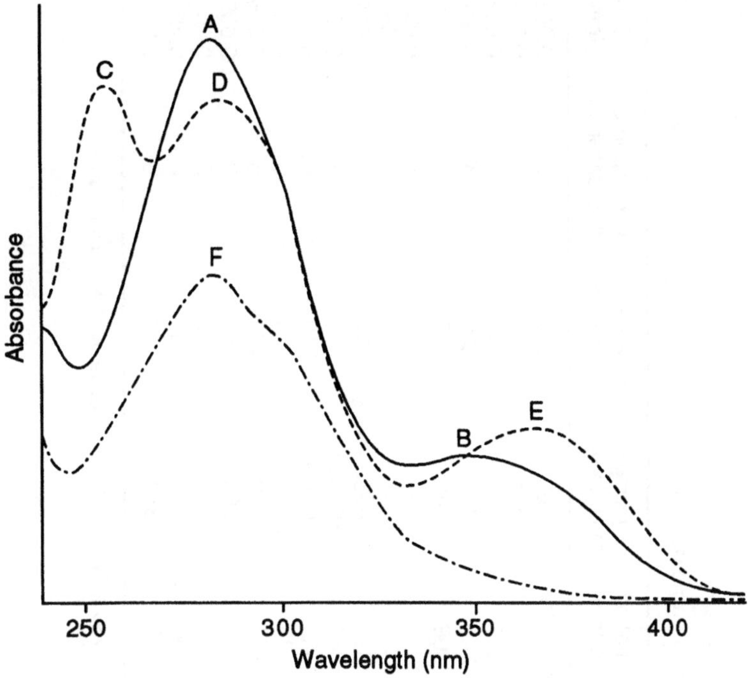

Figure 2.26 Absorption spectra of folic acid and tetrahydrofolic acid (THF). For folic acid in 0.1 M phosphate buffer at pH 7.1 (solid line), λ_{max} of peak A = 282 nm; B = 347 nm. For folic acid in 0.1 M NaOH, pH 13 (broken line), λ_{max} of peak C = 255 nm; D = 283 nm; E = 364 nm. For THF in 0.1 M phosphate buffer at pH 7.1 (discontinuous line), λ_{max} of peak F = 286 nm.

the *p*-aminobenzoyl moiety, such as tetrahydropterin and 6-methyltetrahydropterin, fail to exhibit fluorescence, although the oxidized pterin derivatives exhibit fluorescence.

The pterin derivatives, pteroic acid, PGA and the available derivatives of PGA tested exhibit an excitation maximum at 360–380 nm and an emission maximum at 450–460 nm. It is probable that these fluorescence characteristics result from the presence of the pteridine ring, and that reduction of this ring abolishes the fluorescence.

The fluorescence of PGA depends markedly on the pH of the medium. PGA does not fluoresce at pH 6, but the fluorescence intensity increases in media above or below pH 6. The fluorescence spectra of PGA at pH 9 are shown in Figure 2.27.

2.7.6 DIETARY SOURCES

Polyglutamyl folate is an essential biochemical constituent of living cells, and most foods contribute some folate. Yeast and yeast extract, liver,

Table 2.4 Fluorescence properties of folates and pterin derivatives

Compound	Excitation max. (nm)	Emission max. (nm)	Relative fluorescence	pH of optimum fluorescence	Conc (mM)
THF	305–310	360	1600	3	0.0038
5-Formyl-THF	314	365	32	7	0.05
10-Formyl-THF	313	360	47	7	0.007
5,10-Methenyl-THF	370	470	500	4	0.0088
5-Formimino-THF	308	360	5	7	0.00285
Tetrahydropterin	–	–	0	–	0.05
6-Methyltetrahydropterin	–	–	0	–	0.05
DHF	317	425	32	9	0.011
Folic acid	363	450–460	1	9	0.05
10-Formylfolic acid	364	450–460	140	9	0.05
Pteroic acid	375	450–460	4	9	0.05
Pterin	353	450	120	8	0.025
6-Methylpterin	355	450	1200	8	0.005
6-Carboxaldehydepterin	360	450	22	9	0.05
6-Carboxypterin	360	450	160	8	0.25
p-Aminobenzoylglutamate (PABG)	310	360	2	6	0.05

From Uyeda, K. and Rabinowitz, J.C. (1963) *Analyt. Biochem.*, **6**, 100–8. By permission of Academic Press.

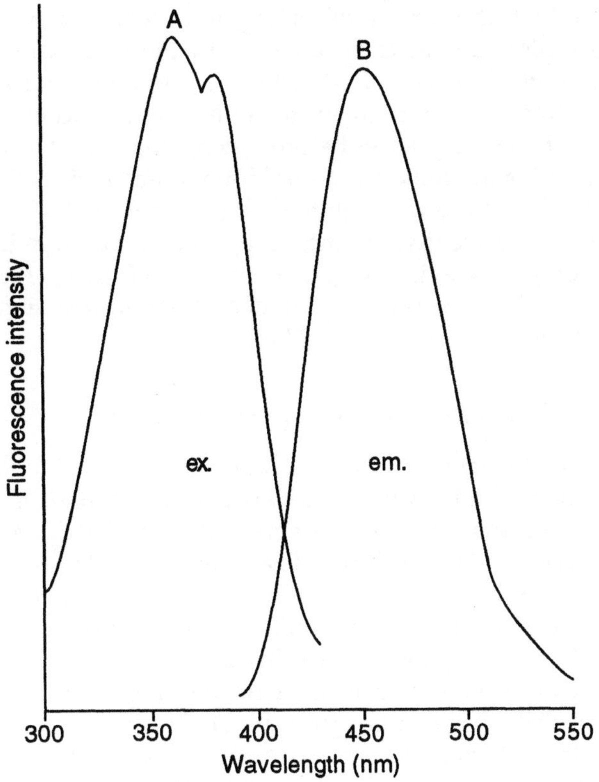

Figure 2.27 Fluorescence excitation and emission spectra of folic acid in 0.1 M phosphate buffer at pH 9.0 (λ_{max} of peak A = 360 nm; B = 450 nm).

wheat bran, beetroot, green leafy vegetables, chick peas and nuts are rich natural sources of folate. Other useful sources include oatmeal, whole-grain cereals, potatoes, eggs, cheese, kidney, muscle meats, fish and fruit. Milk is a rather poor source of the vitamin (see Table 1.1).

The predominant folate vitamers in animal tissues are polyglutamyl forms of THF, 5-methyl-THF and 10-formyl-THF, while plant tissues contain mainly polyglutamyl 5-methyl-THF (Gregory, Sartain and Day, 1984). The folates generally exist in nature bound to proteins (Baugh and Krumdieck, 1971) and they are also bound to storage polysaccharides (various types of starch and glycogen) in foods (Černá and Káš, 1983). At one time the folate in food was classified into two main groups according to its availability to *L. casei*. 'Free' folate referred to the mono-, di- and triglutamates that were assayed by *L. casei* without pretreatment with pteroyl-γ-glutamyl carboxypeptidase (conjugase), whilst 'total' folate was assayed by *L. casei* after treatment with conjugase. It has since been shown that the action of endogenous conjugases present in vegetable samples can cause an increase in the apparent 'free' folate during extraction of the sample (Leichter, Landymore and Krumdieck, 1979). Thus, 'free' (i.e. short-chain) folate is only a valid concept if care is taken to inactivate conjugases before homogenization (Gregory, 1989).

The folate in bovine milk occurs predominantly as 5-methyl-THF, of which about 60% is the monoglutamate (Wagner, 1985). The folate is tightly, but not covalently, bound to a specific minor whey protein under physiological conditions (Ford, Salter and Scott, 1969). Folate-binding proteins have also been found in association with membranes of kidney and liver tissue (Wagner, 1985).

2.7.7 EFFECTS OF FOOD PROCESSING AND STORAGE

The extent and mechanisms of loss of folate in processed foods have yet to be established. The PGA that is added to fortified foods is retained to a greater extent than the less stable reduced derivatives that are naturally present. Thus baking destroyed one-third of the folate naturally present in wheat, but only 11% of added folate (Keagy, Stokstad and Fellers, 1975). The milk ingredients casein, iron (II) and ascorbate, which are capable of lowering the concentration of dissolved oxygen, have all been shown to increase the thermal stability of PGA and 5-methyl-THF (Day and Gregory, 1983). Other reducing agents that occur in foods, such as thiols and cysteine, would also retard oxidation. Heat processing of canned and sealed foods results in a markedly higher folate retention than domestic cooking methods. HTST-pasteurized milk (2–3 s at 92 °C) incurs a 12% loss of total folate compared with a 39% loss after in-bottle sterilization (13–15 min at 119–120 °C). Ultra-HTST sterilization of preheated milk causes only a 7% loss of total folate (Tannenbaum, Young and Archer, 1985). The heat treatment of milk partially denatures the folate-binding proteins and destroys their property of enhancing the intestinal absorption of folate (Gregory, 1982).

2.7.8 BIOCHEMICAL AND PHYSIOLOGICAL FUNCTIONS

THF acts as a cofactor in biochemical reactions involving the mobilization of one-carbon units in intermediary metabolism. Such reactions are essential for the synthesis of the purines (adenine and guanine) and one of the pyrimidines (thymine), which are the base constituents of DNA. The reactions also govern the metabolism of certain amino acids, especially the important methyl donor, methionine.

The principal reactions involving THF and its intermediates in mammalian one-carbon metabolism are depicted in a simplified form in

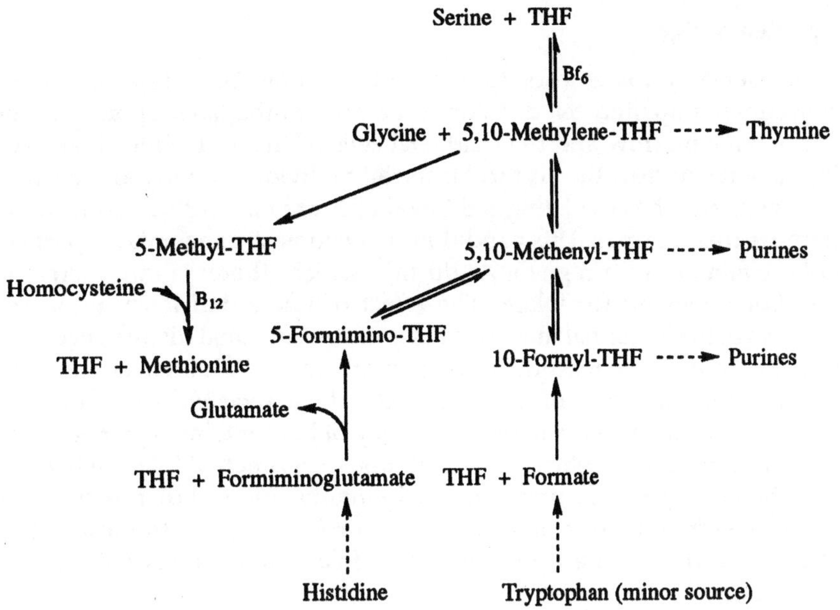

Figure 2.28 A partial summary of the role of tetrahydrofolate (THF) in one-carbon metabolism. All transformations are enzyme catalysed.

Figure 2.28. This particular scheme commences with the vitamin B_6-dependent conversion of serine to glycine, which involves the transfer of the β-hydroxymethyl group (HOH_2C-) of serine to THF and spontaneous cyclization of 10-hydroxymethyl-THF by loss of water to 5,10-methylene-THF. The metabolism of 5,10-methylene-THF can proceed along two main routes. In one route the methylene derivative is reduced to 5-methyl-THF, which then functions as the methyl donor for homocysteine in the biosynthesis of methionine. The second route involves the conversion of the methylene derivative to 5,10-methenyl-THF, which in turn is converted to 10-formyl-THF. The one-carbon fragments of each of these derivatives are utilized in the biosynthesis of the purines and thymine.

Folate metabolism is based on the reversibility of the reactions (where indicated in Figure 2.28) involving the interconversion of the THF derivatives. In mammalian tissues, the β-carbon of serine is the major source of one-carbon units for folate metabolism. Another significant contributor to the one-carbon pool is formiminoglutamate, which is a product of histidine catabolism. Formate, which is derived from the indole ring of tryptophan, constitutes only a minor source of one-carbon units for folate metabolism in mammalian tissues.

Deficiency signs

A deficiency in folate leads to a lack of adequate DNA replication and consequent impaired cell division, especially in the haemopoietic tissue of the bone marrow and the epithelial cells of the gastrointestinal tract. In the bone marrow the erythroblasts fail to divide properly and become enlarged, and the circulating red blood cells are macrocytic and fewer in number than normal. This condition, megaloblastic anaemia, is particularly common in pregnancy, during which there is an increased metabolic demand for folate. The effect of folate deficiency upon cell renewal of the intestinal mucosa causes gastrointestinal disturbances and also has adverse consequences upon overall nutritional status. The biochemical functions of folate are closely associated with those of vitamin B_{12}, and a coincidental deficiency of both vitamins increases the severity of the folate deficiency symptoms. Experimental folate deficiency is difficult to produce under normal circumstances, but the study of patients suffering from malabsorption problems (e.g. tropical sprue; atrophy of the jejenum) or the use of folate antagonists has yielded much clinical information.

Expression of dietary value

No IU for folate activity has been defined, and analytical results are expressed in weight units (μg or mg) of pure crystalline PGA. Folate activity can be assayed biologically in chick or rat growth tests.

Toxicity

Folate is generally considered to have a low acute and chronic toxicity for humans. Gastrointestinal disturbances and neurological symptoms such as altered sleep patterns, malaise and irritability have been reported in a study with healthy volunteers receiving daily doses of 15 mg of PGA (Hunter *et al.*, 1970).

2.7.9 METABOLISM

Although most biological folate is known to be polyglutamyl, the presence of folate conjugases in many raw foods of both plant and animal origin (Gregory, 1989) results in a high proportion of the dietary folate being monoglutamyl when presented to the intestinal mucosa. The buffering action of the food matrix would tend to protect dietary folates against the acidic gastric environment. Ingested polyglutamates, mostly in the reduced tetrahydro form, are hydrolysed by folate conjugases in the mucosal cell to monoglutamates, which are absorbed and transported directly to the liver, where they accumulate. After a slight delay, the liver releases folate (in the form of 5-methyl-THF) into the systemic circulation. On reaching the tissues, the 5-methyl-THF is converted intracellularly into polyglutamate, and then further metabolized to other one-carbon derivatives according to the biochemical requirements. PGA is absorbed largely unchanged in the gut and, on reaching the tissues, is converted to THF via DHF through two successive NADPH hydrogenations. Folate-binding proteins associated with membranes of liver, kidney and intestinal epithelium are believed to participate in the transport of folate molecules into the cell. Soluble intracellular folate-binding proteins have been isolated from mammalian liver and may have a storage role (Wagner, 1985).

2.7.10 BIOAVAILABILITY

Research has shown that the utilization of food folate is incomplete and highly variable (Bailey, 1988; Gregory, 1989). When compared with PGA, dietary folates appeared to be no more than 50% available for humans (Sauberlich *et al.*, 1987). The reduced availability does not seem to be attributable to the degree of conjugation or reduction of the folate molecules, as a synthetic polyglutamate with seven glutamate residues ($PteGlu_7$) and THF were utilized as well as PGA when these compounds were administered orally *per se* (Tamura and Stokstad, 1973). Certain foods contain specific inhibitors of intestinal conjugase activity, causing a decrease in the availability of folate polyglutamatess (Bhandari and Gregory, 1990). Extracts of legumes, tomatoes and orange juice consistently inhibited the conjugase activity, whereas extracts of cereal grain flours, whole egg, milk, cabbage, cauliflower and lettuce caused little inhibition. The food substances that inhibited the conjugase activity did not bind the polyglutamyl folate substrate.

The oxidation products of 5-methyl-THF and 10-formyl-THF (respectively, 5-methyl-5,6-DHF and 10-formylfolic acid) yield essentially full activity when measured using a chick bioassay, which suggests that these compounds would contribute to the folate nutrition of humans.

2.8 VITAMIN B_{12}

2.8.1 HISTORY

A type of anaemia attributed to a digestive disorder was reported by Combe in 1822 and later recognized as pernicious anaemia by Addison in 1849. It was not until 1926 that Minot and Murphy started to cure pernicious anaemia by feeding patients with large amounts of raw liver.

In 1929, Castle showed that the intestinal absorption of the 'antipernicious anaemia principle' in liver (extrinsic factor) required prior binding to a specific protein (intrinsic factor) secreted by the stomach. Research into isolating the active principle from liver was hampered by the difficulty of the only known bioassay, which was the haemopoietic response of patients with pernicious anaemia. Eventually, in 1948, a red crystalline substance having the clinical activity of liver and designated as vitamin B_{12} was isolated almost simultaneously by two independent groups led by Folkers (Merck Company, USA) and E.L. Smith (Glaxo Company, UK). The success of Folkers' group was largely attributable to a microbiological assay developed by Shorb in 1947; Smith used the human bioassay procedure. The structure of vitamin B_{12} was established by Hodgkin using X-ray crystallography in 1955. Its complete chemical synthesis was achieved in 1973, but because of the large number of stages required (over 70) the procedure is of no commercial interest.

2.8.2 STRUCTURE

In accordance with the literature on nutrition and pharmacology, the term vitamin B_{12} is used in this text as the generic descriptor for all cobalamins that exhibit antipernicious anaemia activity. Individual cobalamins will be referred to by their specific names (e.g. cyanocobalamin).

The cobalamin molecule is a six coordination cobalt complex containing a corrin ring system substituted with numerous methyl, acetamide and propionamide radicals (Figure 2.29). Methylene bridges link the pyrrole rings A to B, B to C and C to D but not A to D, which are linked directly. The cobalt atom, which may assume an oxidation state of I, II or III, is linked by four equatorial coordinate bonds to the four pyrrole nitrogens, and by an axial coordinate bond to a 5,6-dimethylbenzimidazole (DMB) moiety, which extends in α-glycosidic linkage to ribose 3-phosphate. The phosphate group is linked to the D ring of the corrin structure via a substituted propionamide chain. The pseudonucleotide (DMB base plus sugar phosphate) is perpendicular to the corrin structure. The remaining axial coordinate bond (X position) links the cobalt atom to a cyano (−CN) group in the case of cyanocobalamin ($C_{23}H_{88}O_{14}N_{14}PCo$, MW = 1355.4) or, depending on the chemical environment, to some other group (e.g. −OH in hydroxocobalamin and $-HSO_3$ in sulphitocobalamin). There are two vitamin B_{12} coenzymes with known metabolic activity in humans, namely methylcobalamin and 5′-deoxyadenosylcobalamin (frequently abbreviated to adenosylcobalamin and also known as coenzyme B_{12}). The methyl or adenosyl ligands of the coenzymes occupy the X position in the corrin structure (Herbert and Colman, 1988). The coenzymes are bound intracellularly to their protein

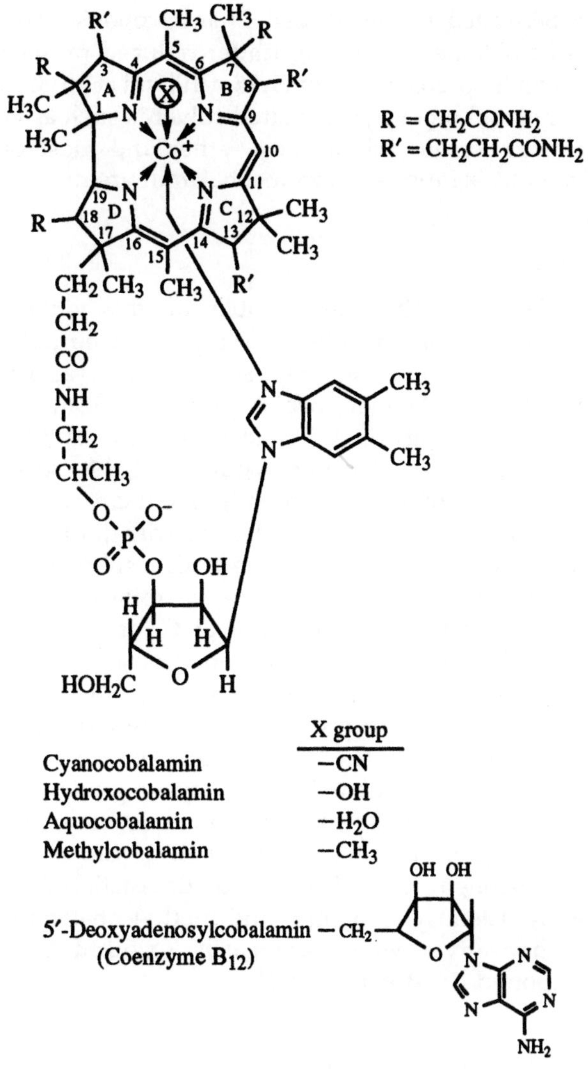

Figure 2.29 Structures of vitamin B_{12} compounds.

apoenzymes through a covalent peptide link, or in milk and plasma to specific transport proteins.

2.8.3 PHYSICAL AND CHEMICAL PROPERTIES

Cyanocobalamin is an artificial product used in pharmaceutical preparations because of its greater stability. It is a tasteless dark red crystalline hygroscopic powder which can take up appreciably more than the 12%

of moisture permitted by the British Pharmacopoeia. The anhydrous material can be obtained by drying under reduced pressure at 105 °C. Cyanocobalamin is soluble in water (1.25 g/100 ml at 25 °C) and in lower alcohols, phenol and other hydroxylated solvents such as ethylene diol; it is insoluble in acetone, chloroform, ether and most other organic solvents. Aqueous solutions of cyanocobalamin are of neutral pH.

2.8.4 STABILITY

Cyanocob(III)alamin is the most stable of the vitamin B_{12}-active cobalamins and is the one mostly used in pharmaceutical preparations and food supplementation. Aqueous solutions of cyanocobalamin are stable in air at room temperature if protected from light. The pH region of optimal stability is 4.5–5 and solutions of pH 4–7 can be autoclaved at 120 °C for 20 min with negligible loss of vitamin activity. The addition of ammonium sulphate increases the stability of cyanocobalamin in aqueous solution. Heating with dilute acid deactivates the vitamin owing to hydrolysis of the amide substituents or further degradation of the molecule. Mild alkaline hydrolysis at 100 °C promotes cyclization of the acetamide side chain at C-7 to form a biologically inactive gamma-lactam or, in the presence of an oxidizing agent, a gamma-lactone (Wong, 1989). The vitamin B_{12} activity in aqueous solutions is destroyed in the presence of strong oxidizing agents and high concentrations of reducing agents, such as ascorbic acid, sulphite and iron (II) salts. On exposure to light, the cyano group dissociates from cyanocobalamin and hydroxocob(III)alamin is formed. In neutral and acid solution hydroxocobalamin exists in the form of aquocobalamin (Gräsbeck and Salonen, 1976). This photolytic reaction does not cause a loss of activity. Adenosylcobalamin and methylcobalamin are reduced cob(I)alamin derivatives which are easily oxidized by light to the hydroxo compound (Hoffbrand, 1979).

2.8.5 SPECTROSCOPIC PROPERTIES

Absorption

Cyanocobalamin dissolved in water exhibits an absorption spectrum with the following maxima (molar absorptivities ε in parentheses) within the UV and visible wavelength range: 278 nm (15 500), 361 nm (28 060) and 551 nm (8740); the $A_1{}^{1\%}_{cm}$ at λ_{max} 361 nm is 207. The absorption spectrum of aquocobalamin, which is formed from cyanocobalamin in neutral or acid solution by exposure to light, is shifted to lower wavelengths to give the following maxima and ε values: 274 nm (20 600), 351 nm (26 500) and 527 nm (8500) (Schneider and Stroinski,

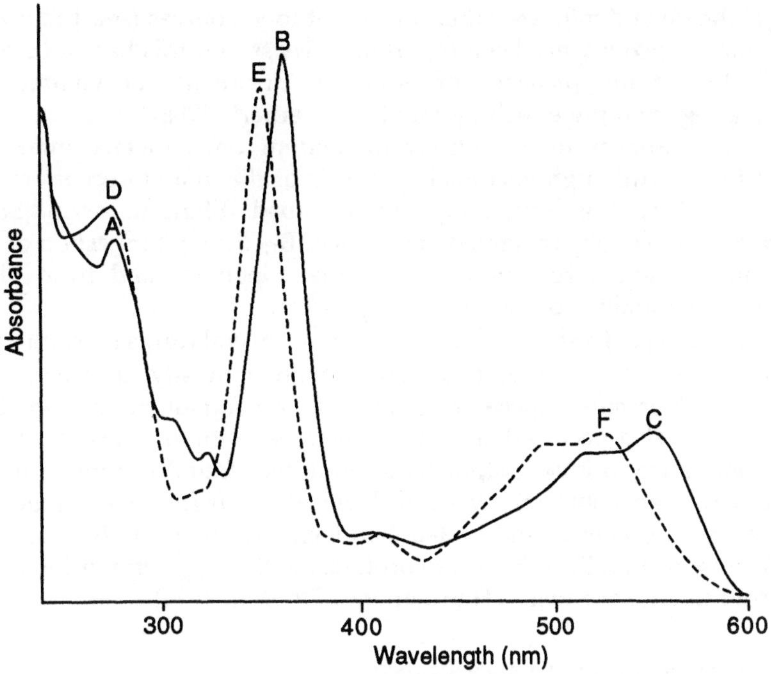

Figure 2.30 Absorption spectra of aqueous solutions (pH 5.8) of cyanocobalamin (solid line) and hydroxocobalamin (actually aquocobalamin) (broken line). For cyanocobalamin, λ_{max} of peak A = 278 nm; B = 361 nm; C = 550 nm. For aquocobalamin, λ_{max} of peak D = 274 nm; E = 351 nm; F = 525 nm.

1987). The spectra of aqueous solutions (pH 5.8) of cyanocobalamin and hydroxocobalamin (actually aquocobalamin) are displayed in Figure 2.30.

2.8.6 DIETARY SOURCES

Naturally occurring vitamin B_{12} originates solely from synthesis by bacteria and other micro-organisms growing in soil or water, in sewage, and in the rumen and intestinal tract of animals. Any traces of the vitamin that may be detected in plants are due to microbial contamination from the soil or manure or, in the case of certain legumes, to bacterial synthesis in the root nodules.

Vitamin B_{12} is ubiquitous in foods of animal origin and is derived from the animal's ingestion of cobalamin-containing animal tissue or microbiologically contaminated plant material, in addition to vitamin absorbed from the animal's own digestive tract. Liver is the outstanding dietary source of the vitamin, followed by kidney and heart. Muscle meats, fish, eggs, cheese and milk are other important food sources (see Table 1.1). Vitamin B_{12} activity has been reported in yeast, but this has since been attributed to the presence of nonactive corrinoids or vitamin B_{12} originating from the enriching medium (Herbert, 1988).

Humans appear to be entirely dependent on a dietary intake of vitamin B_{12}. Although microbial synthesis of the vitamin occurs in the human colon, it is apparently not absorbed (Shinton, 1972). Strict vegetarians may obtain limited amounts of B_{12} through ingestion of the vitamin-containing root nodules of certain legumes and from plant material contaminated with micro-organisms.

Vitamin B_{12} in foods was found to exist in several forms (Farquharson and Adams, 1976). Meat and fish contained mostly adenosyl- and hydroxocobalamins; these compounds, accompanied by methylcobalamin, also occurred in dairy products, with hydroxoxobalamin predominating in milk. Sulphitocobalamin was found in canned meats and fish. Cyanocobalamin was not detected, apart from small amounts in egg white, cheese and boiled haddock. In bovine milk, naturally occurring vitamin B_{12} is bound to proteins, with a high proportion being present in whey proteins (Hartman and Dryden, 1974).

2.8.7 EFFECTS OF FOOD PROCESSING

The cobalamins present in food are generally resistant to thermal processing and cooking in a nonalkaline medium. Vitamin B_{12} losses incurred during the normal oven heating of frozen convenience dinners prior to serving ranged from 0% to 21% in products containing fish, fried chicken, turkey and beef (De Ritter, 1976). A 27–33% loss of vitamin B_{12} expressed per unit of nitrogen occurred during the cooking of beef due to the loss of moisture and fat; the vitamin content of raw and cooked beef was, however, similar on a moisture basis (Bennink and Ono, 1982). Thus there is little loss of the vitamin in the cooking of meat provided that the meat juices are utilized. In the processing of milk, the following losses of vitamin B_{12} have been reported: pasteurization for 2–3 s, 7%; sterilization in the bottle at 120 °C for 13 min, 77%; rapid sterilization at 143 °C for 3–4 s with superheated steam, 10%; evaporation, 70–90%; and spray-drying, 20–35% (Tannenbaum, Young and Archer, 1985). The light-sensitive coenzyme forms of vitamin B_{12} are largely converted to hydroxocobalamin in light-exposed milk, but with no loss of vitamin activity (Farquharson and Adams, 1976).

2.8.8 BIOCHEMICAL AND PHYSIOLOGICAL FUNCTIONS

Vitamin B_{12} is essential for the regeneration of THF in folate metabolism through the coenzymatic action of methylcobalamin in removing the methyl group from 5-methyl-THF and donating it to homocysteine, thus forming methionine (Figure 2.28). Adenosylcobalamin is a coenzyme in the conversion of L-methylmalonyl-CoA to succinyl-CoA, an important intermediary in the tricarboxylic acid cycle. This reaction is a common pathway for the degradation of odd-chain fatty acids and certain amino acids (Herbert, 1987).

Deficiency signs

A deficiency in vitamin B_{12} is manifested by haematological and neurological changes. As previously explained, the inability to synthesize methionine from homocysteine in the absence of cobalamin means that THF cannot be regenerated from the demethylation of 5-methyl-THF. The folate thus becomes trapped in the form of 5-methyl-THF because the formation of this derivative by reduction of 5,10-methylene-THF is thermodynamically irreversible. As shown in Figure 2.28, this situation could lead to the inability to form the other THF derivatives that are necessary for purine and pyrimidine synthesis. In this event a megaloblastic anaemia that is clinically indistinguishable from that induced by folate deficiency results. When this type of anaemia is due to deficiency of vitamin B_{12} it is called pernicious or Addisonian anaemia.

The neurological changes are unrelated to folate deficiency and are caused by the inability to manufacture the lipid component of myelin, which results in a generalized demyelinization of nerve tissue. Neuropathy begins in the peripheral nerves, affecting first the feet and fingers, and then progressing to the spinal cord and brain.

The deficiency disease of pernicious anaemia is due to the lack of absorption of vitamin B_{12} caused by the inability to synthesize intrinsic factor or by some other digestive malfunction. It is rarely, if ever, caused by a lack of dietary vitamin B_{12}. Failure to absorb the vitamin results in clinical vitamin B_{12} deficiency within 3–6 years, whereas a dietary deficiency could take 20 years or more to develop owing to the very low nutritional requirement for the vitamin and the efficiency of the body at conserving the vitamin. The deficiency symptoms are relieved quickly when cobalamin is injected into the bloodstream to bypass the absorption process.

In the event of vitamin B_{12} deficiency, there is a danger of irreversible neurological damage if folic acid supplements are taken without including vitamin B_{12}. This is because the obvious symptoms of anaemia will be alleviated by the folate treatment, but the concomitant nerve degeneration will be undetected. For this reason, prophylactic vitamin supplementation always includes vitamin B_{12} with folic acid.

Expression of dietary value

No IU for vitamin B_{12} activity has been defined, and the assay results are expressed in milligrams, micrograms or nanograms of pure crystalline cyanocobalamin. The measurement of biological activity in preparations containing vitamin B_{12} relies on microbiological assays, there being no animal bioassay.

Toxicity

Vitamin B_{12} is nontoxic, even in doses that exceed the maximum daily adult human requirement by 10 000 times. Excessive intakes above the limited serum- and tissue-available binding capacity tend to be excreted in the urine rather than retained (Herbert and Colman, 1988).

2.8.9 METABOLISM

Ingested cobalamins are released from their peptide bonding to food proteins (if not previously released during cooking) by the action of gastric acid and digestive enzymes in the stomach, and then bind to a specific binding protein (R protein) secreted by the salivary glands. In the mildly alkaline medium of the upper intestine, pancreatic proteases digest the R protein and the released cobalamins are attached to the intrinsic factor, another specific binding protein secreted by the stomach. The intrinsic factor–cobalamin complex is carried down to the ileum, where it attaches to specific receptors on the brush border of the ileal mucosal cell. In crossing the ileal mucosa the intrinsic factor is detached and the cobalamins are attached to plasma transport proteins (transcobalamins) and conveyed to the tissues. Within the cell, the cobalamins are bound to the cobalamin-dependent apoenzymes and converted into their coenzyme forms, adenosyl- and methylcobalamin.

2.8.10 BIOAVAILABILITY

The body is extremely efficient at conserving vitamin B_{12}. Unlike other water-soluble vitamins, vitamin B_{12} is stored protein-bound in the blood and other tissues, notably the liver. There is also an enterohepatic cycle, whereby the vitamin B_{12} that is secreted mainly in the bile into the jejenum can be reabsorbed. The vitamin B_{12} content of cooked meat seems to be readily available, as the vitamin in liver, mutton and chicken is absorbed as completely as a similar amount of cyanocobalamin administered in aqueous solution. In eggs, however, the vitamin is relatively poorly absorbed (FAO/WHO, 1988). The largest amount of vitamin B_{12} that can be physiologically absorbed from any one meal is limited to between about 1.5 and 3.5 μg. Saturation of the intrinsic factor-mediated system at one meal does not preclude absorption of normal amounts of the vitamin some hours later. At an intake of less than 3 μg, between 60% and 80% of vitamin B_{12} is physiologically absorbed; this percentage decreases as the intestinal content of the vitamin increases (FAO/WHO, 1970).

2.9 VITAMIN C

2.9.1 HISTORY

The concept of an antiscorbutic vitamin was postulated by Funk in 1912 after Holz and Fröhlich in 1907 induced scurvy in guinea pigs. By 1924, Zilva had obtained concentrates of the antiscorbutic factor from lemons and showed that the factor possessed strong reducing properties. Isolation of an antiscorbutic 'hexuronic acid' in crystalline form was achieved from cabbage and adrenal glands by Szent-Györgyi in 1928 and from lemon juice by Waugh and King in 1932. The synthesis of an identical substance by Reichstein in 1933 confirmed that the hexuronic acid was the vitamin ascorbic acid.

2.9.2 STRUCTURE

The term vitamin C is used as the generic descriptor for all compounds exhibiting qualitatively the biological activity of ascorbic acid. The principal natural compound with vitamin C activity is L-ascorbic acid (Figure 2.32), which is systematically named L-*threo*-2-hexenono-1,4-lactone ($C_6H_8O_6$, MW = 176.13). The stereochemistry of the 2-hexenono-1,4-lactone structure is shown in Figure 2.31. There are two enantiomeric pairs: namely, L- and D-ascorbic acid, and L- and D-isoascorbic acid. D-Ascorbic acid and L-isoascorbic acid are devoid of vitamin C activity and do not occur in nature. D-isoascorbic acid (commonly known as erythorbic acid) is an epimer of L-ascorbic acid, the structural difference being the orientation of the hydrogen and hydroxyl groups at the fifth carbon atom. The epimer is not found in natural products, apart from its occurrence in certain micro-organisms. Erythorbic acid possesses similar reductive properties to L-ascorbic acid, but possesses only 5% of the antiscorbutic activity of L-ascorbic acid in guinea pigs (Hornig and Weiser, 1976; Pelletier and Godin, 1969). Ascorbic acid 2-phosphate is a stabilized form of ascorbic acid which is used to inhibit enzymatic browning in fruits and vegetables (Sapers *et al.*, 1989).

Ascorbigen (Figure 2.32) is a bound form of ascorbic acid which is formed in cabbage and other brassica through the nonenzymatic

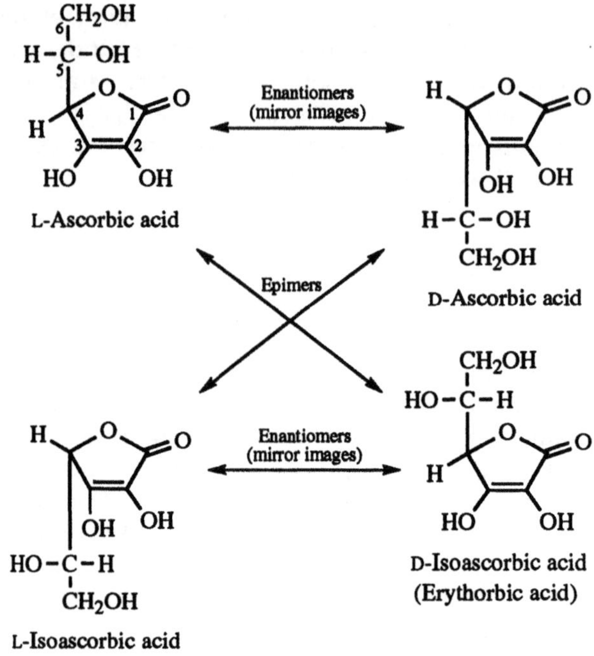

Figure 2.31 Stereoisomers of 2-hexenono-1,4-lactone.

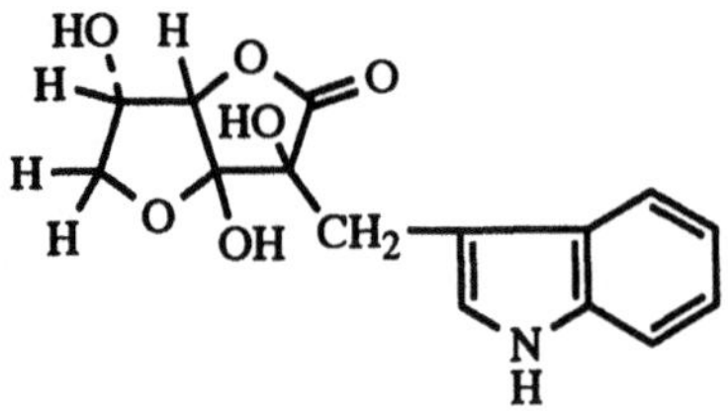

Figure 2.32 Structure of ascorbigen.

reaction between 3-hydroxymethylindole and ascorbic acid (Kiesvaara and Virtanen, 1962). Ascorbic acid is slowly released by hydrolysis of ascorbigen at pH 2 and 37 °C (Kiss and Neukom, 1966).

2.9.3 PHYSICAL AND CHEMICAL PROPERTIES

L-Ascorbic acid is an almost odourless white or very pale yellow crystalline powder with a pleasant sharp taste and a melting point of about 190 °C with decomposition. It is readily soluble in water (33 g/100 ml at 25 °C) less soluble in 95% ethanol (3.3 g/100 ml), absolute ethanol (2 g/100 ml), acetic acid (0.2 g/100 ml) and acetonitrile (0.05 g/100 ml) and insoluble in fat solvents (Seib, 1985). A 5% aqueous solution of L-ascorbic acid has a pH of 2.2–2.55, the acidic nature being due to the facile ionization of the hydroxyl on C-3 ($pK_{a1} = 4.17$); the hydroxyl on C-2 is much more resistant to ionization ($pK_{a2} = 11.79$) (Crawford and Crawford, 1980). Sodium ascorbate is freely soluble in water (62 g/100 ml at 25 °C; 78 g/100 ml at 75 °C) and practically insoluble in ethanol, diethyl ether and chloroform; the pH of an aqueous solution is 5.6–7.0. Ascorbyl palmitate is a stable fat-soluble form of the vitamin which is practically insoluble at 25 °C in water (0.2 g/100 ml), soluble in ethanol (20 g/100 ml) and slightly soluble in diethyl ether. The solubility in vegetable oils at room temperature is very low (30 mg/100 ml) but increases sharply with increasing temperature.

The carbonyl enediol group of ascorbic acid confers strong reducing properties to the molecule, as indicated by its ability to reduce Fehling's or Tollen's solution at room temperature. The redox potential of the first stage at pH 5.0 is $\varepsilon_0^1 = +0.127$ V.

2.9.4 STABILITY

Pure dry crystalline ascorbic acid is stable on exposure to air and daylight at normal room temperature for long periods of time. Commercial vitamin C tablets possess virtually their original potency even after 8 years' storage at 25 °C (Killeit, 1986). Crystalline sodium ascorbate is also very stable, apart from a tendency to turn yellow.

The aerobic oxidation of ascorbic acid in the presence of transition metals is the most important reaction responsible for loss of vitamin C in foods. In the presence of molecular oxygen and trace amounts of transition metals (particularly copper (II) and iron (III)), an intermediate ternary complex is formed which undergoes a single two-electron transfer to yield dehydroascorbic acid and hydrogen peroxide (Seib, 1985; Figure 2.33). The rate of loss of ascorbic acid due to metal-catalysed oxidation is dependent upon the concentration of ascorbic acid, as shown in Figure 2.34. A high hydrogen ion concentration (pH about 1) suppresses the ionization of ascorbic acid, and the fully protonated molecule is relatively slowly attacked by oxygen. Consequently, the rate of oxidation of ascorbic acid accelerates as acidity is decreased from pH 1.5 to 3.5. The photochemical oxidation of ascorbic acid proceeds through the generation of free radicals and is accelerated in the presence of metal ions and oxygen (Hay, Lewis and Smith, 1967). Other reactions of ascorbic acid related to foods have been discussed by Liao and Seib (1987, 1988).

Dehydroascorbic acid is not a true organic acid, as it contains no readily ionizable protons. It exists in aqueous solution as the bicyclic

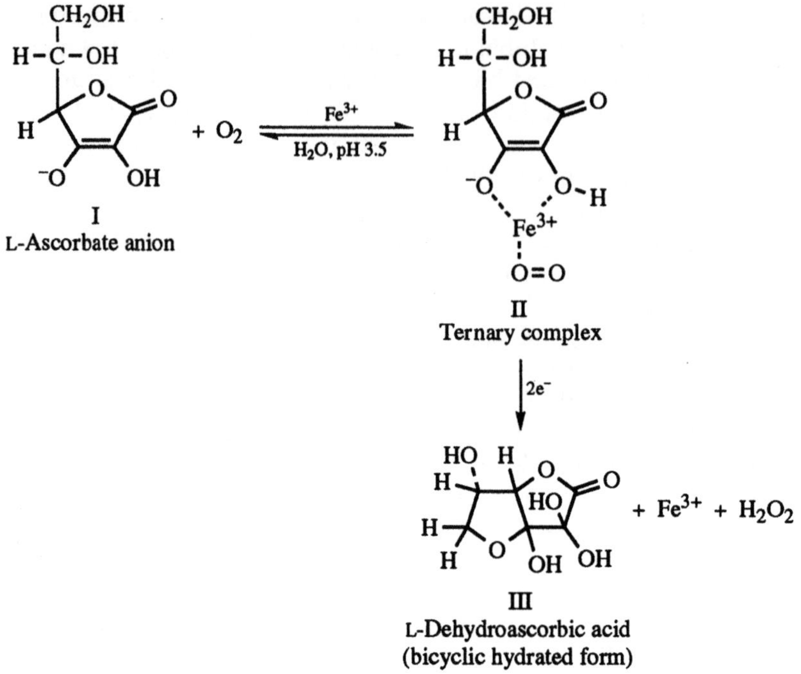

Figure 2.33 Metal-catalysed autoxidation of ascorbic acid.

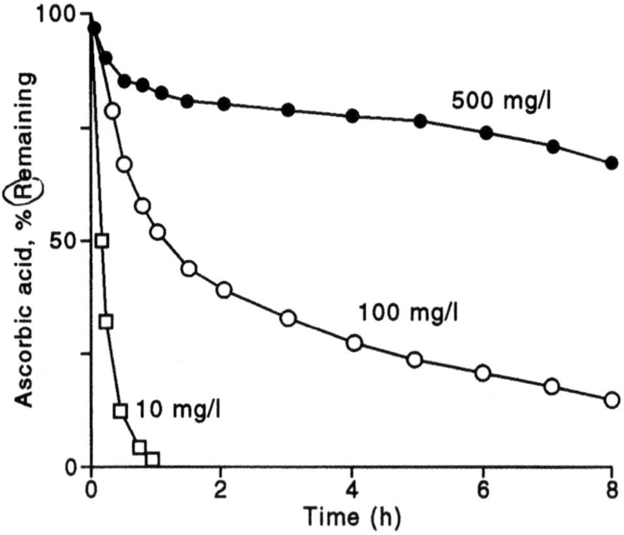

Figure 2.34 Loss of L-ascorbic acid at various concentrations in tap water (from Hornig and Moser, 1981).

hemiketal hydrate rather than as the 2,3-diketo compound and is stable for several days at 4 °C at pH 2.5–5.5. In buffered solution at neutral or alkaline pH, dehydroascorbic acid undergoes a nonreversible oxidation in which the two rings open to give 2,3-diketogulonic acid in a straight-chain structure. Upon standing for 14 h in water at pH 7 and 27 °C, the diketogulonic acid undergoes decarboxylation to give L-*threo*-2-pentulose (Seib, 1985; Figure 2.35). Dehydroascorbic acid is thermolabile, and has a thermal half-life at pH 6 of less than 1 min at 100 °C and 2 min at 70 °C, irrespective of the presence of air (Bender, 1979). Ascorbic acid and dehydroascorbic acid possess equal antiscorbutic activity but diketogulonic acid and its oxidation products are inactive. Thus the total vitamin C content of a biological material is based on the combined levels of ascorbic acid and dehydroascorbic acid.

2.9.5 SPECTROSCOPIC PROPERTIES

Absorption

Ascorbic acid displays an absorption spectrum which is attributable to its enediol structure. The λ_{max} depends on the ionic state of the

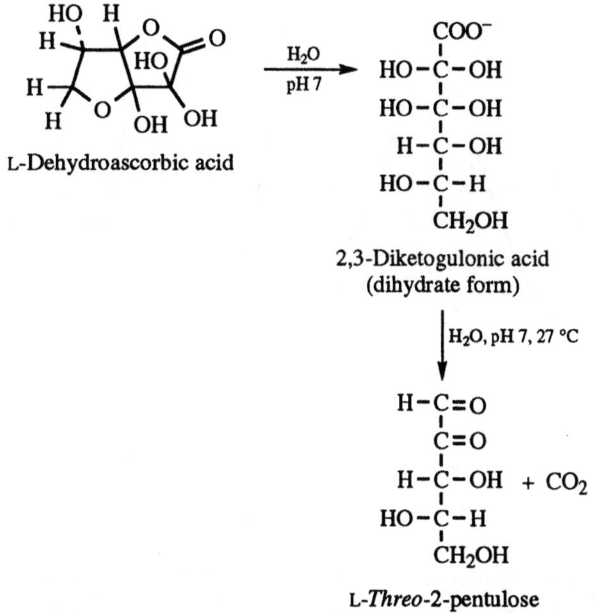

Figure 2.35 Oxidation of dehydroascorbic acid.

molecule and is therefore influenced by the pH of the medium. In acidic solution (pH <2.0) ascorbic acid exists predominantly in the undissociated form, which has a λ_{max} at 244 nm ($A_{1\,cm}^{1\%}$ = 560; *Pharmaceutical Codex*, 1979). Within the pH range 5–10, ascorbic acid exists predominantly as the monoanion, which absorbs maximally at 265 nm ($A_{1\,cm}^{1\%}$ = 940 at pH 6.4) (Lawendel, 1957). At pH 12 and above, where the acid is expected to dissociate fully, λ_{max} occurs at 300 nm (Lau, Luk and Wong, 1986). The absorption spectra of L-ascorbic acid at pH 2.0 and 6.0 are shown in Figure 2.36; also shown is the spectrum of L-dehydroascorbic acid, which has a λ_{max} at 223 nm (Karayannis, Samios and Gousetis, 1977). It is evident from the concentrations of each solution (16 μg/ml for ascorbic acid and 1 mg/ml for dehydroascorbic acid) that the molar absorptivity of the oxidized compound is relatively very weak. The spectra of erythorbic acid at pH 2.0 and 6.0 are virtually identical to those of its epimer, L-ascorbic acid.

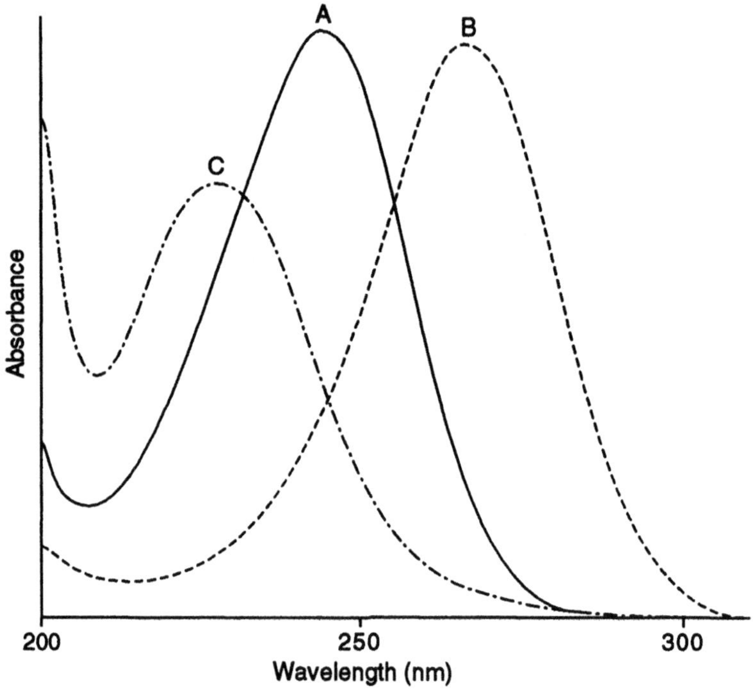

Figure 2.36 Absorption spectra of L-ascorbic acid (16 μg/ml) in 0.1 M phosphate buffer at pH 2.0 (solid line) and pH 6.0 (broken line). L-Dehydroascorbic acid (1 mg/ml) in water at pH 3.1 (discontinuous line). For L-ascorbic acid, λ_{max} of peak A = 244 nm; B = 265 nm. For L-dehydroascorbic acid, λ_{max} of peak C = 223 nm.

2.9.6 DIETARY SOURCES

Fresh fruits (especially citrus fruits and blackcurrants) and green vegetables constitute rich sources of vitamin C. Potatoes contain moderate amounts but, because of their high consumption, represent the most important source of the vitamin in the British diet. Liver, kidney and heart are good sources, but muscle meats and cereal grains do not contain the vitamin (see Table 1.1). Human milk provides enough ascorbic acid to prevent scurvy in breast-fed infants, but preparations of cow's milk are a poor source owing to oxidative losses incurred during processing.

2.9.7 SUPPLEMENTATION OF FOODS

Ascorbic acid is used extensively in the food industry for a variety of purposes. It is added to fruit beverages to inhibit the characteristic pasteurization taste, to enhance the thirst-quenching properties, and to preserve the aroma and colour of the fruit. It is also added to counteract the losses of vitamin C incurred during processing and storage in those drinks that are required to contain a definite amount of the vitamin. The nutritive value of fruit beverages that contain little or no ascorbic acid, such as apple, pineapple and grape juice, is increased by adding the vitamin. The oxidative changes in beer that impair the flavour and aroma, whilst also promoting turbidity, can be retarded by adding ascorbic acid. In wine the addition of ascorbic acid can prevent turbidity through its ability to prevent the oxidation of iron (II) to iron (III). The enzymatic browning that causes problems in fruits and vegetables with a relatively low ascorbic acid content can be prevented by adding the vitamin to the syrup or brine in canned products, or by dipping or spraying the product with aqueous solutions of ascorbic acid before deep freezing. Ascorbic acid is also used as an antibrowning wash for peeled potatoes prior to vacuum packing in bags, and to control the pH of canned tomatoes. In breadmaking, ascorbic acid improves the dough handling, bread texture and loaf volume by increasing the gluten strength through the oxidation of sulphydryl (—SH) groups to intermolecular disulphide (—S—S—) bonds. The oxidation is effected by dehydroascorbic acid, which is formed in the dough by the oxidation of ascorbic acid (Elkassabany, Hoseney and Seib, 1980). Sodium ascorbate is employed as a reducing agent in the curing of bacon and ham to ensure the decomposition of nitrite to nitric oxide in the meat. The nitric oxide released combines with the myoglobin of the muscle tissue to form nitrosomyoglobin, which imparts the characteristic pinkish-red colour of raw bacon and ham. Ascorbate also permits a reduction in the amount of added nitrite and the residual nitrite in the product.

Ascorbyl palmitate is supplied as a proprietary preparation dissolved in lecithin for use as an antioxidant to stabilize fats and oils. The ascorbyl palmitate acts primarily as an oxygen scavenger, whilst the lecithin acts as an emulsifying agent to solubilize the vitamin. One use for this preparation is the prevention of 'white spot' in the British sausage. A synergistic relationship exists between solubilized ascorbyl palmitate and α-tocopherol (vitamin E), and hence the two antioxidants are often used in combination.

Erythorbic acid is cheaper to manufacture on a commercial scale than L-ascorbic acid and, in some countries, it is legal to substitute erythorbate for ascorbate when, for technological reasons, the antioxidant or reducing properties and not the vitamin C activity of the additive is required. (In the UK erythorbate is not permitted as an antioxidant, and it is also prohibited for use with raw and unprocessed meats.)

2.9.8 EFFECTS OF FOOD PROCESSING AND STORAGE

Ascorbic acid is very susceptible to chemical and enzymatic oxidation during the processing, cooking and storage of food. The enzyme ascorbic acid oxidase, which promotes the direct oxidation of ascorbic acid in plant tissues, exhibits maximum activity at 40 °C and is almost completely inactivated at 65 °C (Bender, 1979). Hence rapid heating, such as the blanching of fruits and vegetables or the pasteurization of fruit juices, serves to prevent vitamin loss during post-process storage. Another plant enzyme, phenolase (formerly called polyphenol oxidase), is indirectly responsible for ascorbic acid loss (Coultate, 1989). These enzymes are separated from ascorbic acid in the intact cells but, if the cells are damaged, the enzymes gain access to the vitamin and begin to destroy it. In jam making, when the fruit is boiled with sugar, ascorbic acid is remarkably stable (Olliver, 1967).

Chemical oxidation of ascorbic acid is lowered during processing by carrying out vacuum deaeration and inert gas treatment where feasible. The headspace in containers should be minimized and hermetically sealed systems used. Ascorbic acid is very stable in canned or bottled foods after the oxygen in the headspace has been used up, and provided the food is not subjected to high-temperature storage or exposed to light. The vitamin also keeps well in frozen storage. In contrast to glass containers, plastic bottles and cardboard cartons are permeable to oxygen, so a lowered vitamin C retention is to be expected. Bronze, brass, copper and iron equipment should be avoided, whilst sequestering agents such as ethylenediaminetetraacetic acid (EDTA), polyphosphates and citrates prevent the catalytic action of traces of copper and iron. The sulphites and metabisulphites, which are added to juices or beverages as a source of SO_2, exert a stabilizing effect on ascorbic acid in addition to their role as antimicrobial agents. The addition of food-grade antioxidants such as butylated hydroxyanisole (BHA), butylated hydroxytoluene (BHT) and propyl gallate also protect the vitamin.

Vitamin C in freshly secreted cow's milk is predominantly in the form of ascorbic acid, but this is rapidly oxidized by the dissolved oxygen content. If milk is exposed to light, the oxidation process is greatly accelerated due to the catalytic effect of lumichrome and lumiflavin produced by the photochemical destruction of riboflavin. Losses of vitamin C activity during HTST and ultra-HTST treatment of milk average 20%, but losses incurred during in-bottle sterilization of milk are higher, at 40–79% (Cremin and Power, 1985).

Ascorbic acid can leach away from fruit and vegetables during processing or cooking. This is of little importance with canned, bottled or stewed fruits, where the juice is eaten with the tissue, but may represent a serious loss with vegetables, where the liquor is drained away before serving. If vegetables are steamed or pressure cooked instead of boiled, the leached effect is greatly reduced, but a greater loss of ascorbic acid is to be expected from oxidation. Cold water washing or steeping does not normally leach out a significant amount of the vitamin in whole undamaged fruits and vegetables.

2.9.9 BIOCHEMICAL AND PHYSIOLOGICAL FUNCTIONS

Ascorbic acid acts as an important redox compound in destroying toxic free radicals in cell metabolism (Liao and Seib, 1988). A deficiency of the vitamin causes impaired formation of collagen in the basement membrane of capillaries. The synthesis of collagen involves the enzymatic hydroxylation of proline to hydroxyproline. The latter amino acid, which is not supplied in the diet, is a principal constituent of the collagen fibres. The hydroxylation of lysine is necessary for the subsequent formation of cross-links in the fibres. Experimental evidence suggests that ascorbate acts by maintaining enzyme-bound iron in a loosely bound iron (II) form, the hydroxylase enzymes being rendered inactive if the iron moiety is allowed to oxidize to the more tightly bound iron (III) form (Bates, 1981). Although a wealth of evidence has accumulated showing the role of ascorbate as a redox compound in a variety of enzyme systems, the unique specificity of ascorbate in this role is questionable. Research into collagen metabolism suggests that ascorbate is concerned generally with protein biosynthesis and specifically with collagen biosynthesis (Englard and Seifter, 1986).

Deficiency signs

A deficiency of vitamin C results in scurvy, the symptoms of which are haemorrhages in the gums, skin, bones and joints, and the failure of wound healing.

Expression of dietary value

The IU of vitamin C activity is 0.05 mg of L-ascorbic acid; hence, by definition, 1 g of L-ascorbic acid is equivalent to 20 000 IU (Association of Vitamin Chemists, Inc., 1966). Dehydroascorbic acid possesses full vitamin C activity because it is readily reduced to ascorbic acid in the animal body. Ascorbyl palmitate exhibits the full antiscorbutic activity of ascorbic acid on a molecular weight basis, i.e. 1 g of ascorbyl palmitate is equivalent to the potency of 0.425 g of ascorbic acid. The biological activity of preparations containing vitamin C can be determined by the odontoblast assay in guinea pigs, which measures the length of the mature odontoblast cells in longitudinally sectioned incisors (Bliss and György, 1967). Results obtained by chemical analysis are usually expressed in mg of pure L-ascorbic acid.

Toxicity

Ascorbic acid is generally regarded as being nontoxic (Rivers, 1987). With excessive dietary intakes almost all the ingested amount is excreted in the urine. In healthy individuals, daily dosages of up to at least 1 g may be taken over a period of weeks without the manifestations of toxic symptoms (Hornig and Moser, 1981).

2.9.10 METABOLISM

Many animals can synthesize ascorbic acid by the glucuronic acid pathway, but humans and other primates, in common with guinea pigs and fruit-eating bats, lack the enzyme which catalyses the final step, and thus rely upon their diet to provide the vitamin (Johnson, 1979).

Ascorbic acid is absorbed in the small intestine by an active transport mechanism and assimilated by the tissues. The metabolism follows the pathways of oxidation whereby two electrons are removed in succession to yield firstly the ascorbate free radical and then dehydroascorbate. the latter active compound is then hydrolysed to the inactive 2,3-diketogulonate, and the final degradation products are oxalate and carbon dioxide. A minor pathway is the sulphation of ascorbate to ascorbate2-sulphate, which is unlikely to possess antiscorbutic properties (Bates, 1981).

2.9.11 BIOAVAILABILITY

Information on the availability of vitamin C in foods is limited (Sauberlich, 1985). The average absorption of moderate amounts of vitamin C administered to healthy nonsmoking males was estimated to be 80–90% of the dose (Kallner, Hartmann and Hornig, 1977). There was no significant difference in the intestinal absorption of ascorbate from an orange juice solution and from a solution of synthetic vitamin C (Nelson, Streiff and Cerda, 1975).

REFERENCES

Achuta Murthy, P.N. and Mistry, S.P. (1977) Biotin. *Prog. Fd Nutr. Sci.*, **2**, 405–55.

Alhadeff, L., Gualtieri, T. and Lipton, M. (1984) Toxic effects of water-soluble vitamins. *Nutr. Rev.*, **42**, 33–40.

Andrews, J.S. and Nordgren, R. (1941) The application of the thiochrome method to the thiamin analysis of cereals and cereal products. *Cereal Chem.*, **18**, 686–95.

Ang, C.Y.W. (1979) Stability of three forms of vitamin B_6 to laboratory light conditions. *J. Ass. Off. Analyt. Chem.*, **62**, 1170–3.

Archer, M.C. and Tannenbaum, S.R. (1979) Vitamins. In *Nutritional and Safety Aspects of Food Processing* (ed. S.R. Tannenbaum), Marcel Dekker, Inc., New York, pp. 47–95.

Association of Vitamin Chemists, Inc. (1966) *Methods of Vitamin Assay*, 3rd edn, Interscience Publishers, New York.

Bailey, L.B. (1988) Factors affecting folate bioavailability. *Fd Technol.*, **42**(10), 206–12, 238.

Bates, C.J. (1981) The function and metabolism of vitamin C in man. In *Vitamin C (Ascorbic Acid)* (eds J.N. Counsell and D.H. Hornig), Applied Science Publishers, London, pp. 1–22.

Baugh, C.M. and Krumdieck, C.L. (1971) Naturally occurring folates. *Ann. N.Y. Acad. Sci.*, **186**, 7–28.

Belitz, H.-D. and Grosch, W. (1987) *Food Chemistry*, Springer Verlag, Berlin, pp. 305–19.

Bender, A.E. (1979) The effects of processing on the stability of vitamins in foods. In *Proceedings of the Kellogg Nutrition Symposium*, London, 14–15th Dec., 1978 (ed. T.G. Taylor), MTP Press, Lancaster, pp. 111–25.

Bender, D.A. and Bender, A.E. (1986) Niacin and tryptophan metabolism: the biochemical basis of niacin requirements and recommendations. *Nutr. Abstr. Rev. (Ser. A)*, **56**, 695–719.

Bennink, M.R. and Ono, K. (1982) Vitamin B_{12}, E and D content of raw and cooked beef. *J. Fd Sci.*, **47**, 1786–92.

Benterud, A. (1977) Vitamin losses during thermal processing. In *Physical, Chemical and Biological Changes in Food caused by Thermal Processing* (eds T. Høyem and O. Kvåle), Applied Science Publishers Ltd, London, pp. 185–201.

Bernhart, F.W., D'amato, E. and Tomarelli, R.M. (1960) The vitamin B_6 activity of heat-sterilized milk. *Arch. Biochem. Biophys.*, **88**, 267–9.

Bhandari, S.D. and Gregory, J.F. (1990) Inhibition by selected food components of human and porcine intestinal pteroylpolyglutamate hydrolase activity. *Am. J. Clin. Nutr.*, **51**, 87–94.

Bird, O.D. and Thompson, R.Q. (1967) Pantothenic acid. I. Introduction. In *The Vitamins. Chemistry, Physiology, Pathology, Methods*, 2nd edn, Vol. VII (eds P. György and W.N. Pearson), Academic Press, New York, pp. 209–19.

Bliss, C.I. and György, P. (1967) Ascorbic acid. III. Animal assay. In *The Vitamins. Chemistry, Physiology, Pathology, Methods*, 2nd edn. Vol. VII (eds P. György and W.N. Pearson), Academic Press, New York, pp. 49–51.

Bonjour, J.-P. (1984) Biotin. In *Handbook of Vitamins. Nutritional, Biochemical, and Clinical Aspects* (ed. L. J. Machlin), Marcel Dekker, Inc., New York, pp. 403–35.

Bowman, B.B. and Rosenberg, I.H. (1987) Biotin absorption by distal rat intestine. *J. Nutr.*, **117**, 2121–6.

Bridges, J.W., Davies, D.S. and Williams, R.T. (1966) Fluorescence studies on some hydroxypyridines including compounds of the vitamin B_6 group. *Biochem. J.*, **98**, 451–68.

Brin, M. (1978) Vitamin B_6: chemistry, absorption, metabolism, catabolism, and toxicity. In *Human Vitamin B_6 Requirements*, Food and Nutrition Board, National Research Council. National Academy of Sciences, Washington, DC, pp. 1–20.

Brown, G.M. (1959) Assay and distribution of bound forms of pantothenic acid. *J. Biol. Chem.*, **234**, 379–82.

Carter, E.G.A. and Carpenter, K.J. (1982a) The bioavailability for humans of bound niacin from wheat bran. *Am. J. Clin. Nutr.*, **36**, 855–61.

Carter, E.G.A. and Carpenter, K.J. (1982b) The available niacin values of foods for rats and their relation to analytical values. *J. Nutr.*, **112**, 2091–103.

Černá, J. and Káš, J. (1983) New conception of folacin assay in starch or glycogen containing food samples. *Nahrung*, **27**, 957–64.

Chaykin, S. (1967) Nicotinamide coenzymes. *Annu. Rev. Biochem.*, **36**, 149–70.

Chen, T.-S. and Cooper, R. G. (1979) Thermal destruction of folacin: effect of ascorbic acid, oxygen and temperature. *J. Fd Sci.*, **44**, 713–16.

Chia, C.P., Addison, R. and McCormick, D.B. (1978) Absorption, metabolism, and excretion of 8α- (amino acid) riboflavins in the rat. *J. Nutr.*, **108**, 373–81.

Cooperman, J.M. and Lopez, R. (1984) Riboflavin. In *Handbook of Vitamins. Nutritional, Biochemical, and Clinical Aspects* (ed. L.J. Machlin), Marcel Dekker, Inc., New York, pp. 299–327.

Coultate, T.P. (1989) *Food. The Chemistry of its Components*, 2nd edn, Royal Society of Chemistry, London.

Coursin, D.B. (1954) Convulsive seizures in infants with pyridoxine-deficient diet. *JAMA*, **154**, 406–8.

Crawford, T.C. and Crawford, S.A. (1980) Synthesis of L-ascorbic acid. *Adv. Carbohydr. Chem.*, **37**, 79–155.

Cremin, F.M. and Power, P. (1985) Vitamins in bovine and human milks. In *Developments in Dairy Chemistry*, Vol. III (ed. P.F. Fox), Elsevier Applied Science Publishers, London and New York, pp. 337–98.

Cumming, F., Briggs, M. and Briggs, M. (1981) Clinical toxicology of vitamin supplements. In *Vitamins in Human Biology and Medicine* (ed. M.H. Briggs), CRC Press, Inc., Boca Raton, Florida, pp. 187–243.

Dakshinamurti, K., Paulose, C.S. and Siow, Y.L. (1985) Neurobiology of pyridoxine. In *Vitamin B-6: its Role in Health and Disease* (ed. R.D. Reynolds and J.E. Leklem), Alan R. Liss, Inc., New York, pp. 99–121.

Dalton, K. and Dalton, M.J.T. (1987) Characteristics of pyridoxine overdose neuropathy syndrome. *Acta Neurol. Scand.*, **76**, 8–11.

Day, B.P.F. and Gregory, J.F. (1983) Thermal stability of folic acid and 5-methyltetrahydrofolic acid in liquid model food systems. *J. Fd Sci.*, **48**, 581–7, 599.

De Ritter, E. (1976) Stability characteristics of vitamins in processed foods. *Fd Technol.*, **30**(1), 48–51, 54.

Dunkley, W.L., Franklin, J.D. and Pangborn, R.M. (1962) Effects of fluorescent light on flavor, ascorbic acid, and riboflavin in milk. *Fd Technol.*, **16**(9), 112–18.

Dwivedi, B.K. and Arnold, R.G. (1973) Chemistry of thiamine degradation in food products and model system: a review. *J. Agric. Fd Chem.*, **21**, 54–60.

Ebadi, M. (1978) Vitamin B_6 and biogenic amines in brain metabolism. In *Human Vitamin B_6 Requirements*, Committee on Dietary Allowances, Food and Nutrition Board, National Research Council. National Academy of Sciences, Washington, DC, pp. 129–61.

Edwards, C.H., Booker, L.K., Rumph, C.H., Craven, R. and Ganapathy, S.N. (1971) Utilization of wheat by adult man: excretion of vitamins and minerals. *Am J. Clin. Nutr.*, **24**, 547–55.

Elkassabany, M., Hoseney, R.C. and Seib, P.A. (1980) Ascorbic acid as an oxidant in wheat flour dough. I. Conversion to dehydroascorbic acid. *Cereal Chem.*, **57**, 85–7.

Englard, S. and Seifter, S. (1986) The biochemical functions of ascorbic acid. *Annu. Rev. Nutr.*, **6**, 365–406.

FAO/WHO (1967) Requirements of vitamin A, thiamine, riboflavine and niacin. *World Health Organisation Technical Report Series No. 362*, World Health Organisation, Geneva.

FAO/WHO (1970) Requirements of ascorbic acid, vitamin D, vitamin B-12, folate, and iron. *Report of a Joint FAO/WHO Expert Group*, World Health Organisation, Geneva.

FAO/WHO (1988) Requirements of vitamin A, iron, folate and vitamin B_{12}. *Report of a Joint FAO/WHO Expert Consultation*, Food and Agriculture Organisation of the United Nations, Rome.

Farquharson, J. and Adams, J.F. (1976) The forms of vitamin B-12 in foods. *Br. J. Nutr.*, **36**, 127–36.

Food and Nutrition Board (1989) Water-soluble vitamins. In *Recommended Dietary Allowances*, 10th edn, National Research Council, National Academy Press, Washington, DC, pp. 115–73.

Ford, J.E., Salter, D.N. and Scott, K.J. (1969) The folate-binding protein in milk. *J. Dairy Res.*, **36**, 435–46.

Ghosh, H.P., Sarkar, P.K. and Guha, B.C. (1963) Distribution of the bound form of nicotinic acid in natural materials. *J. Nutr.*, **79**, 451–3.

Gräsbeck, R. and Salonen, E.-M. (1976) Vitamin B-12. *Prog. Fd Nutr. Sci.*, **2**, 193–231.

Gregory, J.F. (1980a) Effects of ε-pyridoxyllysine bound to dietary protein on the vitamin B-6 status of rats. *J. Nutr.*, **110**, 995–1005.

Gregory, J.F. (1980b) Effects of ε-pyridoxyllysine and related compounds on liver and brain pyridoxal kinase and liver pyridoxamine (pyridoxine) 5'-phosphate oxidase. *J. Biol. Chem.*, **255**, 2355–9.

Gregory, J.F. (1982) Denaturation of the folacin-binding protein in pasteurized milk products. *J. Nutr.*, **112**, 1329–38.

Gregory, J.F. (1985) Chemical changes of vitamins during food processing. In *Chemical Changes of Food during Processing* (eds T. Richardson and J. W. Finley), Van Nostrand Reinhold Co., New York, pp. 373–408.

Gregory, J.F. (1988) Methods for determination of vitamin B6 in foods and other biological materials: a critical review. *J. Fd Comp. Anal.*, **1**, 105–23.

Gregory, J.F. (1989) Chemical and nutritional aspects of folate research: analytical procedures, methods of folate synthesis, stability, and bioavailability of dietary folates. *Adv. Fd Nutr. Res.*, **33**, 1–101.

Gregory, J.F. and Feldstein, D. (1985) Determination of vitamin B-6 in foods and other biological materials by paired-ion high-performance liquid chromatography. *J. Agric. Fd Chem.*, **33**, 359–63.

Gregory, J.F. and Hiner, M.E. (1983) Thermal stability of vitamin B6 compounds in liquid model food systems. *J. Fd Sci.*, **48**, 1323–7, 1339.

Gregory, J.F. and Ink, S.L. (1987) Identification and quantification of pyridoxine-β-glucoside as a major form of vitamin B6 in plant-derived foods. *J. Agric. Fd Chem.*, **35**, 76–82.

Gregory, J.F., Ink, S.L. and Sartain, D.B. (1986) Degradation and binding to food proteins of vitamin B-6 compounds during thermal processing. *J. Fd Sci.*, **51**, 1345–51.

Gregory, J.F. and Kirk, J.R. (1977) Interaction of pyridoxal and pyridoxal phosphate with peptides in a model food system during thermal processing. *J. Fd Sci.*, **42**, 1554–7, 1561.

Gregory, J.F. and Kirk, J.R. (1978) Assessment of storage effects on vitamin B_6 stability and bioavailability in dehydrated food systems. *J. Fd Sci.*, **43**, 1801–8, 1815.

Gregory, J.F. and Kirk, J.R. (1981) The bioavailability of vitamin B-6 in foods. *Nutr. Rev.*, **39**, 1–8.

Gregory, J.F., Sartain, D.B. and Day, B.P.F. (1984) Fluorometric determination of folacin in biological materials using high performance liquid chromatography. *J. Nutr.*, **114**, 341–53.

Gregory, J.F., Ristow, K.A., Sartain, D.B. and Damron, B.L. (1984). Biological activity of the folacin oxidation products 10-formylfolic acid and 5-methyl-5,6-dihydrofolic acid. *J. Agric. Fd Chem.*, **32**, 1337–42.

Gregory, J.F., Trumbo, P.R., Bailey, L.B., Toth, J.P., Baumgartner, T.G. and Cerda, J.J. (1991) Bioavailability of pyridoxine-5'-β-D-glucoside determined in humans by stable-isotopic methods. *J. Nutr.*, **121**, 177–86.

Gregory, M.E. (1959) The effect of heat on the vitamin B-6 of milk. 1. Microbiological tests. *J. Dairy Res.*, **26**, 203–14.

Gubler, C.J. (1984) Thiamin. In *Handbook of Vitamins. Nutritional, Biochemical, and Clinical Aspects* (ed. L.J. Machlin), Marcel Dekker, Inc., New York, pp. 245–97.

Guilbert, C.C. and Johnson, S.L. (1977) Investigation of the open ring form of nicotinamide adenine dinucleotide. *Biochemistry*, **16**, 335–44.

Hankes, L.V. (1984) Nicotinic acid and nicotinamide. In *Handbook of Vitamins. Nutritional, Biochemical, and Clinical Aspects* (ed. L.J. Machlin), Marcel Dekker, Inc., New York, pp. 329–77.

Hartman, A.M. and Dryden, L.P. (1974) Vitamins in milk and milk products. In *Fundamentals of Dairy Chemistry*, 2nd edn (eds B.H. Webb, A.H. Johnson and J.A. Alford), AVI Publishing Co., Inc., Westport, CT, pp. 325–441.

Hashmi, M. (1973) *Assay of Vitamins in Pharmaceutical Preparations*, John Wiley & Sons, London and New York.

Hassinen, J.B., Durbin, G.T. and Bernhart, F.W. (1954) The vitamin B-6 content of milk products. *J. Nutr.*, **53**, 249–57.

Hawkes, J.G. and Villota, R. (1989) Folates in foods: reactivity, stability during processing, and nutritional implications. *Crit. Rev. Fd Sci. Nutr.*, **28**, 439–539.

Hay, G.W., Lewis, B.A. and Smith, F. (1967) Ascorbic acid. II. Chemistry. In *The Vitamins. Chemistry, Physiology, Pathology, Methods*, 2nd edn, Vol. I (eds W.H. Sebrell, Jr and R.S. Harris), Academic Press, New York, pp. 307–36.

Herbert, V. (1987) Recommended dietary intakes (RDI) of vitamin B-12 in humans. *Am. J. Clin. Nutr.*, **45**, 671–8.

Herbert, V. (1988) Vitamin B-12: plant sources, requirements, and assays. *Am. J. Clin. Nutr.*, **48**, 852–8.

Herbert, V.D. and Colman, N. (1988) Folic acid and vitamin B-12. In *Modern Nutrition in Health and Disease*, 7th edn (eds M.E. Shils and V.R. Young), Lea & Febiger, Philadelphia, pp. 388–416.

Hilker, D.M. and Somogyi, J.C. (1982) Antithiamins of plant origin: their chemical nature and mode of action. *Ann. N.Y. Acad. Sci.*, **378**, 137–45.

Hoffbrand, A.V. (1979) Nutritional and biochemical aspects of vitamin B_{12}. In *The Importance of Vitamins to Human Health* (ed. T.G. Taylor), MTP Press Ltd, Lancaster, pp. 41–6.

Hoffer, A., Alcock, A.W. and Geddes, W.F. (1943) A rapid method for the determination of thiamine in wheat and flour. *Cereal Chem.*, **20**, 717–29.

Hornig, D.H. and Moser, U. (1981) The safety of high vitamin C intakes in man. In *Vitamin C (Ascorbic Acid)* (eds J.N. Counsell and D.H. Hornig), Applied Science Publishers, London and New Jersey, pp. 225–48.

Hornig, D. and Weiser, H. (1976) Interaction of erythorbic acid with ascorbic acid catabolism. *Int. J. Vitam. Nutr. Res.*, **46**, 40–7.

Horwitt, M.K. (1972) Riboflavin, V. Occurrence in food. In *The Vitamins. Chemistry, Physiology, Pathology, Methods*, 2nd edn, Vol. V (eds W.H. Sebrell, Jr and R.S. Harris), Academic Press, New York, pp. 46–9.

Horwitt, M.K., Harper, A.E. and Henderson, L.M. (1981) Niacin–tryptophan relationship for evaluating niacin equivalents. *Am. J. Clin. Nutr.*, **34**, 423–7.

Hunter, R., Barnes, J., Oakeley, H.F. and Matthews, D.M. (1970) Toxicity of folic acid given in pharmacological doses to healthy volunteers. *Lancet*, **1**, 61–3.

Ink, S.L., Gregory, J.F. and Sartain, D.B. (1986) Determination of pyridoxine β-glucoside bioavailability using intrinsic and extrinsic labeling in the rat. *J. Agric. Fd Chem.*, **34**, 857–62.

Ishii, K., Sarai, K., Sanemori, H. and Kawasaki, T. (1979a) Analysis of thiamine and its phosphate esters by high-performance liquid chromatography. *Analyt. Biochem.*, **97**, 191–5.

Ishii, K., Sarai, K., Sanemori, H. and Kawasaki, T. (1979b) Concentrations of thiamine and its phosphate esters in rat tissues determined by high-performance liquid chromatography. *J. Nutr. Sci. Vitaminol.*, **25**, 517–23.

Johnson, F.C. (1979) The antioxidant vitamins. *CRC Crit. Rev. Fd Sci. Nutr.*, **11**, 217–309.

Kabir, H., Leklem, J.E. and Miller, L.T. (1983) Measurement of glycosylated vitamin B-6 in foods. *J. Fd Sci.*, **48**, 1422–5.

Kallner, A., Hartmann, D. and Hornig, D. (1977) On the absorption of ascorbic acid in man. *Int. J. Vitam. Nutr. Res.*, **47**, 383–8.

Kanno, C., Kanehara, N., Shirafuji, K., Tanji, R. and Imai, T. (1991) Binding form of vitamin B_2 in bovine milk: its concentration, distribution and binding linkage. *J. Nutr. Sci. Vitaminol.*, **37**, 15–27.

Karayannis, M.I., Samios, D.N. and Gousetis, Ch.P. (1977) A study of the molar absorptivity of ascorbic acid at different wavelengths and pH values. *Analyt. Chim. Acta*, **93**, 275–9.

Keagy, P.M., Stokstad, E.L.R. and Fellers, D.A. (1975) Folacin stability during bread processing and family flour storage. *Cereal Chem.*, **52**, 348–56.

Kies, C., Kan, S. and Fox, H.M. (1984) Vitamin B6 availability from wheat, rice and corn brans for humans. *Nutr. Rep. Int.*, **30**, 483–91.

Kiesvaara, M. and Virtanen, A.I. (1962) Synthetic ascorbigen as a vitamin C source for guinea pigs and man. *Acta Chem. Scand.*, **16**, 510–12

Killeit, U . (1986) The stability of vitamins. *Fd Europe*, No. 3, March/April, 21–4.

Kiss, G. and Neukom, H. (1966) Upon the structure of ascorbigens. *Helv. Chim. Acta*, **49**, 989–92 (in German).

Kodicek, E., Braude, R., Kon, S.K. and Mitchell, K.G. (1956) The effect of alkaline hydrolysis of maize on the availability of its nicotinic acid to the pig. *Br. J. Nutr.*, **10**, 51–67.

Kodicek, E., Braude, R., Kon, S.K. and Mitchell, K.G. (1959) The availability to pigs of nicotinic acid in *tortilla* baked from maize treated with lime-water. *Br. J. Nutr.*, **13**, 363–84.

Koetz, R., Amadò, R. and Neukom, H. (1979) Nature of the bound nicotinic acid in wheat bran. *Lebensm.-Wiss. u.-Technol.*, **12**, 346–9.

Koetz, R. and Neukom, H. (1977) Nature of bound nicotinic acid in cereals and its release by thermal and chemical treatment. In *Physical, Chemical and Biological Changes in Food caused by Thermal Processing* (eds T. Høyem and O. Kvåle), Applied Science Publishers Ltd, London, pp. 305–10.

Koziol, J. (1971) Fluorometric analyses of riboflavin and its coenzymes. *Methods Enzymol.*, **18B**, 253–85.

Krehl, W.A., De La Huerga, J., Elvehjem, C.A. and Hart, E.B. (1946) The distribution of niacinamide and niacin in natural materials. *J. Biol. Chem.*, **166**, 53–7.

Kutsky, R.J. (1973) Pantothenic acid. In *Handbook of Vitamins and Hormones*, Van Nostrand Reinhold Company, New York, pp. 104–11.

Lampen, J.O., Bahler, G.P. and Peterson, W.H. (1942) The occurrence of free and bound biotin. *J. Nutr.*, **23**, 11–21.

Lau, O.-W., Luk, S.-F. and Wong, K.-S. (1986) Background correction method for the determination of ascorbic acid in soft drinks, fruit juices and cordials using direct ultra-violet spectrophotometry. *Analyst, Lond.*, **111**, 665–70.

Lawendel, J.S. (1957) Ultra-violet absorption spectra of L-ascorbic acid in aqueous solutions. *Nature*, **180**, 434–5.

Leichter, J., Landymore, A.F. and Krumdieck, C.L. (1979) Folate conjugase activity in fresh vegetables and its effect on the determination of free folate content. *Am. J. Clin. Nutr.*, **32**, 92–5.

Leklem, J.E., Miller, L.T., Perera, A.D. and Peffers, D.E. (1980) Bioavailability of vitamin B-6 from wheat bread in humans. *J. Nutr.*, **110**, 1819–28.

Liao, M.-L. and Seib, P.A. (1987) Selected reactions of L-ascorbic acid related to foods. *Fd Technol.*, **41**(11), 104–7.

Liao, M.-L. and Seib, P.A. (1988) Chemistry of L-ascorbic acid related to foods. *Fd Chem.*, **30**, 289–312.

Lindberg, A.S., Leklem, J.E. and Miller, L.T. (1983) The effect of wheat bran on the bioavailability of vitamin B-6 in young men. *J. Nutr.*, **113**, 2578–86.

McCormick, D.B. (1988a) Thiamin. In *Modern Nutrition in Health and Disease*, 7th edn (eds M.E. Shils and V.R. Young), Lea & Febiger, Philadelphia, pp. 355–61.

McCormick, D.B. (1988b). Riboflavin. In *Modern Nutrition in Health and Disease*, 7th edn (eds M.E. Shils and V.R. Young), Lea & Febiger, Philadelphia, pp. 362–9.

McCormick, D.B. (1988c) Niacin. In *Modern Nutrition in Health and Disease*, 7th edn (eds M.E. Shils and V.R. Young), Lea & Febiger, Philadelphia, pp. 320–75.

McCormick, D.B. (1988d) Vitamin B-6. In *Modern Nutrition in Health and Disease*, 7th edn (eds M.E. Shils and V.R. Young), Lea & Febiger, Philadelphia, pp. 376–82.

McCormick, D.B. (1988e) Pantothenic acid. In *Modern Nutrition in Health and Disease*, 7th edn (eds M.E. Shils and V.R. Young), Lea & Febiger, Philadelphia, pp. 383–7.

McCormick, D.B. (1988f) Biotin. In *Modern Nutrition in Health and Disease*, 7th edn (eds M.E. Shils and V.R. Young), Lea & Febiger, Philadelphia, pp. 436–9.

McRoberts, L.H. (1954) Report on the determination of thiamine in enriched flour. Comparison of fluorometric methods. *J. Ass. Off. Agric. Chem.*, **37**, 757–70.

McRoberts, L.H. (1957) Report on thiamine in enriched cereal and bakery products. *J. Ass. Off. Agric. Chem.*, **40**, 843–53.

Mason, J.B., Gibson, N. and Kodicek, E. (1973) The chemical nature of the bound nicotinic acid of wheat bran: studies of nicotinic acid-containing macromolecules. *Br. J. Nutr.*, **30**, 297–311.

Mason, J.B. and Kodicek, E. (1973) The chemical nature of the bound nicotinic acid of wheat bran: studies of partial hydrolysis products. *Cereal Chem.*, **50**, 637–46.

Merrill, A.H. Jr., Lambeth, J.D., Edmondson, D.E. and McCormick, D.B. (1981) Formation and mode of action of flavoproteins. *Annu. Rev. Nutr.*, **1**, 281–317.

Miller, D.R. and Hayes, K.C. (1982) Vitamin excess and toxicity. In *Nutritional Toxicology*, Vol. I (ed. J.N. Hathcock), Academic Press, New York, pp. 81–133.

Morino, Y. and Nagashima, F. (1986) Methods for isolation and purification of pyridoxal phosphate and derivatives. In *Vitamin B_6 Pyridoxal Phosphate. Chemical, Biochemical, and Medical Aspects*, Part A (eds D. Dolphin, R. Poulson and O. Avramović), John Wiley & Sons, New York, pp. 477–96.

NAS/NRC (1980) Water-soluble vitamins. In *Recommended Dietary Allowances*, 9th edn, National Academy of Sciences/National Research Council, Washington, DC, pp. 72–124.

NAS/NRC (1989) Water-soluble vitamins. In *Recommended Dietary Allowances*,

10th edn, National Academy of Sciences/National Research Council, Washington, DC, pp. 115–73.

Nelson, E.W., Streiff, R.R. and Cerda, J.J. (1975) Comparative bioavailability of folate and vitamin C from a synthetic and a natural source. *Am. J. Clin. Nutr.*, **28**, 1014–19.

Nguyen, L.B. and Gregory, J.F. (1983) Effects of food composition on the bioavailability of vitamin B-6 in the rat. *J. Nutr.*, **113**, 1550–60.

Nguyen, L.B., Gregory, J.F. and Damron, B.L. (1981) Effects of selected polysaccharides on the bioavailability of pyridoxine in rats and chicks. *J. Nutr.*, **111**, 1403–10.

Nguyen, L.B., Gregory, J.F., Burgin, C.W. and Cerda, J.J. (1981). In vitro binding of vitamin B-6 by selected polysaccharides, lignin, and wheat bran. *J. Fd Sci.*, **46**, 1860–2.

Nguyen, L.B., Hiner, M.E., Litherland, S.A. and Gregory, J.F. (1983) Relative biological activity of nonphosphorylated vitamin B-6 compounds in the rat. *J. Agric. Fd Chem.*, **31**, 1282–7.

Nielsen, P., Rauschenbach, P. and Bacher, A. (1986) Preparation, properties, and separation by high-performance liquid chromatography of riboflavin phosphates. *Methods Enzymol.*, **122G**, 209–20.

Obermeyer, H.G., Fulmer, W.C. and Young, J.M. (1944) Cocarboxylase hydrolysis by a wheat phosphatase. *J. Biol. Chem.*, **154**, 557–9.

Olliver, M. (1967) Ascorbic acid. V. Occurrence in foods. In *The Vitamins. Chemistry, Physiology, Pathology, Methods*, 2nd edn, Vol. I (eds W.H. Sebrell, Jr and R.S. Harris), Academic Press, New York, pp. 359–67.

Orr, M.L. and Watt, B.K. (1972) Losses of vitamins and trace minerals resulting from processing and preservation of foods. *Am. J. Clin. Nutr.*, **25**, 647–8.

Paine-Wilson, B. and Chen, T.-S. (1979) Thermal destruction of folacin: effect of pH and buffer ions. *J. Fd Sci.*, **44**, 717–22.

Passmore, R. and Eastwood, M.A. (1986) *Davidson and Passmore Human Nutrition and Dietetics*, 8th edn, Churchill Livingstone, New York.

Pelletier, O. and Godin, C. (1969) Vitamin C activity of D-isoascorbic acid for the guinea pig. *Can. J. Physiol. Pharmacol.*, **47**, 985–91.

Pharmaceutical Codex (1979) 11th edn, Pharmaceutical Press, London.

Polansky, M.M. and Toepfer, E.W. (1969a) Nutrient composition of selected wheats and wheat products. IV. Vitamin B-6 components. *Cereal Chem.*, **46**, 664–74.

Polansky, M.M. and Toepfer, E.W. (1969b) Vitamin B-6 components in some meats, fish, dairy products, and commercial infant formulas. *J. Agric. Fd Chem.*, **17**, 1394–7.

Reed, L.S. and Archer, M.C. (1979) Action of sodium nitrite on folic acid and tetrahydrofolic acid. *J. Agric. Fd Chem.*, **27**, 995–9.

Reed, L.S. and Archer, M.C. (1980) Oxidation of tetrahydrofolic acid by air. *J. Agric. Fd Chem.*, **28**, 801–5.

Reiber, H. (1972) Photochemical reactions of vitamin B_6 compounds, isolation and properties of products. *Biochim. Biophys. Acta*, **279**, 310–15.

Rivers, J.M. (1987) Safety of high-level vitamin C ingestion. *Ann. N.Y. Acad. Sci.*, **498**, 445–54.

Robinson, D.R. (1971) The nonenzymatic hydrolysis of N^5, N^{10}-methenyltetrahydrofolic acid and related reactions. *Methods Enzymol.*, **18B**, 716–25.

Saidi, B. and Warthesen, J.J. (1983) Influence of pH and light on the kinetics of vitamin B_6 degradation. *J. Agric. Fd Chem.*, **31**, 876–80.

Sapers, G.M., Hicks, K.B., Phillips, J.G. *et al.* (1989) Control of enzymatic browning in apple with ascorbic acid derivatives, polyphenol oxidase inhibitors, and complexing agents. *J. Fd Sci.*, **54**, 997–1002, 1012.

Sauberlich, H.E. (1985) Bioavailability of vitamins. *Prog. Fd Nutr. Sci.*, **9**, 1–33.

Sauberlich, H.E., Kretsch, M.J., Skala, J.H., Johnson, H.L. and Taylor, P.C. (1987) Folate requirement and metabolism in nonpregnant women. *Am. J. Clin. Nutr.*, **46**, 1016–28.

Schneider, A. and Stroinski, A. (1987) *Comprehensive B-12. Chemistry, Biochemistry, Nutrition, Ecology, Medicine,* Walter de Gruyter, Berlin and New York, pp. 44–51.

Schroeder, H.A. (1971) Losses of vitamins and trace minerals resulting from processing and preservation of foods. *Am. J. Clin. Nutr.*, **24**, 562–73.

Seib, P.A. (1985) Oxidation, monosubstitution and industrial synthesis of ascorbic acid. *Int. J. Vitam. Nutr. Res.*, Suppl. 27, 259–306.

Shinton, N.K. (1972) Vitamin B-12 and folate metabolism. *Br. Med. J.*, **1**, 556–9.

Shultz, T.D. and Leklem, J.E. (1987) Vitamin B-6 status and bioavailability in vegetarian women. *Am. J. Clin. Nutr.*, **46**, 647–51.

Siegel, L., Melnick, D. and Oser, B.L. (1943) Bound pyridoxine (vitamin B_6) in biological materials. *J. Biol. Chem.*, **149**, 361–7.

Snell, E.E. (1958) Chemical structure in relation to biological activities of vitamin B_6. *Vitams Horm.*, **15**, 77–125.

Snell, E.E. (1986) Pyridoxal phosphate: history and nomenclature. In *Vitamin B_6 Pyridoxal Phosphate. Chemical, Biochemical, and Medical Aspects,* Part A (eds D. Dolphin, R. Poulson and O. Avramović), John Wiley & Sons, New York, pp. 1–12.

Stokstad, E.L.R. and Koch, J. (1967) Folic acid metabolism. *Physiol. Rev.*, **47**, 83–116.

Strohecker, R. and Henning, H.M. (1966) *Vitamin Assay – Tested Methods,* Verlag Chemie, Weinheim.

Tadera, K., Kaneko, T. and Yagi, F. (1986) Evidence for the occurrence and distribution of a new type of vitamin B_6 conjugate in plant foods. *Agric. Biol. Chem.*, **50**, 2933–4.

Tadera, K. and Orite, K. (1991) Isolation and structure of a new vitamin B_6 conjugate in rice bran. *J. Fd Sci.*, **56**, 268–9.

Tamura, T. and Stokstad, E.L.R. (1973) The availability of food folate in man. *Br. J. Haematol.*, **25**, 513–32.

Tannenbaum, S.R., Young, V.R. and Archer, M.C. (1985) Vitamins and minerals. In *Food Chemistry*, 2nd edn (ed. O.R. Fennema), Marcel Dekker, Inc., New York, pp. 477–544.

Tarr, J.B., Tamura, T. and Stokstad, E.L.R. (1981) Availability of vitamin B-6 and pantothenate in an average American diet in man. *Am. J. Clin. Nutr.*, **34**, 1328–37.

Temple, C. Jr and Montgomery, J.A. (1984) Chemical and physical properties of folic acid and reduced derivatives. In *Folates and Pterins,* Vol. 1. *Chemistry and Biochemistry of Folates* (ed. R.L. Blakley and S.J. Benkovic), John Wiley & Sons, New York, pp. 61–120.

Tomarelli, R.M., Spence, E.R. and Bernhart, F.W. (1955) Biological availability of vitamin B_6 of heated milk. *J. Agric. Fd Chem.*, **3**, 338–41.

Trumbo, P.R., Gregory, J.F. and Sartain, D.B. (1988) Incomplete utilization of pyridoxine-β-glucoside as vitamin B-6 in the rat. *J. Nutr.*, **118**, 170–5.

Uyeda, K. and Rabinowitz, J.C. (1963) Fluorescence properties of tetrahydrofolate and related compounds. *Analyt. Biochem.*, **6**, 100–8.

Vanderslice, J.T., Brownlee, S.G., Cortissoz, M.E. and Maire, C.E. (1985) Vitamin B_6 analysis; sample preparation, extraction procedures, and chromatographic separations. In *Modern Chromatographic Analysis of the Vitamins* (eds A.P. De Leenheer, W.E. Lambert and M.G.M. De Ruyter), Marcel Dekker, Inc., New York, pp. 435–75.

Viani, R. and Horman, I. (1974) Thermal behaviour of trigonelline. *J. Fd Sci.*, **39**, 1216–7.

Vimokesant, S., Kunjara, S., Rungruangsak, K., Nakornchai, S. and Panijpan, B. (1982) Beriberi caused by antithiamin factors in food and its prevention. *Ann. N.Y. Acad. Sci.*, **378**, 123–36.

Voigt, M.N. and Eitenmiller, R.R. (1978) Comparative review of the thiochrome, microbial and protozoan analyses of B-vitamins. *J. Fd Protection*, **41**, 730–8.

Wagner, C. (1985) Folate-binding proteins. *Nutr. Rev.*, **43**, 293–9.

Wall, J.S. and Carpenter, K.J. (1988) Variation in availability of niacin in grain products. *Fd Technol.*, **42**(10), 198–202, 204.

Walsh, J.H., Wyse, B.W. and Hansen, R.G. (1981) Pantothenic acid content of 75 processed and cooked foods. *J. Am. Diet. Ass.*, **78**, 140–4.

Weiner, M. and van Eys, J. (1983) *Nicotinic Acid. Nutrient–Cofactor–Drug*, Marcel Dekker, Inc., New York.

Wendt, G. and Bernhart, F.W. (1960) The structure of a sulphur-containing compound with vitamin B_6 activity. *Arch. Biochem. Biophys.*, **88**, 270–2.

Windholz, M. (ed.) (1993) *Merck Index*, 10th edn, Merck & Co., Inc., Rahway, NJ.

Wong, D.W.S. (1989) *Mechanism and Theory in Food Chemistry*, Van Nostrand Reinhold Co., New York, pp. 335–99.

Yagi, K. (1962) Chemical determination of flavins. In *Methods of Biochemical Analysis*, Vol. 10 (ed. D. Glick), John Wiley & Sons, New York, pp. 319–56.

Zapsalis, C. and Beck, R.A. (1985) Vitamins and vitamin-like substances. In *Food Chemistry and Nutritional Biochemistry*, John Wiley & Sons, New York, pp. 189–312.

3 Analytical considerations

3.1 ANALYTICAL REQUIREMENTS

The analytical requirements may be considered from three different viewpoints. In the first case, the chemist in the food manufacturing industry needs to know how much of the vitamin that was added in fortification is actually present in the finished product. In practical terms this case is comparatively simple, as the vitamin will be present in the form of the parent molecule that can be readily extracted, and in a measurable quantity. In routine quality control work the fortified product will be reasonably consistent from batch to batch, and therefore no unforeseen problems associated with the matrix should be encountered. On the other hand, the quality control manager will want a quick and reliable result on a regular basis and with minimum expense per analysis. Hence a facile rapid method with good repeatability is required, preferably a method that determines several vitamins simultaneously and that can be automated.

The other two cases concern the investigator who needs to determine the nutritional value of a food commodity or diet. There are two approaches here. If the investigator is carrying out an animal bioassay, the bioavailability can be calculated as a ratio of standardized biological activity to the total vitamin content. This approach entails the determination, by microbiological or physicochemical means, of all bound forms of the vitamin in addition to the bioassay. If, however, the investigator is not carrying out an animal bioassay, it is desirable to estimate the biological vitamin activity using an appropriate extraction procedure that does not necessarily yield the total vitamin content.

The term 'total' vitamin must be regarded with caution, bearing in mind the diversity of bound forms and the complications of extraction. Thus unbound B_6 vitamers in milk, for example, are readily extracted, whereas Schiff base forms present in meat products require more rigorous methods of extraction. If the vitamers of a particular vitamin respond identically to the analytical end-point (e.g. fluorescence intensity) they need not be determined individually, but if they exhibit different responses it is necessary to separate them chromatographically prior to measurement. HPLC is ideally suited for this purpose, as it combines a high separation power with selective and sensitive measurement. There is also the question of relative biopotency between vitamers, and the problem of the biological availability arises if the vitamin is bound in a conjugated form.

3.2 SCOPE OF ANALYTICAL TECHNIQUES

The analytical techniques that have been routinely applied to the quantitative determination of water-soluble vitamins in foods are physicochemical, microbiological and biospecific assays. The selection of a particular assay technique is influenced by a number of factors. Firstly, the biological potencies of the vitamins vary considerably and this is reflected in the concentrations in which they occur in foods. Thus vitamin C may be found in Brussels sprouts at around 115 mg/100 g, whereas the richest source of vitamin B_{12}, liver, contains only 110 μg/100 g (ox liver), i.e. three orders of magnitude less. This wide variation in concentration immediately imposes limitations upon certain analytical techniques for certain vitamins. For example, ascorbic acid in fruit juices can be assayed quite adequately by simple titration, whereas even the most sensitive physicochemical technique, such as HPLC, cannot accurately measure naturally occurring vitamin B_{12}, even in liver. A further limitation imposed by the variation in concentration is that the simultaneous determination of two or more vitamins may be precluded.

Another factor is the inherent physicochemical and biological properties of the vitamin that may allow (or preclude) a particularly advantageous measurement technique to be exploited. For example, the strong native fluorescence exhibited by riboflavin allows this vitamin to be selectively measured at levels that are well within those that occur naturally in foods. On the other hand, neither pantothenic acid nor biotin possess chromophores or fluorophores, and this rules out HPLC using direct photometric or fluorimetric detection. All of the B-group vitamins can be assayed microbiologically, but there are no known microbiological organisms that have an absolute requirement for ascorbic acid. Other factors that are beyond the control of the analyst are constraints imposed by lack of resources. Taking all of these factors into account, the choice of analytical technique should depend upon what needs to be measured in order to provide the information that will fulfil the overall objective.

3.2.1 THIAMIN

The major form of thiamin in meat products is protein-bound thiamin pyrophosphate (TPP). In cereals and cereal products, including white flour made from wheat, free thiamin predominates, but wheat germ, bran and also white bread contain TPP. For the analysis of these products it is customary to determine the combined thiamin activity of the various forms present. The principal techniques for determining thiamin are direct fluorimetric measurement after conversion to thiochrome, and HPLC with fluorimetric detection of thiochrome.

3.2.2 RIBOFLAVIN

Riboflavin occurs naturally in biological tissues as protein-bound FAD and FMN, while riboflavin itself is the major form in bovine milk. It is usually required to determine the total riboflavin content of the sample, which is defined in the nutritional context as the sum of FAD, FMN and riboflavin. Current techniques for determining total riboflavin are microbiological assay, direct fluorimetry, and HPLC with fluorimetric detection. HPLC can also be used to determine the individual flavins.

3.2.3 NIACIN

The niacin in mature cereal grains exists as a chemically bound form of nicotinic acid, while pulses and other non-cereal plant foods contain mainly free nicotinic acid. In meat the niacin content is mainly in the form of nicotinamide, which is also the form used in fortification. It is customary when employing *in vitro* analytical methods to measure the total niacin (i.e. free plus bound) content of the food sample; however, this provides a gross overestimate of the niacin value of several staple cereal-based foods. A better prediction of available niacin is to measure just the free niacin, yet this may result in a degree of undervaluation because of the apparent partial utilization of the bound nicotinic acid present in mature cereal grains. Nevertheless, the measurement of free niacin would seem to be the more appropriate for cereal products as a means of ensuring an adequate level of enrichment. The terms 'total' and 'free' niacin are defined by the extraction methods employed in the analysis. Both can be measured microbiologically, colorimetrically or by HPLC. HPLC also permits the separate measurement of nicotinamide and nicotinic acid.

Food composition tables express the niacin value as the niacin equivalent content, one niacin equivalent being equal to either 1 mg of available niacin or 60 mg of L-tryptophan. The data are obtained using a chick growth assay. The standard microbiological assay procedure for determining 'total' niacin does not account for tryptophan, because the mild acid digestion used to extract the niacin does not hydrolyse the proteins, and the lactic acid bacterium employed as the test organism cannot utilize peptide-bound tryptophan. Apart from using an animal bioassay, or possibly a protozoan assay, an estimate of the niacin equivalent content would necessitate the determination of L-tryptophan in a separate assay. If the protein content of a particular food sample is known, the tryptophan content can be estimated on the basis that animal and vegetable proteins contain *c.*1.4% and 1.0% tryptophan, respectively (Thompson, 1982).

3.2.4 VITAMIN B_6

Vitamin B_6 exists as pyridoxine (PN), pyridoxal (PL) and pyridoxamine (PM), together with their 5′-phosphorylated derivatives, PNP, PLP and PMP. PNP does not occur to any significant extent in natural products. PN.HCl is used in the fortification of foods. The Schiff base forms of PLP and PL that predominate in foods of animal origin are presumed to be totally available. PN and PNP are virtually absent in animal tissues, one exception being liver tissue, in which they are detectable at very low levels. Plant-derived foods contain mostly PN, a significant proportion of which may be present as PN-glucoside and/or other conjugated forms which appear to be largely unavailable to humans. It has been suggested (Kabir, Leklem and Miller, 1983) that the level of glycosylated vitamin B_6 may be useful as an index of B_6 bioavailability. Total vitamin B_6 activity is usually estimated microbiologically using a turbidimetric yeast assay; the radiometric–microbiological assay is a more recent innovation. With the aid of HPLC, it is possible to measure all of the B_6 vitamers present after non-destructive extraction, including PN-glucoside. HPLC techniques should be capable of separating the inactive metabolite 4-pyridoxic acid, which may be present in foods, from the B_6 vitamers. The various bound forms of vitamin B_6 can be assayed microbiologically or by HPLC using selective extraction procedures.

3.2.5 PANTOTHENIC ACID

The majority of naturally occurring pantothenic acid is in the form of coenzyme A and is routinely determined by microbiological assay after suitable extraction. Biospecific methods of analysis include the radioimmunoassay and the enzyme-linked immunosorbent assay (ELISA).

3.2.6 BIOTIN

Biotin occurs covalently bound to proteins as well as in the free state. In addition to the conventional microbiological assay for determining biotin, biospecific methods have been developed utilizing radiometric protein-binding assays (radioassays) and non-isotopic protein-binding assays.

3.2.7 FOLATE

Folate compounds constitute a large family of pteroylpolyglutamates which differ in the reduction state of the pteridine nucleus, the nature of the single carbon substituent at the N-5 and/or N-10 positions, and the number of glutamate residues. Up to 150 different folate structures are theoretically possible (Baugh and Krumdieck, 1971), although less than 50 principal folates exist in most animal and plant tissues (Gregory, 1989). Naturally occurring folates exist in protein-bound form, the predominant vitamers being polyglutamyl forms of tetrahydrofolic acid (THF), 5-methyl-THF and 10-formyl-THF (Gregory, 1984). THF is extremely susceptible to oxidation but the presence of substituent groups in the N-5 position greatly increases the oxidative stability. Folic acid (pteroylmonoglutamic acid, PGA) is used in fortification because of its comparative stability.

The multiplicity and diversity of natural folates, their instability and their existence at low concentration in biological tissues poses a formidable obstacle to the separation, identification and quantification of these compounds. The study of folates is further complicated by their association with enzymes capable of modifying or degrading them during sample preparation. Attempts to determine intact pteroylpolyglutamates in biological tissues have involved fractionation of tissue extracts by column chromatography and comparison of elution profiles with those of authentic folate standards. The effluent fractions are then further characterized and quantified by differential microbiological assay both before and after treatment with conjugase (Krumdieck, Tamura and Eto, 1983). Stokstad, Shin and Tamura (1977) described such a technique in which food extracts were subjected to preliminary gel chromatography on Sephadex G-15. This technique separates the folate analogues into a monoglutamate fraction and a polyglutamate fraction on the basis of molecular size. Both fractions were then rechromatographed by anion exchange chromatography through diethylaminoethyl cellulose (DEAE-cellulose) columns using gradient elution. The technique was applied to the analysis of cabbage (Chan, Shin and Stokstad, 1973), soybeans and bovine milk (Shin *et al.*, 1975) and romaine lettuce (Batra, Wagner and Stokstad, 1977). Perry (1971) applied a similar technique, but without the gel filtration step, to the study of folate analogues in normal mixed diets.

The methods described above for determining intact folates are powerful analytical tools, but they cannot possibly yield complete and accurate qualitative and quantitative information about all of the folates present in a biological sample. The methods also suffer from being slow and extremely laborious. The simplest approach for determining the chain length of pteroylpolyglutamates would be to cleave the C-9–N-10 bond and separate the *p*-aminobenzoylpolyglutamates ($PABAGlu_n$) by ion exchange or gel chromatography. Converting the folates to a common chemical form differing only in polyglutamyl chain length would reduce the number of potential compounds to a level readily manageable by column chromatographic techniques, whilst also eliminating the need for enzyme treatment and microbiological assay. Methods using this simplified approach have been published, but the direct oxidation or reductive procedures originally employed have since been found to be inconsistent (Krumdieck, Tamura and Eto, 1983). A quantitative conversion of all naturally occurring folates to $PABAGlu_n$ has been achieved by prior conversion of 5- and 10-formyl-THFs to 5-

methyl-THFs, followed by standard Zn/HCl reductive cleavage. The $PABAGlu_n$ fragments were converted to azo dyes by coupling their diazonium salts with naphthylethylene diamine, and the dye compounds were then separated according to glutamate chain length by polyacrylamide gel chromatography (Brody, Shane and Stokstad, 1979). Several variations of the cleavage procedure have been proposed, including a differential procedure by which the chain lengths of specific pools of folates are ascertained. More recently, HPLC has been applied to the separation of the azo dye derivatives of $PABAGlu_n$ (Krumdieck, Tamura and Eto, 1983).

For most food analysis purposes, the determination of the chain length of folate polyglutamates is not required, and the folates are determined as their monoglutamyl forms after enzymatic deconjugation. The microbiological assay of total folate activity is the most widely used and accepted procedure. The radioassay and non-isotopic protein-binding assay represent current biospecific techniques. HPLC assays permit the determination of the major folate vitamers that occur in foods.

3.2.8 VITAMIN B_{12}

Vitamin B_{12} occurs intracellularly in the living tissues of animals in the form of the two coenzymes, adenosylcobalamin and methylcobalamin, which are covalently bound to their protein apoenzymes. In milk, these coenzymes are bound noncovalently to specific transport proteins. Hydroxocobalamin is present in animal-derived foods, especially in milk, as a result of the photo-oxidation of the coenzyme forms. Cyanocobalamin is a synthetic stable form of the vitamin used in fortification. The potential vitamin B_{12} activity of a food sample is represented by the total cobalamin content, regardless of the ligand attached. The determination of total vitamin B_{12} may be performed by microbiological assay or by radioassay. Supplemental vitamin B_{12} (cyanocobalamin) may be determined by a non-isotopic protein-binding assay.

3.2.9 VITAMIN C

The classic titrimetric method using 2,6-dichlorophenolindophenol accounts for ascorbic acid but not dehydroascorbic acid. Analytical methods for total vitamin C include colorimetry and fluorimetry, in which ascorbic acid is oxidized to dehydroascorbic acid and then reacted with a chemical reagent to form a coloured or fluorescent compound. Total vitamin C can also be determined by HPLC using absorbance or electrochemical detection after reduction of dehydroascorbic acid to ascorbic acid, or using fluorescence detection after oxidation or ascorbic acid and derivatization of the dehydroascorbic acid formed.

3.3 THE GENERAL ANALYTICAL PROCEDURE

The general analytical procedure for determining water-soluble vitamins in foods can be broken down into six main stages, namely sampling, extraction, clean-up, measurement, calculation of results, and interpretation of data. Other factors to be considered are maintenance of sample integrity, storage of the sample pending analysis, and preparation of the sample for analysis. The International Union of Pure and Applied Chemistry (IUPAC) has prepared a document intended to furnish concepts, terms and definitions in the field of analytical chemistry with the emphasis on sampling (Horwitz, 1990). The term 'sample' should be used with an appropriate modifier to indicate its position in the hierarchical scheme depicted in Figure 3.1 (e.g. 'laboratory sample' and 'test sample'). Once analytical work begins, the term 'sample' should be avoided and 'test' used instead, as in 'test portion'.

All operations with vitamin solutions and vitamin-containing materials should be carried out in subdued light or in low-actinic amber glassware. A dedicated laboratory fitted with gold fluorescent tubes which exclude radiation wavelengths of less than 500 nm is the ideal. Several of the water-soluble vitamins are rapidly destroyed by alkali, and glassware should be acid-washed before rinsing to prevent inactivation of vitamins by surface films of alkaline detergents.

3.3.1 SAMPLING

A major problem encountered in food analysis is the heterogeneity of foods. Pomeranz and Meloan (1978) referred to a macroheterogeneity (among various units of a lot) and microheterogeneity (within various parts of a unit). The latter is especially important in vitamin assays. Thus, thiamin and nicotinic acid are concentrated in the aleurone and scutellum tissues of the wheat kernel, whilst the starchy endosperm is relatively devoid of these vitamins. The uneven distribution of fat in meat makes it necessary to express analytical values on a fat-free basis. Heterogeneity may also be a problem in vitamin-enriched foods such as breakfast cereals, in which the distribution of vitamins applied by spray-drying is frequently far from uniform. It is evident that the 'concentration' of a nutrient is actually a mean value with an associated uncertainty. Therefore, before a food sample can be analysed, consideration must be given to obtain a representative sample in order to reduce this

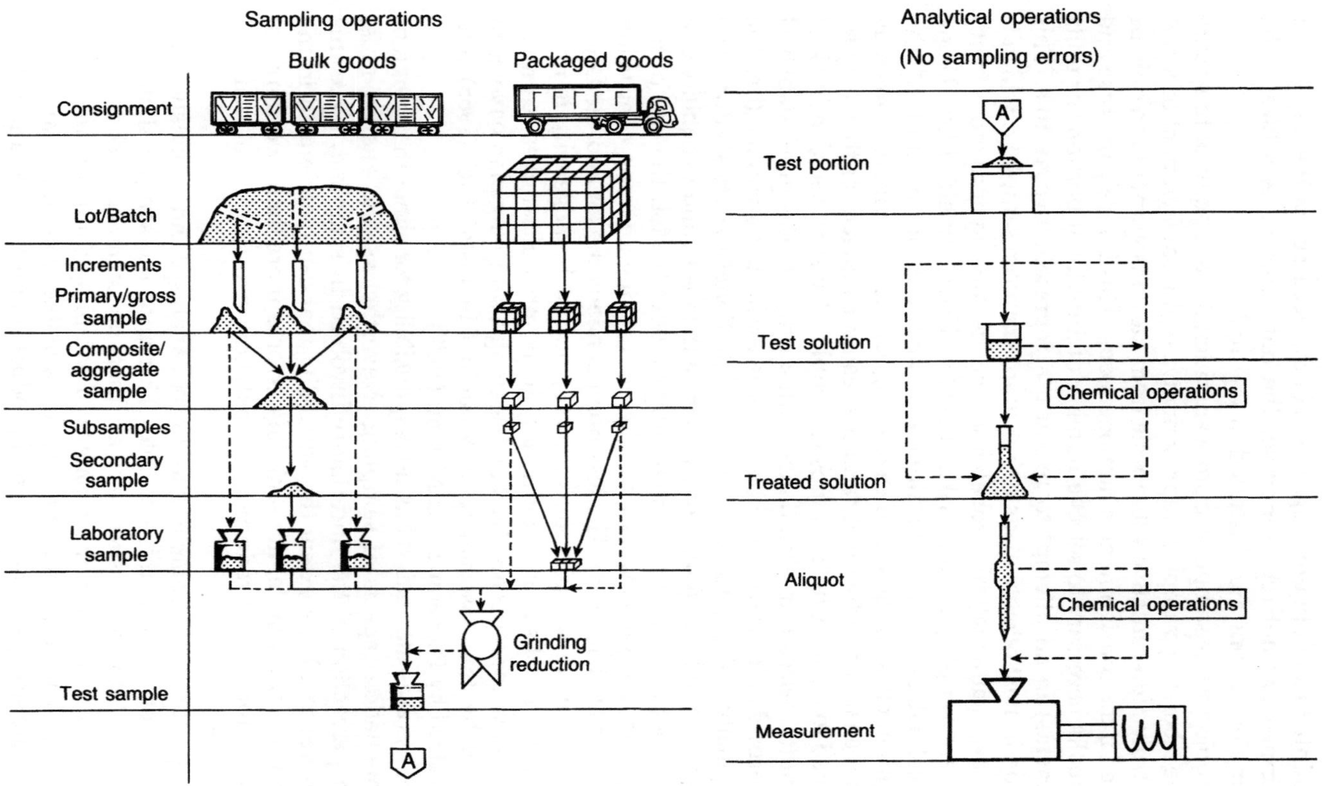

Figure 3.1 The relationships of the operations involved in sampling and analysis. The lower 'A' of the sampling operations continues with the upper 'A' of the analytical operations. From Horwitz (1990). © 1990 IUPAC.

uncertainty to a minimum. Regardless of the accuracy of the analysis, if the samples are not representative, the data may be worthless. The sampling operations are illustrated in Figure 3.1.

The objective of sampling from a nutritional standpoint is to ensure that the laboratory sample is representative of the consignment or lot. A single truly representative subsample from the consignment can only be obtained if the consignment is homogeneous. This is rarely the case and it is usually necessary to select a number of individual portions or units (increments) in an attempt to produce a representative sample. This selection is most reliably made using simple random sampling, which is based on mathematical probability and is not synonymous with haphazard sampling (Kratochvil and Taylor, 1981; Garfield, 1989). Using statistical tables of random numbers, any portion or unit of the consignment has an equal chance of being selected. The increments may be either analysed individually and the results averaged, or they may be combined to form a single composite sample. The analysis of individual increments, selected in accordance with a properly designed statistical plan, provides information about between-sample variability (i.e. the homogeneity of the lot) at the expense of additional analytical effort. The number of samples required for estimating the mean and variability of a particular lot depends upon the homogeneity of the lot, the size of the lot, and the risk one is willing to take on reaching a wrong conclusion (Elkins and Dudek, 1985). The less homogeneous the lot and the larger the lot, the more samples are required, but lot homogeneity is more important than lot size in determining the number of samples required. The statistical concepts involved in designing a sampling plan have been discussed by the Association of Vitamin Chemists, Inc. (1966) and summarized by Pomeranz and Meloan (1978).

In many cases the analyst has no responsibility for either the design or implementation aspects of sampling. Nevertheless, the analyst must have a perception of the uncertainty involved in sampling, since this determines to a large extent the variability that can be tolerated in the analysis. If, for example, the sampling error is more than two-thirds of the total error, then a reduction in analytical error is only of marginal importance.

Ideally, the food sample should be analysed immediately after selection, but rarely is this possible. Therefore the sample should be packed and stored in such a way that no significant changes in composition occur from the moment of sampling until the analysis is completed. This calls for the use of suitable containers and low-temperature storage for non-canned products to protect the sample from moisture loss or gain, chemical decomposition, contamination and microbial spoilage.

In preparing a laboratory food sample for analysis, the non-edible portions must first be removed, noting the weight proportion of non-edible to edible portions. The sample must then be treated in such a manner as to prevent changes in composition so that a representative portion can be taken for the actual analysis. In practice, both of these criteria are difficult to achieve, the latter particularly if only a small amount of sample is used in the determination. Apparently homogeneous materials such as single-phase liquids and powders, as well as heterogeneous materials, should be mixed thoroughly immediately before taking the portion for analysis. Dry particulate material can be reduced in volume by quartering the thoroughly mixed sample, discarding two opposite quarters, remixing the remaining material, and repeating the process until the sample is reduced to a desired size. Commodities such as meat and fish products and raw vegetables can be finely chopped using a food processor, while products containing liquid, such as canned fruit or fruit beverages, can be blended in a high-speed blender. Care must be taken not to chop sausages or sandwich meats too finely in the food processor, or the fat will liquefy and separate. Blending must not be excessively vigorous or prolonged, as aeration and heat generation can promote oxidation and decomposition of vitamins. Non-canned products held in the frozen state pending analysis should be thawed overnight at 4 °C, and then stored in the dark and brought to room temperature before opening the container. Raw and unblanched fruit or vegetables selected for vitamin C analysis should be blended directly with the acid stabilizing solution used in the assay to prevent enzymatic oxidation of ascorbic acid by the action of liberated ascorbic acid oxidase. For cooked or blanched samples or for canned produce, the stabilizing solution can be added immediately after chopping or blending. Techniques have been described for preparing various types of food commodities for analysis (Association of Vitamin Chemists, Inc., 1966).

3.3.2 EXTRACTION

Generally speaking, the B-group vitamins occur naturally as coenzymes in animal and plant tissues tightly bound to their protein apoenzymes. Plant tissues may also contain storage forms of certain vitamins (e.g. vitamin B_6) bound to carbohydrates, while the vitamins in milk are bound to specific transport proteins. In addition, many of the vitamins are integral parts of complex molecules, such as FAD, NAD and coenzyme A. It is essential for a successful assay that the vitamins be extracted from their bound forms in a form that can be utilized by assay micro-organisms or measured by biospecific assay or chemical/physico-chemical techniques. The extraction stage serves to homogenize the sample, isolate the vitamin from its parent coenzyme molecule, release the vitamin from its association with protein or carbohydrate, eliminate as far as is possible known interfering substances, and destroy any indigenous enzyme activity. There is no common extraction method for all of the water-soluble vitamins and, to further complicate the situation, the state of combination of a given vitamin often varies with different tissues. The appropriate method of extraction depends upon the following criteria: (1) the analytical information required; (2) the type of food under test (different bound forms of vitamins are often found in meat, plant and dairy products); (3) the selectivity and specificity of the analytical method to be used; and (4) the stability of the vitamin towards heat and extremes of pH. Many of the vitamins are extracted most efficiently by acid or alkaline hydrolysis at elevated temperature (121 °C) in an autoclave. Vitamins that are unstable under such conditions can be extracted by enzymatic digestion. Much valuable information can be obtained regarding the nature of the various bound and free forms of vitamins by the use of selective extraction techniques. Further aspects of the extraction stage are discussed in Chapter 4.

3.3.3 CLEAN-UP

The extracts prepared by hydrolysis and/or enzymatic treatment of the test material may require further purification (clean-up) before they can be subjected to analysis. The extent of the clean-up depends upon the ratio of analyte to interfering substances, and also upon the sensitivity and selectivity of the analytical technique. Colorimetric, titrimetric and spectrophotometric techniques have rather poor specificity and require extensive sample clean-up. Direct fluorimetric techniques are rather more specific, while chromatographic techniques, particularly HPLC, have relatively high specificity. Microbiological assays are subject to interference from many substances, although these can usually be diluted out owing to the high sensitivity of such techniques. It is frequently necessary, however, to remove lipoidal material prior to microbiological assay.

Deproteinization

The soluble denatured protein present in acid hydrolysates of food samples can be precipitated by adjusting the pH of the hydrolysate to 4.5 (near the isoelectric point of most proteins in solution) and then removed by simple filtration through a suitable paper. This technique is particularly useful in microbiological assays, as it also removes lipoidal material from low-fat samples together with any unhydrolysed starch, which might otherwise cause interference. The deproteinization of sample extracts prior to assay by HPLC is effected by treatment with dilute trichloroacetic acid, perchloric acid or some other deproteinizing agent, followed by filtration or centrifugation.

Solvent extraction

For high-fat samples (e.g. meat, eggs, cheese, wheat germ, maize, soya beans) it is often necessary to remove the fat by preliminary Soxhlet extraction with either diethyl ether or light petroleum ether to prevent interference from lipids in microbiological assays. This step also prevents the formation of oily emulsions which may hinder complete extraction of the vitamin to be determined. Sample extracts can be defatted prior to HPLC analysis by extraction with a suitable fat solvent (e.g. dichloromethane) using a separating funnel. In the AOAC fluorimetric method for thiamin, extraction of the oxidized vitamin (thiochrome) into isobutanol constitutes an effective purification step as well as providing a means of concentrating the sample.

Dialysis

This is a size-exclusion technique which has found useful application in isolating pantothenic acid from proteins following enzymatic digestion of autoclaved food samples as a means of liberating the vitamin from coenzyme A (Walsh, Wyse and Hansen, 1979). In this simple process, the food digest–enzyme mixture is transferred with water washings into a short length of semipermeable dialysis tubing, which is tied securely at both ends and immersed in a relatively large volume of distilled water. Large molecules (molecular weight >10 000) are retained, but smaller molecules, including free pantothenic acid, diffuse through the tubing into the more dilute surrounding medium, which is stirred continuously to maintain the concentration difference. After 8 h, all of the pantothenic acid has diffused out of the food digest–enzyme mixture, and the water extract is assayed microbiologically or by radioimmunoassay.

Ion exchange chromatography

Acid-hydrolysed extracts of food samples prepared for the fluorimetric determination of thiamin can be purified by passing through a cation exchange column, which retains the positively charged thiamin molecules and allows unretained anions and non-ionized solutes to be washed off with distilled water. The thiamin is then eluted using hot acidified potassium chloride solution, during which process the thiamin is exchanged for potassium ions. The same principle, using gravity-flow or preparative HPLC columns, can be applied for purifying sample extracts prior to the determination of thiamin and other ionized vitamins by HPLC.

Solid-phase extraction (SPE)

This has found widespread application for purifying sample extracts prior to analysis by HPLC. The technique uses small disposable prepacked chromatographic cartridges, usually containing a reversed-phase C_{18} material, although the full range of silica-based polar and nonpolar stationary phases encountered in HPLC column packings is commercially available. The average silica particle size is typically 40 μm (Bond Elut and Bakerbond) or 60 μm (Sep-Pak) and allows easy elution under low pressure. The small mean pore diameter (typically 60 Å) excludes proteins of molecular weight higher than 15–20 000, and the large surface area confers a high sample-loading capacity. The SPE cartridges may be operated under positive pressure using a hand-held syringe or under negative pressure using a vacuum manifold. The latter technique is preferable, as multiple samples can be processed simultaneously, and the solvent flow rates can be precisely controlled with the aid of a vacuum gauge.

Purification of the sample extract can be effected in two ways, after first conditioning the cartridge with an appropriate solvent in order to solvate the functional groups of the sorbent. In the matrix removal mode, the sample extract is simply passed through the cartridge. Molecules with relatively hydrophobic properties, such as lipids, pigments and proteins, will be retained, while the polar water-soluble vitamins will pass through the sorbent. In the sample clean-up mode, the sorbent retains the analyte and allows impurities to pass through the sorbent. The cartridge is washed with an appropriate solvent, which selectively elutes the impurities, and the purified analyte is finally eluted with the minimum volume of a solvent that is just strong enough to displace the analyte from the sorbent. Concentration of the sample extract is achieved in the clean-up mode if the elution volume is less than the volume of sample extract applied to the cartridge.

3.3.4 MEASUREMENT

The measurement techniques suitable for determining water-soluble vitamins in foods can be divided into animal growth assays, microbiological assays, physicochemical methods and biospecific methods. Animal growth assays involve the feeding of experimental animals (usually young rats) with a specially purified basal diet, which provides for all their nutritional requirements except for the vitamin being determined. The animals receiving such a diet fail to grow and gain weight. By comparing growth rate when known amounts of the required vitamin are added to the basal diet with the growth rate when known quantities of the food under investigation are added, it is possible to deduce the vitamin content of the test food. Animal assays are only satisfactory in the hands of experienced workers, the procedure is lengthy and expensive, and a large number of specially selected animals are required from the statistical angle. Animal assays have been reviewed by Bliss and György (1967) and their purpose is discussed in Chapter 1. They will not be considered further, apart from their mention in comparative studies. The principal *in vitro* techniques are outlined below to illustrate their scope and applicability as a preview to their discussion in subsequent chapters.

Physicochemical methods

Titrimetric methods provide a rapid and simple means of determining vitamin C in fruits and fruit juices. Both the dichlorophenolindophenol (DCPIP) titration for ascorbic acid and the *N*-bromosuccinimide titration for total vitamin C (ascorbic plus dehydroascorbic acids) can be performed potentiometrically to overcome the end-point difficulty encountered with coloured solutions.

Voltammetry is a highly sensitive but not very selective technique for determining electroactive compounds that can be oxidized or reduced at a charged electrode surface. The technique has found commercial application for the determination of several water-soluble vitamins in pharmaceutical preparations, but is limited in food analysis to the determination of ascorbic acid and erythorbic acid. Voltammetry is widely used in the form of the electrochemical detector in HPLC, which provides high sensitivity and high selectivity for the determination of several vitamins.

Absorption spectroscopy is limited to those vitamins that possess a strong chromophore, and hence pantothenic acid and biotin are excluded. Direct UV spectrophotometry has been applied to the routine determination of ascorbic acid in fruit beverages after correction for background absorption. The technique has not found application for the B-group vitamins because of the need for extensive purification of the sample extract. An adequate purification can, however, be readily achieved using HPLC (see later) which, with photometric detection, can be regarded as a specialized spectrophotometric technique. Absorbance measurement at λ_{max} provides a rapid and accurate means of determining the concentration of a solution of authentic crystalline vitamin in the absence of interfering substances using published $A_{1\,cm}^{1\%}$ values. The technique is of indirect value in food analysis for establishing the precise concentrations of standard vitamin solutions used for HPLC applications.

Colorimetry involves the reaction of the vitamin with a reagent to produce a coloured complex whose optical density is measured photometrically. Such techniques have found high utility for analysing vitamin pharmaceutical preparations but, in most cases, they lack the necessary sensitivity and specificity for application to food analysis. A colorimetric method using cyanogen bromide has been adopted by the AOAC for the determination of niacin in foods and feeds, and a semi-automated continuous-flow technique based upon the manual method has been adopted by the AOAC for the analysis of cereal products. Vitamin C can be determined in foods as the 2,4-dinitrophenylhydrazine derivative after oxidation of ascorbic acid to dehydroascorbic acid.

Fluorimetry is more sensitive and more selective than absorption spectroscopy and has been applied to the determination of thiamin after conversion to thiochrome; to riboflavin directly or after conversion to lumiflavin; to vitamin B_6 directly (pyridoxine only) or after conversion to 4-pyridoxic acid lactone; and to vitamin C after conversion to a quinoxaline derivative. All of these manual fluorimetric techniques require some means of purifying the test extract to remove interfering substances. Fluorimetry is best utilized as a means of detection in HPLC using pre- or post-column conversion of non-fluorescent vitamins to fluorescent compounds.

Continuous-flow analysis using a segmented flow technique has been utilized to automate the analytical stages of official fluorimetric methods for thiamin, riboflavin and vitamin C, and the colorimetric method for niacin. A nonsegmented flow technique (flow-injection analysis) has found application for the determination of ascorbic acid. Such techniques are very similar to the corresponding manual versions, but the time-consuming preparation of sample extracts still remains, so the full capabilities of the automatic stages cannot be exploited.

Gas chromatography (GC) has been applied to the determination of thiamin as its thiazole degradation product using the nitrogen–phosphorus detector (NPD) or flame photometric detector (FPD); nicotinamide as 3-cyanopyridine using the flame ionization detector (FID); vitamin B_6 as the trifluoroacetate derivatives of PN, PL and PM using the electron capture detector (ECD); pantothenic acid as the pantoyl lactone using FID; and ascorbic acid as its trimethylsilyl ether derivative using FID. The GC methods published for vitamin C are obsolete, since the mediocre packed-column efficiency and the non-selective measurement technique (FID) cannot compete with modern HPLC methods. The use of high-resolution open-tubular capillary columns coupled with selective detectors would greatly enhance the performance of GC assays.

High-performance liquid chromatography (HPLC) provides a greater chromatographic selectivity than GC and, being non-destructive, can be used as a preparative purification method as well as a quantitative technique. HPLC is particularly useful for the determination of thiamin and riboflavin, which can be extracted together and chromatographed either simultaneously or successively using fluorescence detection (after derivatization of thiamin to thiochrome). HPLC techniques have also been published for determining niacin using absorption detection, and all of the B_6 vitamers can be separated and quantified using fluorescence detection after post-column derivatization of weakly fluorescent vitamers. The nutritionally important folate compounds can be separated and quantified either by absorption detection or fluorimetric detection following post-column oxidation of certain forms to highly fluorescent pterin products. Many HPLC procedures have been published for determining vitamin C using a variety of chromatographic modes and absorption, fluorimetric (after pre- or post-column derivatization) or electrochemical detection. Various combinations of water-soluble vitamins coextracted from a particular food can also be determined simultaneously. HPLC is not generally applicable to the determination of pantothenic acid, biotin and vitamin B_{12} in food, owing to their low indigenous levels and/or the lack of a suitable detection system.

Microbiological methods

Microbiological methods have been developed for all of the B-group vitamins and continue to be preferred for niacin, vitamin B_6, biotin, pantothenic acid and folate. Vitamin B_{12} is usually assayed microbiologically but, because it is present at such low levels, it occasionally gives problems.

Biospecific methods

Commercial radioassay kits are available for the determination of several vitamins, and those for biotin, folate and vitamin B_{12} have been applied with varying degrees of success to food analysis. Non-isotopic protein-binding assays have more recently been developed for these three vitamins. Radioimmunoassay and ELISA techniques have been utilized for the determination of pantothenic acid. Also included among biospecific methods are enzymatic methods for determining ascorbic acid.

3.4 METHOD VALIDATION

Vitamin determinations in foods are difficult to perform because of the complex nature of the food matrix, the low levels of vitamins, and the existence of the vitamins in various bound forms. These difficulties constitute potential sources of error and consequently call for validated methods of analysis. A candidate method for validation is best selected on the basis of its performance characteristics (precision, accuracy, detection limit, etc.) obtained by a peer laboratory in a carefully designed method-testing programme (Taylor, 1986). In addition, the method should be rugged, i.e. not easily subject to interference or minor variations under routine conditions.

In validating a method, the two most important performance parameters are precision and accuracy. These parameters depend upon the laboratory environment and facilities, analyst expertise, and factors that are inherent in the sample or analyte itself. Such factors include the concentration, integrity and stability of the analyte, and the types and nature of interfering substances in the sample matrix. Factors within the method itself are also implicated, including the sampling procedure, sample preparation and clean-up, and the measurement technique.

Precision is an estimate of the variability of a method and deals only with random errors that cannot be eliminated. Imprecisions arise from sample inhomogeneity, improper extraction procedures, instrument sources and the inherent variability of the sample itself. These errors follow the normal distribution curve, and hence can be expressed in units of standard deviation. Factors concerned with precision include repeatability, reproducibility and outlying values (outliers). Repeatability refers to the within-laboratory precision and is determined from a set of replicate results obtained simultaneously or in quick succession by one operator using the same equipment throughout. Reproducibility refers to the between-laboratory precision and is determined from results obtained by a number of analysts in different laboratories. The precision of a method can be ascertained by analysing sets of replicate samples containing low, medium and high levels of the analyte. Precision is usually expressed as the coefficient of variation (CV) or relative standard deviation (RSD), which are synonymous terms for the standard deviation expressed as a percentage of the mean value. The CV is often independent of concentration or amount of analyte over a range of values of one order of magnitude or less, and hence the CV facilitates comparison of variabilities at different concentrations. When the CV begins to increase rapidly with lower concentration or amount, it determines the limit of reliable measurement.

Accuracy describes the nearness of the determined value to the true value and takes into account systematic non-random errors or bias. Such errors include drift and improper calibration produced by the measurement system, report generation errors, and errors introduced by interfering compounds. For a method to be truly accurate it must be able to measure the true content of the desired analyte despite the presence of interfering substances in the original sample; these include related vitamers if individual vitamins are to be determined. In other words, the method must be specific. It is impossible to determine with absolute certainty the true value of a nutrient in a natural food product, so there is no actual method of measuring the systematic error. If a certified standard reference material (SRM) were available whose compositional properties simulated those of the samples of interest, its 'correct' measurement could imply 'correct' measurement of the samples, provided that the laboratory analytical system is in a state of statistical control (Taylor, 1981). Unfortunately, very few SRMs are presently available that are suitable for validating vitamin assays. Accuracy can only be assessed by comparing the results with those obtained using a method that is different in principle to the method under evaluation. If two independent methods give the same result, it is more probable that the measured value is near to the true value than that both methods have the same systematic error by chance.

The accuracy of a method can be maximized by adding a suitable internal standard at the earliest step possible in the procedure. If a suitable internal standard cannot be found, then an external standard must be used. For the analysis of fortified food commodities, an unfortified 'matrix' sample (if available) can be spiked with a known amount of analyte and analysed alongside the test samples. An unspiked matrix sample is included as a blank for determining the indigenous level of analyte (if any). The spiked matrix sample, after blank correction, constitutes an external standard and accounts for analyte losses incurred during the analysis. The matrix sample (blank corrected) can also be used in the preparation of a standard curve.

3.4.1 COLLABORATIVE STUDIES

The most acceptable way of validating a candidate method is through an interlaboratory collaborative study such as that described by Horwitz (1984). The collaborative study serves to confirm the performance characteristics obtained from the peer laboratory, and to define the criteria for accepting a method after testing. The role of collaborative testing in the validation of a candidate method has been discussed by Taylor (1986), who emphasized the importance of conducting the test under statistical control. Problems with the collaborative testing of microbiological methods have been outlined by Mälkki (1986). A method is considered to have been successfully validated when all participants in the study can obtain results comparable with those of the peer laboratory, and when no unexplainable outlying results are obtained. When the candidate method has been validated and standardized by an organization such as the Association of Official Analytical Chemists

(AOAC) in the USA or the International Organization for Standardization (ISO), it becomes a standard test method.

Specific performance characteristics are not inherent to an analytical method, even if the method has been successfully validated, because there is no way to predict whether a given analyst will duplicate that experience or obtain better or worse results. A successful validation merely means that the method is capable of producing useful data for its stated application. The performance characteristics of a collaborative study or the reported statistics of the peer laboratory should not be used to support any claims for the reliability of data obtained using the method at any other time.

3.4.2 QUALITY ASSURANCE

A valid method is necessary, but not sufficient, for the production of reliable data; for instance, a degree of skill is required on the part of the analyst. Data obtained by a valid method used in a well-defined quality assurance programme should allow the assignment of limits of uncertainty that can be used to judge the reliability of the data (Taylor, 1983).

Quality assurance is the broad management concept of maintaining the ability of a laboratory to furnish reliable information (Horwitz, Kamps and Boyer, 1980). A quality assurance programme encompasses the entire laboratory operation from sampling to application of the analytical result. The analytical chemist is usually confronted with the problem of having too few data with which to apply statistical analysis to a set of results, and hence other techniques for verifying how a method behaves in actual practice must be used. A laboratory that routinely performs a particular determination should periodically analyse a working standard sample (house standard) along with routine samples, and monitor such analyses using a statistical control chart. The working standard consists of a relatively large amount of a homogeneous product such as non-fat dry milk or flour, which is dispensed into small sealed bottles and stored under conditions that inhibit deterioration. In the absence of a suitable working standard, previously analysed samples, on which several analyses have been performed, can be used instead.

The sample itself can serve as the matrix for recovery studies to ensure that at least the added analyte is recovered in a satisfactory amount (ideally between 95% and 105%). The sample is first analysed to determine the indigenous level of the analyte. Known amounts of the authentic analyte, from one-half to several times the amount present, are incorporated into portions of the sample or added at as early a stage in the procedure as possible. The spiked samples should be analysed in replicate and in a random order together with appropriate blanks.

Results of unspiked samples should fall on or close to the regression line of the spiked samples. Recovery data provide useful information regarding the completeness and precision of the extraction process, but the recovery of exogenously added vitamin does not necessarily reflect the extraction efficiency of the indigenous vitamin.

3.4.3 AOAC METHODS OF ANALYSIS

Microbiological AOAC methods exist for riboflavin, niacin, vitamin B_6, pantothenic acid, folic acid and cobalamin, although not all of these methods are directly applicable to foods. Of the various AOAC physicochemical methods, thiamin and riboflavin are determined fluorimetrically, the former after conversion to thiochrome; niacin is determined colorimetrically by reaction with cyanogen bromide; vitamin C in fruit and vegetable juices is determined by the DCPIP titration, while in other foods it is determined fluorimetrically after conversion to a quinoxaline derivative.

REFERENCES

Association of Vitamin Chemists, Inc. (1966) *Methods of Vitamin Assay*, 3rd edn, Interscience Publishers, New York, pp. 1–20.

Batra, K.K., Wagner, J.R. and Stokstad, E.L.R. (1977) Folic acid compounds in romaine lettuce. *Can. J. Biochem.*, **55**, 865–8.

Baugh, C.M. and Krumdieck, C.L. (1971) Naturally occurring folates. *Ann. N.Y. Acad. Sci.*, **186**, 7–28.

Bliss, C.I. and György, P. (1967) Animal assays for vitamins. In *The Vitamins. Chemistry, Physiology, Pathology, Methods*, 2nd edn, Vol. VI (eds P. György and W. N. Pearson), Academic Press, New York, pp. 1–23.

Brody, T., Shane, B. and Stokstad, E.L.R. (1979) Separation and identification of pteroylpolyglutamates by polyacrylamide gel chromatography. *Analyt. Biochem.*, **92**, 501–9.

Chan, C., Shin, Y.S. and Stokstad, E.L.R. (1973) Studies of folic acid compounds in nature. III. Folic acid compounds in cabbage. *Can. J. Biochem.*, **51**, 1617–23.

Elkins, E.R. and Dudek, J.A. (1985) Sampling for vitamin analyses. In *Methods of Vitamin Assay*, 4th edn (eds J. Augustin, B.P. Klein, D. Becker and P.B. Venugopal), John Wiley & Sons, New York, pp. 135–51.

Garfield, F.M. (1989) Sampling in the analytical scheme. *J. Ass. Off. Analyt. Chem.*, **72**, 405–11.

Gregory, J.F. (1984) Determination of folacin in foods and other biological materials. *J. Ass. Off. Analyt. Chem.*, **67**, 1015–19.

Gregory, J.F. (1989) Chemical and nutritional aspects of folate research: analytical procedures, methods of folate synthesis, stability, and bioavailability of dietary folates. *Adv. Fd Nutr. Res.*, **33**, 1–101.

Horwitz, W. (1984) Report of the committee on collaborative interlaboratory studies. *J. Ass. Off. Analyt. Chem.*, **67**, 432–40.

Horwitz, W. (1990) Nomenclature for sampling in analytical chemistry (Recommendations 1990). *Pure Appl. Chem.*, **62**, 1193–208.

Horwitz, W., Kamps, L.R. and Boyer, K.W. (1980) Quality assurance in the analysis of foods for trace constituents. *J. Ass. Off. Analyt. Chem.*, **63**, 1344–54.

Kabir, H., Leklem, J.E. and Miller, L.T. (1983) Relationship of the glycosylated vitamin B_6 content of foods to vitamin B_6 bioavailability in humans. *Nutr. Rep. Int.*, **28**, 709–16.

Kratochvil, B. and Taylor, J.K. (1981) Sampling for chemical analysis. *Analyt. Chem.*, **53**, 924A–6A, 928A, 930A, 932A, 934A, 936A, 938A.

Krumdieck, C.L., Tamura, T. and Eto, I. (1983) Synthesis and analysis of the pteroylpolyglutamates. *Vitams Horm.*, **40**, 45–104.

Mälkki, Y. (1986) Collaborative testing of methods for food analysis. *J. Ass. Off. Analyt. Chem.*, **69**, 403–4.

Perry, J. (1971) Folate analogues in normal mixed diets. *Br. J. Haematol.*, **21**, 435–41.

Pomeranz, Y. and Meloan, C.E. (1978) *Food Analysis: Theory and Practice*, AVI Pub. Co. Inc., Westport, CT., pp. 11–20.

Shin, Y.S., Kim, E.S., Watson, J.E. and Stokstad, E.L.R. (1975) Studies of folic acid compounds in nature. IV. Folic acid compounds in soybeans and cow milk. *Can. J. Biochem.*, **53**, 338–43.

Stokstad, E.L.R., Shin, Y.S. and Tamura, T. (1977) Distribution of folate forms in food and folate availability. In *Folic Acid. Biochemistry and Physiology in Relation to the Human Nutrition Requirement*, Food and Nutrition Board, National Research Council, National Academy of Sciences, Washington, D.C., pp. 56–68.

Taylor, J.K. (1981) Quality assurance of chemical measurements. *Analyt. Chem.*, **53**, 1588A, 1589A, 1591A, 1592A, 1596A.

Taylor, J.K. (1983) Validation of analytical methods. *Analyt. Chem.*, **55**, 600A–2A, 604A, 608A.

Taylor, J.K. (1986) Role of collaborative and cooperative studies in evaluation of analytical methods. *J. Ass. Off. Analyt. Chem.*, **69**, 398–400.

Thompson, J.N. (1982) Trace analysis of vitamins by liquid chromatography. In *Trace Analysis*, Vol 2 (ed J.F. Lawrence), Academic Press, New York, pp. 1–67.

Walsh, J.H., Wyse, B.W. and Hansen, R.G. (1979) A comparison of microbiological and radioimmunoassay methods for the determination of pantothenic acid in foods. *J. Fd Biochem.*, **3**, 175–89.

Extraction of the water-soluble vitamins

4

4.1 OBJECTIVES

A discussion of the extraction process begins with establishing the analytical objective. If the investigator needs to know the nutritional value of a food sample, but is not carrying out an animal bioassay, it is desirable to use an extraction process that allows only the biologically available fraction of the total amount of vitamin present to be measured. On the other hand, if the investigator is carrying out an animal bioassay, the additional *in vitro* determination of the total vitamin content of the food source allows the bioavailability of the vitamin to be calculated. The extraction procedure in the *in vitro* assay must be capable of releasing the bound forms of the vitamin for subsequent quantification. This creates the problem of ensuring that the extraction procedure is powerful enough to break the bonds linking the vitamin to protein or to carbohydrate, and yet does not cause significant thermal or chemical destruction of the vitamin during the process. The vitamins have little in common with each other in terms of their physical and chemical properties, and there is no universal extraction process that adequately fulfils either of the above analytical objectives. The problem is further compounded by the complex and variable nature of the food matrix. The analytical results must therefore be interpreted on the basis of knowledge of the sample and the extraction process employed.

A third objective is the determination of added vitamin in fortified foods for quality control purposes. In this case the vitamin to be determined will be present as the parent molecule, which is relatively easy to extract. Under these circumstances, it may be possible to use a procedure that can extract two or more vitamins simultaneously.

The first requirement in an extraction method is to liberate the vitamins from their parent coenzyme molecules, and from their association with proteins or carbohydrates, in a form that can be utilized by assay micro-organisms or measured by biospecific or physicochemical techniques. This is often achieved most efficiently by vigorous acid hydrolysis at 15 lb/in^2 steam pressure (121 °C) in an autoclave, provided that the vitamin is stable under such conditions. This treatment denatures proteins and hydrolyses starch to soluble sugars; it also hydrolyses phosphorylated forms of vitamin B_6 to the free vitamers. The denatured protein can be subsequently removed by centrifugation or filtration. Alternatively, an enzymatic procedure may be employed, utilizing papain and α-amylase to break down protein and starch, respectively. Enzymatic digestion is necessary to liberate thiamin from its phosphorylated forms, and for releasing bound forms of vitamins (pantothenic acid and folates) that are destroyed by acid or alkaline treatment. The commercial enzyme preparations used are crudely purified natural materials and may contain appreciable amounts of vitamins. Blank determinations must be run in parallel with the extracted samples to allow correction for the vitamin content of the enzyme preparation. The enzyme must be added in sufficient quantity to overcome the effects of naturally occurring inhibitors. Bacterial action during the enzymatic digestion can be inhibited by overlaying the digest with toluene, which can later be evaporated off.

The use of different extraction procedures probably introduces the greatest statistical variation when comparing samples analysed by different methods. For the analysis of fortified foods, the efficiency of extracting the supplemental vitamin(s) can be assessed by adding a known amount of pure vitamin to the sample immediately before homogenization, and calculating the recovery. Because exogenously added free vitamin behaves differently to indigenous bound vitamin, the true efficiency of extracting vitamin(s) from non-fortified foods cannot be reliably assessed from recovery data, and extraction efficiency should be the subject of further research.

4.2 EXTRACTION PROCEDURES USED FOR THE INDIVIDUAL VITAMINS

4.2.1 THIAMIN

The extraction procedure generally used for the determination of total thiamin by fluorimetry, GLC, HPLC and microbiological assay involves hot acid digestion to liberate the thiamin and thiamin phosphate esters from their association with proteins, followed by enzymatic hydrolysis of the phosphate esters to free thiamin. Acid digestion is accomplished by autoclaving the sample at 121 °C for 30 min with 0.1 N HCl. The bound forms of thiamin present in foods of animal origin are stable under these conditions, but vitamin losses occur during the digestion of grain products, which contain mostly free thiamin, and a lower autoclaving temperature of 108 °C is required. Higher concentrations of acid are likely to decompose thiamin.

A commercial diastatic enzyme preparation of fungal origin (e.g. Takadiastase, Claradiastase or Mylase) is highly suitable for the hydrolysis step, such preparations containing phosphatase activity in addition to α-amylase and other enzymes. The enzyme treatment can be omitted for the analysis of those grain products that do not contain phosphorylated thiamin. For proteinaceous samples (e.g. meat and milk), the proteolytic enzyme papain is sometimes added to the diastase in order to dissolve the proteins that have been denatured during the previous acid digestion. The commercial availability of diastatic enzymes has been a problem, and Defibaugh (1987) has evaluated selected enzymes for suitability as substitutes in thiamin assays.

For the analysis of milk, the extraction procedure simply entails precipitation of the protein by acidification at room temperature to below the isoelectric point of casein (pH 4.8), followed by filtration. Woodrow, Torrie and Henderson (1969) showed that a pH range of 4.2–4.8 facilitated a rapid and effective filtration; below pH 4.0 the precipitated particles were too fine. This protein precipitation procedure will extract the free and protein-bound thiamin naturally present. The biologically inactive thiamin monophosphate (TMP) will be coextracted but, as this phosphorylated compound is insoluble in isobutanol, it will not be assayed by the AOAC fluorimetric method (AOAC, 1990a).

4.2.2 RIBOFLAVIN

The approach taken for the determination of total riboflavin using direct fluorimetry is dictated by the relative fluorescence intensities of the three flavins. FMN and riboflavin exhibit equal fluorescence intensity on a molar basis, whereas the fluorescence of FAD is much less intense. It is therefore necessary to release the flavins from their intimate association with proteins, and to completely convert the FAD to FMN and riboflavin. Further conversion of FMN to free riboflavin is not essential. Both of these requirements are readily accomplished (for noncovalently bound flavins) by autoclaving the sample at 121 °C for 30 min with dilute mineral acid (usually 0.1 N HCl) at a pH of <3. The bound flavins are released on denaturation of the proteins and any enzymes that might be present are inactivated. During acid digestion some of the FMN is hydrolysed to riboflavin, and a small but measurable fraction of the FMN is converted to the isomeric 2′-, 3′- and 4′-phosphates (Nielsen, Rauschenbach and Bacher, 1986).

The above acid treatment also serves as the extraction procedure for the microbiological assay, since the assay organism, *Lactobacillus casei*, responds to the products of acid digestion (FMN, riboflavin and the various isomeric riboflavin monophosphates) to give the total vitamin B_2 activity.

HPLC applications are complicated by the fact that the FMN and riboflavin liberated during the acid treatment are chromatographically separated. Consequently, there are two extraction approaches in the determination of total riboflavin by HPLC. The first approach is to convert all of the FMN to riboflavin, and then to calculate total riboflavin based on measurement of the riboflavin peak. The second approach is to calculate FMN and riboflavin separately, and to report the summated results as total riboflavin.

In the first approach, the further conversion of FMN to riboflavin can only be achieved by enzymatic hydrolysis. For this purpose a standardized diastatic enzyme preparation (e.g. Takadiastase or Claradiastase) has been generally employed. Watada and Tran (1985) reported that Mylase was as effective as Takadiastase, the latter being unobtainable at that time. These are relatively inexpensive and crude preparations that contain varying degrees of phosphatase activity. Potential errors caused by the indigenous riboflavin content of the enzyme are reduced by adding the same amount of enzyme to samples and standards or preparing a reagent blank in the same way as the sample. In practice, the complete enzymatic conversion of FMN to riboflavin may not always be achieved, the degree of hydrolysis depending upon the source and batch-to-batch phosphatase activity of the enzyme and upon the incubation conditions (Lumley and Wiggins, 1981; Hasselmann *et al.*, 1989; Ollilainen *et al.*, 1990). It is therefore essential to ascertain the conversion efficiency by checking for the presence of an FMN peak. If the conversion is incomplete, it is necessary to sum the height or area of the FMN and riboflavin peaks.

In the second approach, the enzymatic digestion step is omitted, thus avoiding the possibilities of incomplete hydrolysis of FMN and the introduction of further interfering substances, as well as saving time. A disadvantage of this approach is that commercial preparations of FMN required for standards in the quantification vary in purity from 53% to 71% (Russell and Vanderslice, 1992), and correction needs to be made to compensate for the lack of purity. It should be noted that this approach does not yield the original FMN content of the food sample, as the FMN peak in the acid extract originates largely from hydrolysed FAD.

For the analysis of milk, eggs and dairy products, it is common practice to determine the riboflavin specifically on the assumption that free or loosely bound riboflavin is the predominant naturally occurring flavin present. In this case, the acid and enzyme digestion steps necessary to hydrolyse the protein-bound FAD and FMN in other foods can be omitted. The entire procedure simply entails precipitation of the protein by acidification to pH 4.2–4.8 (as described for thiamin), filtration, and fluorescence measurement of the filtrate either directly or by HPLC.

For the determination of intact noncovalently bound FMN and FAD in foods or tissues, special non-hydrolytic extraction procedures are required to liberate these phosphorylated flavins from their association with protein. The most common of these procedures is treatment of the homogenized sample with ice-cold trichloroacetic acid (TCA) solution, although there is evidence of FAD instability under these conditions (Russell and Vanderslice, 1990). Commercial diastase preparations can be used to hydrolyse starch before deproteinization, provided that a high concentration of phosphate (e.g. 1 M KH_2PO_4) is present to ensure the complete inhibition of phosphatase activity (Koziol, 1971).

At present there is no satisfactory chemical procedure for determining the amount of covalently bound flavins in foodstuffs or tissues. Conventional acid and enzymatic hydrolysis techniques are incapable of breaking the peptide bond linking the protein apoenzyme to the flavin prosthetic group. This is perhaps fortuitous when the nutritional value of food samples is under assessment, as there is evidence that these covalent flavoproteins are largely unavailable to the host as a source of riboflavin. For the biochemist interested in the analysis of enzyme preparations, the flavin peptides (e.g. the 8α-*N*(3)-histidyl FAD of succinate dehydrogenase) can be isolated by proteolytic digestion with trypsin and chymotrypsin, following protein denaturation and removal of noncovalently bound flavins by treatment with TCA (Singer and Edmondson, 1980).

4.2.3 NIACIN

Current techniques for determining niacin are colorimetry, HPLC and microbiological assays. The terms 'total' and 'free' niacin are defined by the extraction methods employed in the analysis. Total niacin generally refers to the niacin that is extractable by autoclaving the sample with alkali or 1 N acid; free niacin is frequently defined as the niacin extractable by autoclaving with 0.1 N acid (Gregory, 1985), but several other extraction procedures have been published. Autoclaving with 1 N (0.5 M) H_2SO_4 for 30 min at 121 °C, as applied to non-cereal foods in the AOAC colorimetric procedure (AOAC, 1990b), liberates nicotinamide from its coenzyme forms; the treatment is also sufficient to release any bound nicotinic acid that may be present (Hepburn, 1971). Cereal products are autoclaved with $Ca(OH)_2$ solution, which readily liberates the nicotinic acid from its chemically bound forms. During the autoclaving with 1 N acid or $Ca(OH)_2$ solution, the liberated nicotinamide is hydrolysed to nicotinic acid. Wall and Carpenter (1988) reported that autoclaving with $Ca(OH)_2$ solution, as used in the AOAC colorimetric method for cereal products (AOAC, 1990b), resulted in a lower niacin activity for immature sweetcorn compared with the results obtained using a rat growth assay. Carpenter and co-workers showed that boiling the immature sweetcorn in water before alkaline hydrolysis resulted in similar niacin values to those obtained using the rat assay. This preliminary cooking step released the nicotinamide from the pyridine nucleotides and therefore prevented the latter from alkali attack. Roy and Merten (1983) found that autoclaving meat samples with 1 N HCl in the presence of urea resulted in a significant increase in the niacin content when compared to extraction with 1 N acid alone. This suggests the release of niacin from non-ester conjugates by the acid–urea combination, possibly from amide-linked forms.

Hepburn (1971) observed that extraction of wheat products with water and dilute acid yielded niacin contents that tended to increase with both time and temperature of treatment. This indicates that, although bound niacin is reported to resist hydrolysis under such mild conditions, gradual breakdown does occur during extraction. Hepburn therefore decided to use the least stringent conditions possible for estimating free niacin, namely suspension of the samples in distilled water with continuous stirring for 30 min. Niacin values so obtained tended to be lower than those obtained after autoclaving with 0.1 N acid, but results were consistent in replication. Furthermore, niacin added in enrichment mixtures appeared to be fully recovered by the method. Other extraction techniques used to estimate free niacin have included blending with 50% aqueous ethanol (Carter and Carpenter, 1981) and boiling (Ghosh, Sarkar and Guha, 1963) or autoclaving (Vidal-Valverde and Reche, 1991) with 0.1 N HCl. The latter authors found that treatment of the acid hydrolysate with Takadiastase was absolutely necessary in the case of legume samples because of the high starch content.

For the determination of added nicotinic acid or nicotinamide as a colour fixative in fresh meat (this practice is not permitted in the UK and has been prohibited in Japan since 1982), meat samples have been extracted by boiling with 96% ethanol (Gorin and Schütz, 1970) and blending with water (van Gend, 1973; Takatsuki *et al.*, 1987; Hamano *et al.*, 1988), acetonitrile (Tanaka *et al.*, 1989), methanol (Oishi *et al.*, 1988) or methanol after addition of a small amount of phosphoric acid (Tsunoda *et al.*, 1988). To extract the added nicotinamide from fortified foods, Rees (1989) heated the samples with 2 N H_2SO_4 on a boiling water bath for 30 min. In contrast to autoclaving with 1 N H_2SO_4 for 30 min, which completely hydrolyses the amide function, this somewhat milder acid treatment caused only a 6% conversion of nicotinamide to nicotinic acid.

4.2.4 VITAMIN B_6

Heating food samples with dilute mineral acid under autoclaving conditions liberates the B_6 vitamers from their Schiff base forms, and also hydrolyses phosphorylated forms to the free vitamers. Dilute solutions of B_6 vitamers are stable in hot dilute acid if protected from light. Acid hydrolysis is used in microbiological assays for the determination of 'total' vitamin B_6 in food extracts, and is necessary because the assay organism *Saccharomyces carlsbergensis* utilizes only the non-phosphorylated forms of the vitamin (Morris, Hughes and Mulder, 1959). Present extraction techniques are based largely on the investigations reported by Atkin *et al.* (1943) and Rabinowitz and Snell (1947a). Both groups found that autoclaving samples with 0.055 N HCl for up to 5 h gave an efficient extraction for a wide range of foods, but not for cereals, which required a higher concentration of acid. This requirement was correctly attributed to the presence of an unidentified bound form of vitamin B_6, now known to be PN-glucoside. The efficiency of extraction depended not only upon the strength of the acid, but also upon the volume of acid used. Another factor to consider is that PL is liberated from PLP much more rapidly than PM is liberated from PMP (Rabinowitz and Snell, 1947b). The possibility of interaction between PL or PLP with amino acids during the extraction procedure of Rabinowitz and Snell (autoclaving with 0.055 N HCl at 20 lb pressure for 5 h) was investigated by Rabinowitz, Mondy and Snell (1948). No loss of activity for *S. carlsbergensis* was observed when PL or PLP was autoclaved in the presence of a relatively high concentration of glutamic acid, which indicated that transamination does not occur under these conditions.

There is no single set of conditions that can quantitatively extract vitamin B_6 from both plant and animal products. In the AOAC microbiological method (AOAC, 1990c), plant products are autoclaved with 0.44 N HCl for 2 h at 121 °C, and animal products are autoclaved with 0.055 N HCl for 5 h at 121 °C. Polansky, Reynolds and Vanderslice (1985) proposed that food composites be autoclaved with 0.2 N HCl for 5 h at 121 °C. Polansky, Murphy and Toepfer (1964) reported that, for whole wheat samples, autoclaving with 0.055 N HCl, instead of 0.44 N HCl, gave a similar PL value, but lower values of PN and PM. Conversely, autoclaving meat products with 0.44 N HCl, instead of 0.055 N HCl, gave approximately the same PN and PL values, but only about half of the PM (Polansky and Toepfer, 1969). The superiority of the lower concentration of acid for extraction of vitamin B_6 from animal products does not result from destruction of the vitamin by the stronger acid, since subsequent enzymatic hydrolysis of 2 N acid hydrolysates liberated as much B_6 as the direct enzyme treatment (Rubin and Scheiner, 1946). Rather, it is due to the incomplete liberation of the vitamin by the more concentrated acid; the optimum release occurs between pH 1.5 and 2.0, with a maximum at pH 1.7–1.8 (Rubin, Scheiner and Hirschberg, 1947). To satisfy these critical pH conditions, one must always ensure that the acid is added in amounts that exceed the buffering capacity of the sample. Analyses based on acid hydrolysis would tend to overestimate the biologically available vitamin B_6 in those plant-derived foods that contain significant quantities of β-glucoside conjugates.

Recent advances in HPLC permit the simultaneous separation of all six B_6 vitamers, plus pyridoxic acid, when used in conjunction with an extraction procedure that preserves the integrity of the vitamers. Treatment of samples with deproteinizing agents such as metaphosphoric, perchloric, trichloroacetic or sulphosalicylic acid at room temperature readily hydrolyses Schiff bases whilst preserving the phosphorylated vitamers. These acids do not hydrolyse PN-glucoside, and hence results obtained using these extractants provide a better estimate of available vitamin B_6 than results obtained using acid hydrolysis. The high efficiency of extraction using these acidic reagents is partly due to the conversion of the pyridine bases to quaternary ammonium salts, thereby increasing their solubility in water. Their use as extracting agents also prevents enzymatic interconversion of B_6 vitamers following homogenization of samples. In such procedures it is usually necessary to remove excess reagent, which might otherwise interfere with the analytical chromatography. TCA can be removed by extraction with diethyl ether, perchloric acid by reaction with 6 M KOH and precipitation as insoluble potassium perchlorate, and sulphosalicylic acid by chromatography on an anion exchange column. An extraction procedure using 5% sulphosalicylic acid has been successfully applied to such complex foods as pork, beef, dry milk and cereals (Vanderslice *et al.*, 1980). Recoveries of B_6 vitamers added to samples were 95–105% for all vitamers except for PNP, where the recovery was 85%.

Free B_6 vitamers are extractable from foods by homogenization in 0.01 M sodium acetate buffer, pH 6.8 (Addo and Augustin, 1988). Selective hydrolysis of phosphorylated B_6 vitamers and PN-glucoside can be achieved enzymatically by incubation with acid phosphatase and *ß*-glucosidase, respectively. None of the extraction processes described above will hydrolyse the peptide-bound ε-pyridoxyllysine and its 5′-phosphate derivative, which exhibit 75–80% stability when subjected to 6 N HCl at 105 °C for 48 h (Gregory, Ink and Sartain, 1986).

Kabir, Leklem and Miller (1983) examined the vitamin B_6 value of 22 varied foods using the level of glycosylated vitamin B_6 as an index of availability. Homogenized food samples were stirred in duplicate flasks with 0.1 M phosphate buffer (pH 6.8) for 2 h at room temperature, after which the pH was adjusted to 5.0 with 1 N HCl. To one of the duplicate flasks was added *ß*-glucosidase; the other flask received no enzyme. All flasks were then incubated at 37 °C for 2 h with shaking. Enzyme action was stopped by addition of 1 N HCl to all flasks, followed by steaming for 5 min. The extracts, after pH adjustment, dilution and filtration, were assayed microbiologically using *S. carlsbergensis* as the test organism. In addition, the total vitamin B_6 of each food was determined microbiologically following acid hydrolysis. The percentage of glycosylated vitamin B_6 in each sample was calculated as follows:

$$\%\ \text{Glycosylated vitamin } B_6 = (G - F)/T \times 100$$

where G = mg B_6/g sample treated with *ß*-glucosidase
F = mg B_6/g sample without enzyme
T = mg total B_6/g sample as determined after acid hydrolysis

Ekanayake and Nelson (1986) devised an *in vitro* method for estimating available vitamin B_6 in processed model foods using a two-stage enzymatic digestion (pepsin/pancreatin) of the food matrix, followed by treatment of the hydrolysate with acidified methanol, and determination of the hydrolysed vitamers by HPLC. The results obtained showed good correlation with the available vitamin B_6 content as determined by rat bioassay. The method was applied to the analysis of natural foods (Ekanayake and Nelson, 1988).

Gregory and Sartain (1991) determined the amounts of free and glycosylated forms of vitamin B_6 in plant-derived foods by homogenization with 5% sulphosalicylic acid and purification by anion exchange chromatography. Portions of the purified extracts were then subjected to the following treatments. (1) Direct analysis by ion interaction HPLC allowed the quantification of PN-glucoside, PMP, PL, PN and PM. The early-eluting PLP was not quantified in this chromatographic run, as it was subject to interference from a cluster of peaks which rendered its accurate measurement difficult or impossible. (2) Extracts treated simultaneously with acid phosphatase and β-glucosidase provided differential information regarding the content of PLP, PMP, PN-glucoside and PN oligosaccharides. (3) Extracts treated with 6 M KOH, followed by the combined enzymes, yielded differential information concerning saponifiable esterified PN-glucosides. Alternatively, autoclaving for 2 h in the presence of 0.44 N HCl could be used to determine total vitamin B_6 (measured as PL, PN and PM). Gregory and Sartain pointed out that this treatment does not completely hydrolyse the glycosylated forms of vitamin B_6 in rice bran, and would lead to an underestimation of the vitamin B_6 value.

4.2.5 PANTOTHENIC ACID

Pantothenic acid exists in animal and plant tissues largely as coenzyme A and other bound forms, which are available to animals used in bioassays (rat and chick) but not to the organisms used in microbiological assays. Consequently, some sort of hydrolytic procedure must be applied to liberate the bound pantothenic acid if the total pantothenate content of a food sample is to be measured by a microbiological assay. It is also necessary to liberate pantothenic acid in radioimmunoassay and ELISA methods, as only the free vitamin has affinity for the binding sites on the antibody. Neither acid nor alkaline hydrolysis can be used, since the vitamin is degraded by such treatments, and the hydrolysis products do not act as growth factors for the microbiological test organism *Lactobacillus plantarum* (Association of Vitamin Chemists, Inc., 1966). The only practicable alternative is enzymatic hydrolysis, and this was successfully accomplished through the simultaneous action of intestinal alkaline phosphatase and an avian liver enzyme (Novelli, Kaplan and Lipmann, 1949). This double enzyme combination liberates practically all of the pantothenic acid from coenzyme A, making it available for microbiological or biospecific assay; it does not release the pantothenic acid from acyl carrier protein (Wyse *et al.*, 1985). The alkaline phosphatase splits the coenzyme A molecule between the phosphate-containing moiety and pantetheine, while the liver enzyme breaks the link in pantetheine between the pantothenic acid and β-mercaptoethylamine moieties.

4.2.6 BIOTIN

Bound forms of biotin, including biocytin, cannot be utilized by *Lactobacillus plantarum*, the organism usually employed in microbiological assays, and strong acid hydrolysis at elevated temperature is required to completely liberate biotin from natural materials (Thompson, Eakin and Williams, 1941). Animal tissues require more stringent hydrolysis conditions than do plant tissues, because the latter contain a higher proportion of free water-extractable biotin (Lampen, Bahler and Peterson, 1942). On the basis of experimental studies with meat and meat products (Schweigert *et al.*, 1943) and feedstuffs of animal origin (Scheiner and De Ritter, 1975), maximum liberation of biotin in animal-derived products is obtained by autoclaving with 6 N H_2SO_4 for 2 h at 121 °C. This procedure promotes losses of biotin in plant materials, which are extracted most efficiently by autoclaving with 4 N H_2SO_4 for 1 h at 121 °C (Lampen, Bahler and Peterson, 1942) or with 2 N H_2SO_4 for 2 h at 121 °C (Scheiner and De Ritter, 1975). Because of the differences in extractability between animal and plant tissues, a single extraction procedure to cover all food commodities must be a compromise, and no such procedure has been universally adopted. Representative methods for extracting foods of any type entail autoclaving with 2 N H_2SO_4 at 121 °C for 2 h (Lampen, Bahler and Peterson, 1942; Strohecker and Henning, 1966) or 3 N H_2SO_4 at 121 °C for 1 h (Shull, Hutchings and Peterson, 1942) or 30 min (Barton-Wright, 1952; Bell, 1974).

Hydrolysis with 6 N H_2SO_4 destroys the synthetic sodium salt of biotin added to feed premixes. A suggested procedure used for feed premixes with potencies up to 1 g/lb entailed the addition of 50 ml of 0.1 N NaOH and 250 ml of water to 5 g of sample, shaking vigorously, and then standing for 30 min at room temperature with occasional swirling (Scheiner, 1966).

Sulphuric acid, rather than hydrochloric acid, is invariably used for sample hydrolysis, as the biotin content of dilute (30 ng/ml) solutions was almost completely destroyed by autoclaving with 2 N HCl (Axelrod and Hofmann, 1950). Evidence from differential microbiological assay pointed to the oxidation of biotin to a mixture of the biotin sulphoxide and sulphone derivatives, possibly caused by trace impurities (e.g. chlorine) in the acid. This loss of vitamin activity does not necessarily occur when autoclaving actual food samples, as many natural products are capable of preventing this oxidation (Langer and György, 1968). Finglas, Faulks and Morgan (1986) reported no loss of biotin from liver using 3 N HCl.

An alternative to acid hydrolysis is digestion with the proteolytic enzyme papain (György, 1967). Bitsch, Salz and Hötzel (1989) compared the efficiency of papain digestion, after treatment with liquid nitrogen and homogenization with conventional acid hydrolysis, in releasing the biotin from a variety of food samples (wheat flour, oat flakes, whole milk and pork liver). No significant differences in biotin content were obtained between extraction methods using either a microbiological assay with *L. plantarum* or a radiometric protein-binding assay. The results indicated that enzymatic hydrolysis with papain, after treatment of the sample with liquid nitrogen and homogenization, was capable of quantitatively releasing protein-bound biotin from both plant and animal tissues. Similar experiments on human plasma within the same study revealed slightly enhanced biotin values obtained with the microbiological assay in relation to the protein-binding assay. In plasma, biotin exists mainly as protein-bound biocytin which, when released from the plasma proteins, is bound to the avidin protein used in the protein-binding assay. If papain digestion is ineffective in hydrolysing biocytin, as reported by Wright *et al.*, (1952), one would expect the microbiological values to be low in relation to the protein-binding assay values, since *L. plantarum* responds only to free biotin. These results for plasma therefore suggest that biotin was, in fact, released from biocytin by papain digestion under the conditions used.

4.2.7 FOLATE

The predominant naturally occurring folate compounds in most biological tissues are polyglutamyl forms of tetrahydrofolate (THF), 5-methyl-THF and 10-formyl-THF (Gregory, 1984), containing typically from five to seven glutamate residues in gamma-peptide linkage (Gregory, 1989). 5-Formyl-THF is a minor form of the vitamin in most tissues, but thermal food processing and/or thermal extraction procedures can cause extensive conversion to this compound from 10-formyl-THF (Gregory, 1989). Folic acid is probably not a significant naturally occurring form, but it is often found in small quantities as an oxidation product of THF in samples stored under conditions permitting exposure to oxygen (Gregory, 1984). The folates generally exist in nature bound to proteins (Baugh and Krumdieck, 1971) and they may also be bound to starch and glycogen in foods (Černá and Káš, 1983). The determination of total folate in food may be performed by microbiological assay using *Lactobacillus casei*, by radiometric or non-isotopic protein-binding assay, or by HPLC. The liberation of protein-bound folates must be conducted under relatively mild conditions, owing to the susceptibility of certain folates, particularly unsubstituted tetrahydrofolic acid, to oxidation and extremes of pH.

The primary requirements for extracting folate from food samples are (1) liberation of protein-bound folate, and (2) deconjugation of polyglutamyl folates. Liberation of folate from polysaccharides is another requirement for starchy foods. Two distinct approaches for extracting folate have evolved from the many published research studies, both of which merit discussion. The first approach is a two-step procedure involving a thermal treatment to denature proteins, followed by enzymatic deconjugation with conjugase. The second approach is entirely enzymatic and utilizes a proteolytic enzyme to liberate protein-bound folate, α-amylase to break down starch, and deconjugation with conjugase.

A complication in the extraction of folates is the thermal conversion of 10-formyl-THF to 5-formyl-THF. Such a conversion is undesirable in the radiometric competitive binding assay (radioassay) conducted at pH 9.3, since the folate-binding protein does not exhibit significant affinity for 5-formyl-THF, and the analysis of samples containing this isomer formed during thermal extraction or processing will underestimate folate activity. The extraction procedure employed for radioassays should therefore minimize the conversion of 10- to 5-formyl-THF. The situation is different in HPLC assays, in which the thermal conversion is carried out intentionally by prolonged heating of the test material as a means of simplifying the quantification of formyl tetrahydrofolates.

Thermal extraction and enzymatic deconjugation

The inclusion of an antioxidant (usually ascorbic acid) is essential in preventing the destruction of labile folates during heat treatment (Malin, 1975). Wilson and Horne (1983) reported that at neutral pH the presence of ascorbate actually induced thermal degradation and interconversion of folates during extraction at 100 °C. This was attributed, at least in part, to the action of formaldehyde produced by the degradation of ascorbate. It was later reported (Wilson and Horne, 1984) that the use of a pH 7.85 extraction buffer containing ascorbate (101 mM) and 2-mercaptoethanol (200 mM) eliminated these problems, probably through removal of the formaldehyde by reaction with the thiol compound. Little or no conversion of 10-formyl-THF to 5-formyl-THF occurred using the pH 7.85 buffer containing ascorbate and 2-mercaptoethanol.

Gregory *et al.* (1990) compared the merits of extraction procedures employing acetate buffer (pH 4.9) containing 50 mM ascorbate (Gregory, Sartain and Day, 1984), phosphate buffer (pH 7.0) containing 50 mM ascorbate, or mixed HEPES/CHES buffers (pH 7.85) containing 101 mM ascorbate and 200 mM 2-mercaptoethanol (Wilson and Horne, 1984). In a preliminary experiment, the pH of the buffer (pH 4.9 versus 7.0) did not consistently affect the recovery of radiolabelled mono- and poly-glutamyl folates added to various food homogenates. However, radio-labelled folates from the livers of rats previously dosed with tritium-labelled folate were more effectively extracted at pH 7.0 and 7.85 than at 4.9. Microbiological assay of total folate in beef liver and green peas extracted with pH 4.9, 7.0 or 7.85 buffers indicated the superiority of the pH 7.85 buffer. In all experiments, the completeness of extraction was improved when the residue from the first extraction was suspended in a new portion of buffer and recentrifuged. The results obtained supported the superiority of the Wilson and Horne extraction buffer, and indicated the need for a second extraction in the analysis of many foods, regardless of the extraction method used. The improved efficiency of extraction at the higher pH might be at least partly explained by the increased ionization of the polyglutamyl folate molecule, which would tend to promote dissociation from anionic sites of the sample matrix.

Three enzymes have been used in folate deconjugation, each differing in its pH optimum and mode of action. Conjugase from chicken pancreas exhibits a neutral pH optimum and yields a folate diglutamate end-product; hog kidney conjugase exhibits an acidic pH optimum (pH 4.5–4.9) and yields a monoglutamate end-product; human plasma conjugase also exhibits a pH optimum of 4.5 and yields a monoglutamate (Gregory, 1989). Deconjugation to monoglutamyl folates is obligatory in HPLC procedures, where chromatographic retention is governed by polyglutamyl chain length, and therefore either hog kidney or human plasma conjugase may be used. Competitive binding assays also require deconjugation to monoglutamyl folates, because of the dependency of the binding affinity on the polyglutamyl chain length (Shane, Tamura and Stokstad, 1980). For microbiological assay using *L. casei*, Phillips and Wright (1983) reported that folate values obtained using hog kidney were consistently higher than values obtained using chicken pancreas and, for this reason, the use of hog kidney enzyme was recommended. Conversely, Pedersen (1988) found that deconjugation with hog kidney compared with chicken pancreas did not give higher results of measurable folate, and preferred the use of chicken pancreas. These conflicting data are probably attributable to differences in conjugase preparation methods, incubation times with conjugase, pH, and other treatment procedures (Kirsch and Chen, 1984).

In a detailed study of the properties and efficacy of hog kidney conjugase, Engelhardt and Gregory (1990) noted that a variety of foods caused detectable inhibition of enzyme activity. However, the use of hog kidney conjugase was judged to be appropriate for the various assay methods, provided that the proper combination of enzyme concentration and incubation time is determined for each type of sample to be assayed, and for each batch of enzyme preparation.

Enzymatic extraction and deconjugation

Martin *et al.* (1990) published a triple enzyme digestion procedure using chicken pancreas conjugase, α-amylase and protease in the microbiological determination of total folate in foods. Ground food samples were homogenized in phosphate buffer (pH 6.8) containing 56.8 mM ascorbate, and diluted aliquots were placed in a boiling water bath for 5 min to gelatinize starch before α-amylase treatment. After cooling, conjugase and α-amylase were added, plus two drops of toluene to layer the tubes, and the capped tubes were incubated at 37 °C for 4 h.

Protease solution and two drops of toluene were then added, and the capped tubes were incubated overnight at 37 °C. It was necessary to add the protease after the action of conjugase and α-amylase to prevent it from deactivating these enzymes. After the second incubation period all extracts were steamed in an autoclave for 5 min at 100 °C to remove the toluene and inactivate the enzymes. The triple enzyme treatment increased measurable folate from several foods when compared to levels found after digestion with chicken pancreas enzyme *per se*. Both protease and α-amylase appeared to be necessary for the complete liberation of bound folate, since increased folate values were also observed using just protease or α-amylase in addition to chicken pancreas conjugase (De Souza and Eitenmiller, 1990). The role of α-amylase in releasing folate bound to starch by physical adsorption was reported by Černá and Káš (1983). According to Pedersen (1988), specific amylase addition is of little benefit if chicken pancreas is used, as the latter was shown to contain equally high amounts of amylases as did α-amylase or amyloglucosidase sources.

Treatment of dairy products

Protein-binding assays invariably use a specific folate-binding protein (FBP) obtained from milk. An initial heating step is therefore essential to denature indigenous FBP when analysing milk and other dairy products by protein-binding assay. For analysis of dairy products by HPLC, folates were extracted by adjusting the pH to 4.5 with glacial acetic acid, centrifuging to remove precipitated proteins, and adding to the supernatant 10% ascorbate and 1 M mercaptoethanol so that the final concentrations of each were 0.1% and 0.01 M, respectively. The supernatant was incubated with a hog kidney conjugase preparation at 37 °C in a sealed tube for 2 h, and then centrifuged and filtered (Holt, Wehling and Zeece, 1988).

4.2.8 VITAMIN B_{12}

The extraction procedure preceding the determination of total vitamin B_{12} in foodstuffs by microbiological or protein-binding assay has the dual purpose of liberating protein-bound cobalamins and converting the labile naturally occurring forms to the stable cyanocobalamin or sulphitocobalamin. The conversion of cobalamins to cyanocobalamin is ideal, as sample measurements can be compared with a cyanocobalamin standard, and the results expressed directly in the official weight units of pure crystalline cyanocobalamin. The simplest approach is to heat the homogenized sample with a buffer solution containing cyanide or sulphite. The heat treatment denatures the proteins, inactivates the enzymes and accelerates the conversion of liberated cobalamins to either cyanocobalamin or sulphitocobalamin.

Proteolytic digestion with papain has been proposed for releasing the cobalamins from liver homogenates prior to heating with sodium metabisulphite (Shenoy and Ramasarma, 1954). This procedure is not recommended, as Voigt, Eitenmiller and Ware (1979) have demonstrated that enzymatic treatment of some materials (e.g. tomato juice and orange juice) causes nonspecific stimulation of *Lactobacillus delbrueckii*.

4.2.9 VITAMIN C

Ascorbic acid is rapidly oxidized by air, and also by ascorbic acid oxidase, to dehydroascorbic acid, and finally to the biologically inactive form, diketogulonic acid. It is therefore essential to stabilize the natural forms of vitamin C during the extraction stage of the sample preparation. A number of acids in dilute solution have been studied for use as extraction agents for vitamin C. Metaphosphoric acid, trichloroacetic acid and perchloric acid are effective protein denaturants and will therefore inactivate ascorbic acid oxidase. These acids will provide a medium below pH 4, which favours the stability of ascorbic acid and dehydroascorbic acid. The stability of vitamin C solutions is not merely a function of pH, but depends also on the nature of the acid. Metaphosphoric acid and oxalic acid prevent catalysis of the oxidation of ascorbic acid by copper(II) or iron(III) ions, whereas other acids at similar pH values do not share this property (Ponting, 1943). Overall, metaphosphoric acid in freshly prepared 3–6% aqueous solution is the most effective agent for extracting and stabilizing ascorbic acid in animal and plant materials. Extracting solutions should be made up in pure water and deoxygenated by bubbling in nitrogen before use.

REFERENCES

Addo, C. and Augustin, J. (1988) Changes in the vitamin B_6 content in potatoes during storage. *J. Fd Sci.*, **53**, 749–52.

AOAC (1990a) Thiamine (vitamin B_1) in milk-based infant formula. Fluorometric method. Final action 1962. In *AOAC Official Methods of Analysis*, 15th edn (ed. K. Helrich), Association of Official Analytical Chemists, Inc., Arlington, VA, 986.27.

AOAC (1990b) Niacin and niacinamide in drugs, food and feeds. Colorimetric method. Final action 1962. In *AOAC Official Methods of Analysis*, 15th edn (ed. K. Helrich), Association of Official Analytical Chemists, Inc., Arlington, VA, 961.14.

AOAC (1990c) Vitamin B_6 (pyridoxine, pyridoxal, pyridoxamine) in food extracts. Microbiological method. Final action 1975. In *AOAC Official Methods of Analysis*, 15th edn (ed. K. Helrich), Association of Official Analytical Chemists, Inc., Arlington, VA, 961.15.

Association of Vitamin Chemists, Inc. (1966) *Methods of Vitamin Assay*, 3rd edn, Interscience Publishers, New York, pp. 197–208.

Atkin, L., Schultz, A.S., Williams, W.L. and Frey, C.N. (1943) Yeast microbiological methods for determination of vitamins. Pyridoxine. *Ind. Engng Chem. Analyt. Edn*, **15**, 141–4.

Axelrod, A.E. and Hofmann, K. (1950) The inactivation of biotin by hydrochloric acid. *J. Biol. Chem.*, **187**, 23–8.

Barton-Wright, E.C. (1952) *The Microbiological Assay of the Vitamin B-Complex and Amino Acids*, Sir Isaac Pitman & Sons Ltd, London, pp. 63–7.

Baugh, C.M. and Krumdieck, C.L. (1971) Naturally occurring folates. *Ann. N.Y. Acad. Sci.*, **186**, 7–28.

Bell, J.G. (1974) Microbiological assay of vitamins of the B group in foodstuffs. *Lab. Pract.*, **23**, 235–42, 252.

Bitsch, R., Şalz, I. and Hötzel, D. (1989) Biotin assessment in foods and body fluids by a protein binding assay (PBA). *Int. J. Vitam. Nutr. Res.*, **59**, 59–64.

Carter, E.G.A. and Carpenter, K.J. (1981) Bound niacin in sorghum and its availability. *Nutr. Res.*, **1**, 571–9.

Cerná, J. and Kás, J. (1983) New conception of folacin assay in starch or glycogen containing food samples. *Nahrung*, **27**, 957–64.

Defibaugh, P.W. (1987) Evaluation of selected enzymes for thiamine determination. *J. Ass. Off. Analyt. Chem.*, **70**, 514–17.

De Souza, S. and Eitenmiller, R. (1990) Effects of different enzyme treatments on extraction of total folate from various foods prior to microbiological assay and radioassay. *J. Micronutr. Anal.*, **7**, 37–57.

Ekanayake, A. and Nelson, P.E. (1986) An *in vitro* method for estimating biologically available vitamin B_6 in processed foods. *Br. J. Nutr.*, **55**, 235–44.

Ekanayake, A. and Nelson, P.E. (1988) Applicability of an *in vitro* method for the estimation of vitamin B_6 biological availability. *J. Micronutr. Anal.*, **4**, 1–15.

Engelhardt, R. and Gregory, J.F. (1990) Adequacy of enzymatic deconjugation in quantification of folate in foods. *J. Agric. Fd Chem.*, **38**, 154–8.

Finglas, P.M., Faulks, R.M. and Morgan, M.R.A. (1986) The analysis of biotin in liver using a protein-binding assay. *J. Micronutr. Anal.*, **2**, 247–57.

Ghosh, H.P., Sarkar, P.K. and Guha, B.C. (1963) Distribution of the bound form of nicotinic acid in natural materials. *J. Nutr.*, **79**, 451–3.

Gorin, N. and Schütz, G.P. (1970) Comparison of a microbiological and a spectrophotometric method for the determination of nicotinic acid in fresh meat. *J. Sci. Fd Agric.*, **21**, 423–5.

Gregory, J.F. (1984) Determination of folacin in foods and other biological materials. *J. Ass. Off. Analyt. Chem.*, **67**, 1015–19.

Gregory, J.F. (1985) Chemical changes of vitamins during food processing. In *Chemical Changes in Food during Processing* (eds T. Richardson and J.W. Finley), Van Nostrand Rheinhold Co., New York, pp. 373–408.

Gregory, J.F. (1989) Chemical and nutritional aspects of folate research: analytical procedures, methods of folate synthesis, stability, and bioavailability of dietary folates. *Adv. Fd Nutr. Res.*, **33**, 1–101.

Gregory, J.F., Ink, S.L. and Sartain, D.B. (1986) Degradation and binding to food proteins of vitamin B_6 compounds during thermal processing. *J. Fd Sci.*, **51**, 1345–51.

Gregory, J.F. and Sartain, D.B. (1991) Improved chromatographic determination of free and glycosylated forms of vitamin B_6 in foods. *J. Agric. Fd Chem.*, **39**, 899–905.

Gregory, J.F., Sartain, D.B. and Day, B.P.F. (1984) Fluorometric determination of folacin in biological materials using high performance liquid chromatography. *J. Nutr.*, **114**, 341–53.

Gregory, J.F., Engelhardt, R., Bhandari, S.D., Sartain, D.B. and Gustafson, S.K. (1990) Adequacy of extraction techniques for determination of folate in foods and other biological materials. *J. Fd Comp. Anal.*, **3**, 134–44.

György, P. (1967) Biotin. In *The Vitamins. Chemistry, Physiology, Pathology, Methods*, 2nd edn, Vol. VII (eds P. György and W.N. Pearson), Academic Press, New York, pp. 303–12.

Hamano, T., Mitsuhashi, Y., Aoki, N. and Yamamoto, S. (1988) Simultaneous determination of niacin and niacinamide in meats by high-performance liquid chromatography. *J. Chromat.*, **457**, 403–8.

Hasselmann, C., Franck, D., Grimm, P., Diop, P.A. and Soules, C. (1989) High-performance liquid chromatographic analysis of thiamin and riboflavin in dietetic foods. *J. Micronutr. Anal.*, **5**, 269–79.

Hepburn, F.N. (1971) Nutrient composition of selected wheats and wheat products. VII. Total and free niacin. *Cereal Chem.*, **48**, 369–72.

Holt, D.L., Wehling, R.L. and Zeece, M.G. (1988) Determination of native folates in milk and other dairy products by high-performance liquid chromatography. *J. Chromat.*, **440**, 271–9.

Kabir, H., Leklem, J. and Miller, L.T. (1983) Measurement of glycosylated vitamin B_6 in foods. *J. Fd Sci.*, **48**, 1422–5.

Kirsch, A.J. and Chen, T.-S. (1984) Comparison of conjugase treatment procedures in the microbiological assay for food folacin. *J. Fd Sci.*, **49**, 94–8.

Koziol, J. (1971) Fluorometric analyses of riboflavin and its coenzymes. *Methods Enzymol.*, **18B**, 253–85.

Lampen, J.O., Bahler, G.P. and Peterson, W.H. (1942) The occurrence of free and bound biotin. *J. Nutr.*, **23**, 11–21.

Langer, B.W. Jr and György, P. (1968) Biotin. VIII. Active compounds and antagonists. In *The Vitamins. Chemistry, Physiology, Pathology, Methods*, 2nd edn, Vol. II (eds W.H. Sebrell, Jr and R.S. Harris), Academic Press, New York, pp. 294–322.

Lumley, I.D. and Wiggins, R.A. (1981) Determination of riboflavin and flavin mononucleotide in foodstuffs using high-performance liquid chromatography and a column-enrichment technique. *Analyst. Lond.*, **106**, 1103–8.

Malin, J.D. (1975) Folic acid. *World Rev. Nutr. Dietetics*, **21**, 198–223.

Martin, J.I., Landen, W.O. Jr, Soliman, A.-G.M. and Eitenmiller, R.R. (1990) Application of a tri-enzyme extraction for total folate determination in foods. *J. Ass. Off. Analyt. Chem.*, **73**, 805–8.

Morris, J.G., Hughes, D.T.D. and Mulder, C. (1959) Observations on the assay of vitamin B_6 with *Saccharomyces carlsbergensis* 4228. *J. Gen. Microbiol.*, **20**, 566–75.

Nielsen, P., Rauschenbach, P. and Bacher, A. (1986) Preparation, properties, and separation by high-performance liquid chromatography of riboflavin phosphates. *Methods Enzymol.*, **122G**, 209–20.

Novelli, G.D., Kaplan, N.O. and Lipmann, F. (1949) The liberation of pantothenic acid from coenzyme A. *J. Biol. Chem.*, **177**, 97–107.

Oishi, M., Amakawa, E., Ogiwara, T. *et al.* (1988) Determination of nicotinic acid and nicotinamide in meats by high performance liquid chromatography and conversion of nicotinamide in meats during storage. *J. Fd Hygiene Soc. Japan*, **29**, 32–7.

Ollilainen, V., Mattila, P., Varo, P., Koivistoinen, P. and Huttunen, J. (1990) The HPLC determination of total riboflavin in foods. *J. Micronutr. Anal.*, **8**, 199–207.

Pedersen, J.C. (1988) Comparison of γ-glutamyl hydrolase (conjugase; EC 3.4.22.12) and amylase treatment procedures in the microbiological assay for food folates. *Br. J. Nutr.*, **59**, 261–71.

Phillips, D.R. and Wright, A.J.A. (1983) Studies on the response of *Lactobacillus casei* to folate vitamin in foods. *Br. J. Nutr.*, **49**, 181–6.

Polansky, M.M., Murphy, E.W. and Toepfer, E.W. (1964) Components of vitamin B_6 in grains and cereal products. *J. Ass. Off. Analyt. Chem.*, **47**, 750–3.

Polansky, M.M., Reynolds, R.D. and Vanderslice, J.T. (1985) Vitamin B_6. In *Methods of Vitamin Assay*, 4th edn (eds J. Augustin, B.P. Klein, D. Becker and P.B. Venugopal), John Wiley & Sons, New York, pp. 417–43.

Polansky, M.M. and Toepfer, E.W. (1969) Vitamin B_6 components in some meats, fish, dairy products, and commercial infant formulas. *J. Agric. Fd Chem.*, **17**, 1394–7.

Ponting, J.D. (1943) Extraction of ascorbic acid from plant materials. *Ind. Engng Chem. Analyt. Edn*, **15**, 389–91.

Rabinowitz, J.C., Mondy, N.I. and Snell, E.E. (1948) The vitamin B_6 group. XIII. An improved procedure for determination of pyridoxal with *Lactobacillus casei. J. Biol. Chem.*, **175**, 147–53.

Rabinowitz, J.C. and Snell, E.E. (1947a) Vitamin B_6 group. Extraction procedures for the microbiological determination of vitamin B_6. *Ind. Engng Chem. Analyt. Edn*, **19**, 277–80.

Rabinowitz, J.C. and Snell, E.E. (1947b) The vitamin B_6 group. XII. Microbiological activity and natural occurrence of pyridoxamine phosphate. *J. Biol. Chem.*, **169**, 643–50.

Rees, D.I. (1989) Determination of nicotinamide and pyridoxine in fortified food products by HPLC. *J. Micronutr. Anal.*, **5**, 53–61.

Roy, R.B. and Merten, J.J. (1983) Evaluation of urea-acid system as medium of extraction for the B-group vitamins. Part II. Simplified semi-automated chemical analysis for niacin and niacinamide in cereal products. *J. Ass. Off. Analyt. Chem.*, **66**, 291–6.

Rubin, S.H. and Scheiner, J. (1946) The availability of vitamin B_6 in yeast to *Saccharomyces carlsbergensis. J. Biol. Chem.*, **162**, 389–90.

Rubin, S.H., Scheiner, J. and Hirschberg, E. (1947) The availability of vitamin B_6 in yeast and liver for growth of *Saccharomyces carlsbergensis. J. Biol. Chem.*, **167**, 599–611.

Russell, L.F. and Vanderslice, J.T. (1990) A comprehensive review of vitamin B_2 analytical methodology. *J. Micronutr. Anal.*, **8**, 257–30.

Russell, L.F. and Vanderslice, J.T. (1992) Non-degradative extraction and simultaneous quantitation of riboflavin, flavin mononucleotide, and flavin adenine dinucleotide in foods by HPLC. *Fd Chem.*, **43**, 151–62.

Scheiner, J. (1966) Extraction of added biotin from animal feed premixes. *J. Ass. Off. Analyt. Chem.*, **49**, 882–3.

Scheiner, J. and De Ritter, E. (1975) Biotin content of feedstuffs. *J. Agric. Fd Chem.*, **23**, 1157–62.

Schweigert, B.S., Nielsen, E., McIntire, J.M. and Elvehjem, C.A. (1943) Biotin content of meat and meat products. *J. Nutr.*, **26**, 65–71.

Shane, B., Tamura, T. and Stokstad, E.L.R. (1980) Folate assay: a comparison of radioassay and microbiological methods. *Clin. Chim. Acta.*, **100**, 13–19.

Shenoy, K.G. and Ramasarma, G.B. (1954) Extraction procedure and determination of the vitamin B_{12} content of some animal livers. *Arch. Biochem. Biophys.*, **51**, 371–8.

Shull, G. M., Hutchings, B.L. and Peterson, W.H. (1942) A microbiological assay for biotin. *J. Biol. Chem.*, **142**, 913–20.

Singer, T.P. and Edmondson, D.E. (1980) Structure, properties, and determination of covalently bound flavins. *Methods Enzymol.*, **66E**, 253–64.

Strohecker, R. and Henning, H.M. (1966) *Vitamin Assay. Tested Methods*, Verlag Chemie, Weinheim, pp. 173–8.

Takatsuki, K., Suzuki, S., Sato, M., Sakai, K. and Ushizawa, I. (1987) Liquid chromatographic determination of free and added niacin and niacinamide in beef and pork. *J. Ass. Off. Analyt. Chem.*, **70**, 698–702.

Tanaka, A., Iijima, M., Kikuchi, Y., Hoshino, Y. and Nose, N. (1989) Gas chromatographic determination of nicotinamide in meats and meat products as 3-cyanopyridine. *J. Chromat.*, **466**, 307–17.

Thompson, R.C., Eakin, R.E. and Williams, R.J. (1941) The extraction of biotin from tissues. *Science*, **94**, 589–90.

Tsunoda, K., Inoue, N., Iwasaki, H., Akiya, M. and Hasebe, A. (1988) Rapid simultaneous analysis of nicotinic acid and nicotinamide in foods, and their behaviour during storage. *J. Fd Hyg. Soc. Japan*, **29**, 262–6.

Vanderslice, J.T., Maire, C.E., Doherty, R.F. and Beecher, G.R. (1980) Sulfosalicyclic acid as an extraction agent for vitamin B_6 in food. *J. Agric. Fd Chem.*, **28**, 1145–9.

van Gend, H.W. (1973) An automated colorimetric method for the determination of free nicotinic acid in minced meat. *Z. Lebensmittelunters. u.-Forsch.*, **153**, 73–7.

Vidal-Valverde, C. and Reche, A. (1991) Determination of available niacin in legumes and meat by high-performance liquid chromatography. *J. Agric. Fd Chem.*, **39**, 116–21.

Voigt, M.N., Eitenmiller, R.R. and Ware, G.O. (1979) Comparison of protozoan and conventional methods of vitamin analysis. *J. Fd Sci.*, **44**, 729–34.

Wall, J.S. and Carpenter, K.J. (1988) Variation in availability of niacin in grain products. *Fd Technol.*, **42**(10), 198–202, 204.

Watada, A.E. and Tran, T.T. (1985) A sensitive high-performance liquid chromatography method for analyzing riboflavin in fresh fruits and vegetables. *J. Liquid Chromat.*, **8**, 1651–62.

Wilson, S.D. and Horne, D.W. (1983) Evaluation of ascorbic acid in protecting labile folic acid derivatives. *Proc. Natl Acad. Sci. USA*, **80**, 6500–4.

Wilson, S.D. and Horne, D.W. (1984) High-performance liquid chromatographic determination of the distribution of naturally occurring folic acid derivatives in rat liver. *Analyt. Biochem.*, **142**, 529–35.

Woodrow, I.L., Torrie, K.M. and Henderson, G.A. (1969) A rapid method for the determination of riboflavin in dried milk products. *J. Inst. Can. Technol. Aliment.*, **2**, 120–2.

Wright, L.D., Cresson, E.L., Leibert, K.V. and Skeggs, H.R. (1952) Biological studies of biocytin. *J. Am. Chem. Soc.*, **74**, 2004–6.

Wyse, B.W., Song, W.O., Walsh, J.H. and Hansen, R.G. (1985) Pantothenic acid. In *Methods of Vitamin Assay*, 4th edn (eds J. Augustin, B.P. Klein, D. Becker and P.B. Venugopal), John Wiley & Sons, New York, pp. 399–416.

Physicochemical methods (excluding HPLC) for determining thiamin, riboflavin, niacin, vitamin B_6, pantothenic acid and vitamin C

5

5.1 TITRIMETRIC METHODS FOR VITAMIN C

5.1.1 TITRATION WITH 2,6-DICHLOROPHENOLINDOPHENOL

The method is based upon the reduction of the dye 2,6-dichlorophenolindophenol (DCPIP) with ascorbic acid in an acid solution (Figure 5.1). In the oxidized form, DCPIP is purplish-blue in neutral or alkaline solution, and pink in an acid solution; the reduced leuco compound is colourless. The procedure entails titrating a standardized solution of the dye into an acid extract of the sample. The pink end-point signals the presence of excess unreduced dye. In the absence of interfering

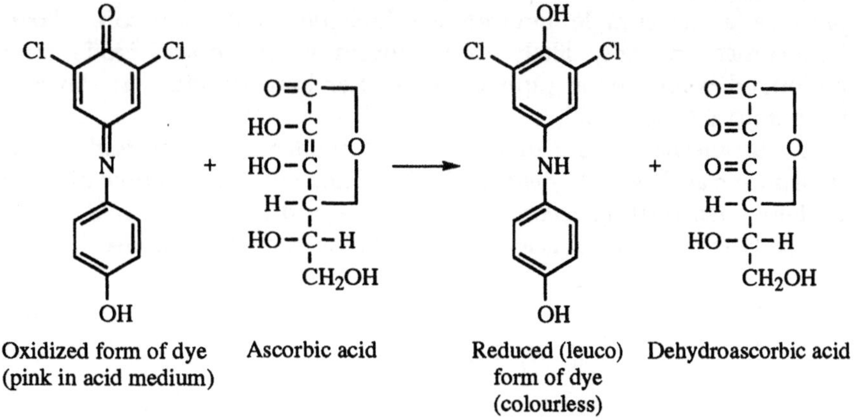

Figure 5.1 Reduction of 2,6-dichlorophenolindophenol (DCPIP) dye with ascorbic acid in an acid medium.

substances, the capacity of the extract to reduce the dye is directly proportional to the ascorbic acid content. Dehydroascorbic acid does not participate in the redox reaction, so the method does not yield the total vitamin C activity of a sample if this compound is present in significant quantities.

The titrimetric method gives results that generally agree with the biological estimation of ascorbic acid in raw and canned fruit and vegetables and their juices, which usually contain negligible amounts of dehydroascorbic acid. Significant quantities of dehydroascorbic acid may be produced under some conditions of processing and during storage of certain foods, in which case the vitamin C value will be underestimated (Olliver, 1967). The simplicity of the method makes it a suitable routine assay in fruit juice manufacture, although the procedure must be modified to analyse highly coloured extracts such as blackcurrant juice. It can also be used to assay vitamin C in vegetables and in aqueous extracts of dry foodstuffs when great accuracy is not required (Strohecker and Henning, 1966).

Unless suitable measures are taken, substances other than ascorbic acid, which have reduction potentials lower than that of the DCPIP indicator, will react with the dye and give a falsely high result for the vitamin C content of the sample. Substances known to interfere in the assay include sulphydryl compounds (e.g. glutathione and cysteine), phenols, sulphites, metal ions (copper (I), iron (II) and tin (II)) and reductones such as reductic acid (Figure 5.2). Sulphites are a common cause of difficulty because of their use as a preservative of foodstuffs. Metal ions are not normally present in sufficient concentration to cause a significant interference. However, iron (II) and tin (II) ions can be leached from non-lacquered cans containing fruit drinks and juices and, in combination with the traces of naturally occurring oxalic acid, can produce a measurable interference (Pelletier and Morrison, 1966). Reductones are only likely to be found in processed foods after prolonged boiling or in canned foods after long standing at elevated temperature (Roe, 1967).

The titrimetric method involves a preliminary extraction with metaphosphoric acid, which yields a clear solution, whilst also precipitating proteins, deactivating ascorbic acid oxidase and preventing catalysis of the oxidation of ascorbic acid by copper (II) or iron (III) ions. The titration

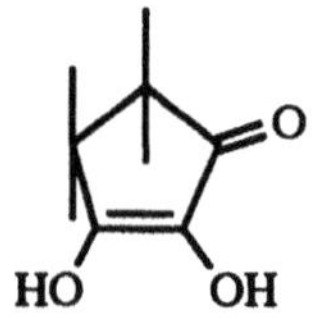

Figure 5.2 Reductic acid.

should be performed rapidly (within 1–2 min) in the pH range 3–4, taking the first definite end-point. At pH 3–4 the reduction of DCPIP by ascorbic acid is rapid, and by sulphydryl and phenol compounds relatively slow (Roe, 1967). The method has been adopted as Final Action for the determination of ascorbic acid in vitamin preparations and juices by the Association of Official Analytical Chemists (AOAC, 1990a). The AOAC procedure is as follows.

A 1 mg/ml standard solution of ascorbic acid is prepared by dissolving immediately before use 50 mg of pure L-ascorbic acid in 50 ml of extracting solution (8% v/v acetic acid and 3% w/v metaphosphoric acid in water). A 0.025% w/v solution of DCPIP (sodium salt) in dilute sodium bicarbonate solution is standardized daily by titrating against 2 ml of standard ascorbic acid added to 5 ml of extracting solution. The dye as made up in alkaline solution is blue, but in an acid medium, such as the extracting solution used in this determination, it is pink. The end-point is therefore a colour change from colourless to pink. A blank titration is carried out using 7 ml of extracting solution plus a volume of water equal to the volume of DCPIP used in the standardization titration. After subtracting the blank titre (usually about 0.1 ml) from the standardization titre, the concentration of DCPIP solution is calculated as mg ascorbic acid equivalent to 1.0 ml of the dye solution.

For the analysis of fruit and vegetable juices, an aliquot (>100 ml) of the filtered juice is added to an equal volume of extracting solution, and the total volume is designated as V ml. Sample aliquots (Y ml) containing about 2 mg of ascorbic acid and blank solutions are titrated against the standardized DCPIP solution. The concentration of ascorbic acid in the sample is calculated thus:

$$\text{mg ascorbic acid per g (or per ml) of sample} = (X - B) \times (F/E) \times (V/Y)$$

where

X = average titre (ml) for sample titration
B = average titre (ml) for sample blank titration
F = mg ascorbic acid equivalent to 1.0 ml dye solution, i.e. mg ascorbic acid in aliquot of standard solution titrated divided by the average corrected titre for the standardization titration
E = amount (g or ml) of sample
V = volume (ml) of initial assay solution
Y = volume (ml) of sample aliquot titrated

The following modifications of the titrimetric method have been published to eliminate the interference from other reducing compounds which may be present.

The reducing action of sulphite can be prevented by pretreatment with acetone to form the sulphite addition compound. In the case of fruit juices or beers, which contain sulphites and metabisulphites as a source of sulphur dioxide, a 25% concentration of acetone is added to the sample, which is then placed in the dark for 5 min before the titration is carried out (Henshall, 1981).

The interference from reductones present in caramelized foods, fermented foods and stored dehydrated vegetables can be eliminated by treating the sample solution with an 8% concentration of formaldehyde at pH 2.0, and then titrating. This value constitutes a blank which may then be subtracted from the 'apparent' ascorbic acid value obtained from an untreated sample. This technique was derived from the observation of Mapson (1943) that ascorbic acid combines rapidly with formaldehyde at pH 2.0, and hence is quickly removed from the DCPIP reaction, whereas reductones are only slowly removed and at a linear rate. At pH 1.5 formaldehyde condenses rapidly with sulphides, sulphites and thiol compounds, whilst the reaction with ascorbic acid is very slow. A procedure was therefore established for titrating with DCPIP in the presence of interfering sulphur compounds (Roe, 1967).

In the analysis of canned fruit juices and drinks, any interfering iron (II) or tin (II) ions which may be present can be removed by aeration in the presence of the chelating agent EDTA. The EDTA chelates the iron (III) and tin (IV) ions resulting from the aerial oxidation, and thereby prevents them from oxidizing the ascorbic acid (Pelletier and Morrison, 1966).

If the solution to be titrated is itself coloured, Strohecker and Henning (1966) suggested adding 10 ml of diethyl ether when the end-point is thought to have been reached. If, after vigorously shaking the mixture, the colour of the ethereal layer is violet–pink, the titration is already complete and excess of DCPIP is present. If the solution has a different colour or is colourless, an equal volume of sample solution is titrated with a volume of DCPIP solution 1.0 ml greater than before. The mixture is again shaken with 10 ml of ether. If the colour of the ether layer is violet–pink, the end-point lies between the two titration figures and can be determined fairly accurately by closer 'bracketing'. In the event of pigments being present that are soluble in ether, Strohecker and Henning (1966) suggested extracting a large volume of the sample solution with ether in a separating funnel, and titrating portions of the aqueous layer.

The assay may be performed using potentiometric titration instead of visual titration to overcome the end-point difficulty encountered with coloured solutions. Spaeth, Baptist and Roberts (1962) described a procedure in which manual potentiometric measurements were made with a pH meter using standard calomel and platinum electrodes to establish the titration curve (Figure 5.3). An automatic titrator was set to

35 mV above the baseline potential, and the standard and test solutions were titrated to ±10 mV of this arbitrary end-point.

A kinetic–spectrophotometric method using stopped-flow techniques has been described for the determination of ascorbic acid based on its reaction with DCPIP (Karayannis and Farasoglou, 1987).

5.1.2 TITRATION WITH *N*-BROMOSUCCINIMIDE

The method is based on the selective oxidation of ascorbic acid to dehydroascorbic acid by *N*-bromosuccinimide (Barakat, El-Wahab and El-Sadr, 1955). The technique relies on the fact that *N*-bromosuccinimide oxidizes ascorbic acid to dehydroascorbic acid before it liberates iodine from potassium iodide. The iodine is liberated from the potassium iodide before most of the other reducing substances have time to react with the *N*-bromosuccinimide. When all the ascorbic acid in the solution has been oxidized, the slightest excess of *N*-bromosuccinimide added will liberate the iodine, which is detected by the starch indicator.

The method is applicable to whole fruits and fruit juices, but is unable to provide a clear distinct end-point for cereals and milk products. The correlation of results obtained titrimetrically and by HPLC is good for

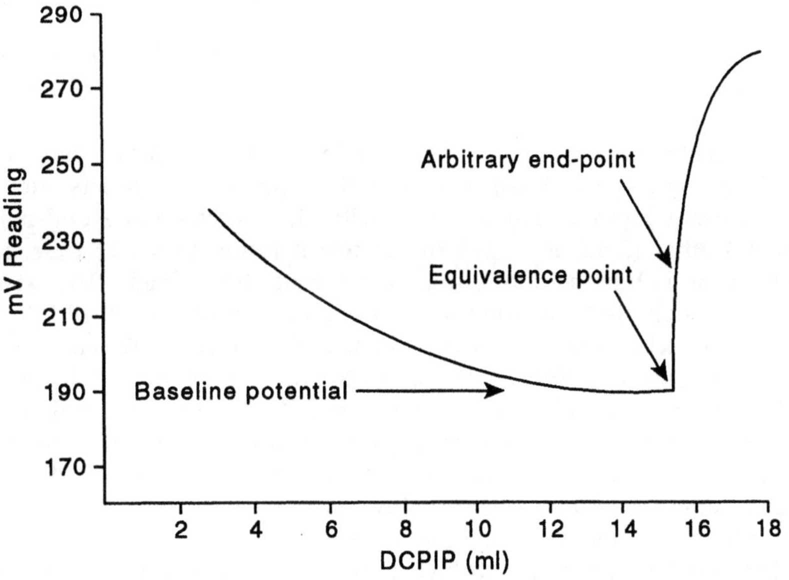

Figure 5.3 Titration curve of ascorbic acid with 2,6-dichlorophenolindophenol (DCPIP). Reprinted with permission from Spaeth, E.E., Baptist, V.H. and Roberts, M. (1962) Rapid potentiometric determination of ascorbic acid. *Analyt. Chem.*, **34**, 1342. Copyright (1962) American Chemical Society.

many common fruits, but tomatoes, and particularly limes, give falsely high vitamin values by the titrimetric method (Pachla and Kissinger, 1976). Reductones and iron salts that interfere in the DCPIP titrimetric method do not interfere with the *N*-bromosuccinimide reaction. The only reducing substances known to be oxidized before the liberation of iodine are sulphur compounds (sulphite, sulphide, thiosulphate and thiourea).

The following method published by Barakat, El-Wahab and El-Sadr (1955) is applicable to fruits.

The juice from the squeezed fruit is directly received in a known volume of 20% TCA, which stabilizes the ascorbic acid and also precipitates the proteins. To a known volume of the filtered solution in a 50-ml conical flask is added 5 ml of 4% potassium iodide solution, 2 ml of 3% acetic acid and two drops of starch indicator. This solution is titrated against a 0.01% w/v aqueous solution of *N*-bromosuccinimide added from a microburette. The end-point is reached when the last drop of the *N*-bromosuccinimide solution added produces a permanent violet colour. The amount of ascorbic acid in the solution is calculated thus:

$$\text{mg ascorbic acid} = V \times C \times 0.9882$$

where

V = volume (ml) of *N*-bromosuccinimide solution used in the titration

C = concentration of *N*-bromosuccinimide solution in mg/ml

0.9882 = the molar ratio of ascorbic acid and *N*-bromosuccinimide

The method of Barakat, El-Wahab and El-Sadr (1955) has been modified by Evered (1960) to deal with pigmented materials such as blackcurrant juice, which interfere with the starch–iodine end-point. Diethyl ether (3 ml) is added to the test solution in a test tube, and potassium iodide solution and acetic acid are added. The starch indicator is omitted. The tube is shaken vigorously after each addition of *N*-bromosuccinimide, and the aqueous/ether layers are allowed to separate. The end-point is indicated by the first appearance of the brown colour of liberated iodine in the ether layer. The *N*-bromosuccinimide is standardized using the same procedure, but titrating against a standard ascorbic acid solution. A blank titration is also carried out to determine the volume of *N*-bromosuccinimide solution necessary to impart a definite brown colour to the ether layer.

The interference from sulphite in the *N*-bromosuccinimide titration causes a problem in the analysis of juices and squashes which contain metabisulphite as preservative. This difficulty can be overcome by complexing the bisulphite with acetone before the titration (Sarwar, Iqbal and Zaidi, 1975).

The masking of end-points in the Barakat method can be avoided by titrating potentiometrically.

5.2 VOLTAMMETRIC METHODS FOR VITAMIN C

5.2.1 PRINCIPLES OF VOLTAMMETRY

Voltammetry is an electroanalytical technique which can be applied to the quantitative determination of oxidizable or reducible compounds. The technique is based on the principle that, when a voltage beyond a certain critical value is applied to a polarizable electrode immersed in an electrolyte solution, any electroactive solute in contact with the electrode will undergo electrolysis and produce an electric current (faradaic current). The technique is known as polarography if a dropping mercury electrode (DME) is employed. The fundamental principles of voltammetry can be explained in terms of classical direct current (DC) polarography.

In DC polarography, a current–potential curve (polarogram) for a solute undergoing oxidation in a stationary solution is obtained by applying a slow linear voltage ramp (typically 1–50 mV/s) in a positive direction to the electrolytic cell. At a certain threshold potential, electrolysis of the solute will begin to occur at the electrode, and a small anodic (negative) current will flow. As the potential is made still more positive, the current increases sharply until a point is reached at which the solute is oxidized as fast as it arrives at the electrode surface by diffusion from the bulk of the solution. At this point the current becomes independent of the applied potential, and the rise in current will flatten out to form a plateau. The limiting current flowing at this plateau (the diffusion current) is proportional to the bulk concentration of the electroactive solute, and hence quantification is based on the measurement of the wave height, i.e. the difference between the diffusion current and the residual current (Figure 5.4). In the case of a solute undergoing reduction, the potential is applied in a negative direction, which causes the cathodic (positive) current to increase in a similar sigmoidal fashion. Qualitative information can be obtained because the potential at which the current reaches half the total wave height (half-wave potential, $E_{1/2}$) is characteristic for each solute in a given electrolyte solution and electrode system. If more than one electroactive compound is present in the solution, the recorded polarogram consists of superimposed polarographic waves of the individual compounds. The optimum potential for a chemical species undergoing electrochemical oxidation or reduction decreases linearly with an increase of pH, and therefore the reduction process becomes more difficult while the oxidation process becomes easier (Riley and Watson, 1987).

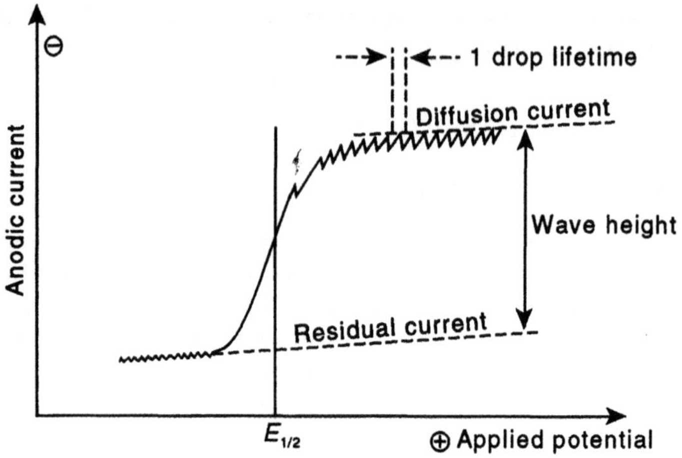

Figure 5.4 Diagram of a polarographic wave for a species undergoing electrochemical oxidation. The oscillations are caused by the decay of the capacitative current during the lifetime of each drop.

The polarogram obtained by DC polarography is less than ideal because of the oscillations resulting from the continual growing and dislodging of the mercury drops at the DME. Moreover, the sensitivity is limited to approximately 10^{-4} M (Hart, 1984), owing to interference from the capacity current arising from the double layer charging of the drop. Modern voltammetric instrumentation is designed to eliminate signals that interfere with the measurement of the faradaic current. This is achieved by using a three-electrode system (working, reference and auxiliary electrodes) operated with potentiostatic control. Among the reference electrodes are the saturated calomel electrode (SCE) and silver–silver chloride electrode; the auxiliary electrode is normally made from platinum wire. The DME has the unique advantage of presenting a constantly renewed electrode surface for the required electrode reaction, but it suffers from mechanical instability and limited anodic range (to about 0.2 V) owing to the mercury itself becoming oxidized. Popular alternatives for use in oxidation reactions are the carbon paste and vitreous (glassy) carbon electrodes, which extend the anodic range to about +2 V (Hart, 1984). The major practical problem with solid electrode voltammetry is the maintenance of a uniform electrode surface, which is prone to contamination (Fleet and Fouzder, 1979).

Improved voltammetric techniques have been discussed by Flato (1972) and include linear sweep voltammetry, differential pulse voltammetry and alternating current (AC) polarography. Each of these techniques has found application in the determination of ascorbic acid in foods. In linear sweep voltammetry, the slowly varying scan potential used in DC polarography is replaced by a fast sweep at 100 mV/s and higher. The technique is referred to as cathode ray voltammetry when an oscilloscope rather than a recorder is utilized, but the use of nomenclature associated with the readout device is best avoided (Bond, 1980). In differential pulse voltammetry, the voltammogram is obtained by superimposing a fixed-height potential pulse at regular intervals on the slowly varying voltage ramp. The flow of current is sampled after the capacitive contribution has decayed. The signal is displayed as a clearly defined peak whose height and location (half-width or half-peak potential, $E_{p/2}$) provide the quantitative and qualitative information for the analyte. In AC polarography, the signal arising from capacitive current is eliminated by measuring only that portion of the AC current which maintains a specific phase relationship with the applied potential. The signal is also displayed as a peak, which allows substances whose half-wave potentials differ by as little as 0.04 V to be distinguished from one another. In those techniques which employ a DME, the data are obtained on a single mercury drop or are drop-synchronized, and therefore the annoying oscillations produced on the DC polarogram are not present.

5.2.2 APPLICABILITY

Voltammetric methods have found commercial application in the determination of thiamin, riboflavin, pyridoxine, nicotinamide, folic acid and ascorbic acid in pharmaceutical preparations such as multivitamin tablets, which contain these vitamins in relatively high concentrations (Söderhjelm and Lindquist, 1976; Ballantine and Woolfson, 1980; Hart, 1986). Using such methods, the active ingredient can frequently be determined in the presence of insoluble excipients, thus eliminating the need for time-consuming extraction steps and calculations of recovery.

Voltammetry is more difficult to apply to the analysis of foods, owing to the presence of macromolecules and electroactive substances that interfere with the measurement. The natural occurrence of the B-group vitamins as protein-bound coenzymes in biological tissues, rather than as their parent compounds, further complicates their determination by voltammetry. Published voltammetric applications with respect to the determination of water-soluble vitamins in foods are limited almost exclusively to ascorbic acid and erythorbic acid.

The voltammetric determination of ascorbic acid is based upon the fast reversible oxidation at an electrode to produce dehydroascorbic acid with the loss of two electrons and two protons. The dehydroascorbic acid is then rapidly and irreversibly hydrated to form an electroinactive product (Figure 5.5.) (Perone and Kretlow, 1966). Only those electroactive compounds whose oxidation potentials are higher than that of

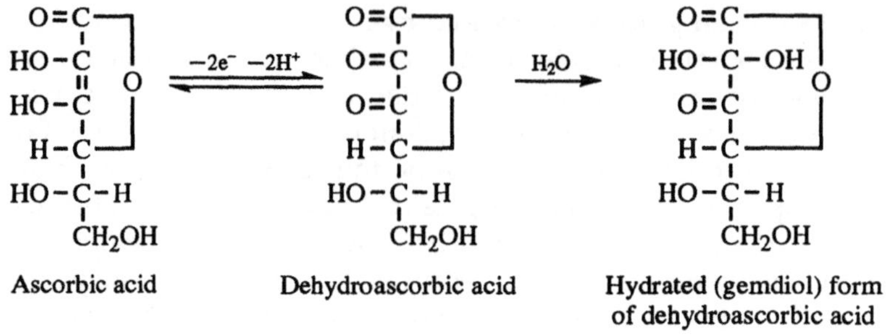

Figure 5.5 The electrochemical oxidation of ascorbic acid.

ascorbic acid will not be measured, so the lower the applied voltage, the greater the specificity. The linear decrease of optimum potential with an increase of pH has been demonstrated for ascorbic acid (Santhanam and Krishnan, 1961). Voltammetric analysis does not yield total vitamin C activity, as it does not account for dehydroascorbic acid.

Lindquist (1975) applied linear sweep voltammetry at a carbon paste electrode to determine ascorbic acid in fresh fruits, vegetables and beverages. The samples were extracted with 6% metaphosphoric acid and analysed after dilution with 3% metaphosphoric acid and addition of sodium acetate to a level of 3%. The method was compared with the DCPIP titrimetric procedure and yielded mostly lower results, owing to the better selectivity. Owen and Franklin Smyth (1975) used a cathode ray polarograph to analyse fruit juices and solid foodstuffs that were diluted or extracted with acetate buffer, pH 4.7.

Ratzkowski and Korol (1977) applied AC polarography to simultaneously determine ascorbic acid and erythorbic acid in foods, using a 0.25 M NaOH/2% metaphosphoric acid electrolyte (pH 11.5) and an applied voltage range of −0.75 to +0.25 V. No problems of decomposition were encountered when all reagents were deaerated with nitrogen before use, despite the high pH of the electrolyte. Three anodic waves were recorded which corresponded to erythorbic acid (−0.26 V), ascorbic acid (−0.18 V) and an additive coinciding peak (−0.11 V). A concentration of each epimer 20 times that of the other was separable, and levels down to 5 μg/ml could be assayed in foods. Recoveries of ascorbic acid and erythorbic acid added to the food samples ranged from 85% to 105%.

Lau, Shiu and Chang (1985) applied differential pulse polarography to the determination of ascorbic acid in vegetables and fruits using a 2 M acetate buffer (pH 4.5) as the electrolyte. Samples were extracted with a mixture of 1% oxalic acid, 2% TCA and 1% sodium sulphate, and then filtered. Oxalic acid was used as an extractant in preference to metaphosphoric acid because a much higher anodic peak was obtained.

A calibration graph was linear for ascorbic acid concentration up to 20 mg/litre. The results agreed closely with results obtained by the AOAC microfluorimetric method, but the polarographic procedure was more sensitive. Lechien *et al.* (1982) applied differential pulse voltammetry at a carbon paste electrode to determine ascorbic acid in fruit juices diluted with 0.1 M acetate buffer, pH 4.7.

Lau, Shiu and Chang (1985) studied the interference effects of a number of common cations and anions on the determination of ascorbic acid using differential pulse polarography. Na^+, K^+, Mg^{2+}, Ca^{2+}, Fe^{2+}, Cu^{2+}, Al^{3+}, Cl^-, NO_3^-, CO_3^{2-}, SO_4^{2-} and HPO_4^{2-} did not interfere with the determination. Fe^{3+} interfered at a mole ratio (foreign ion/ascorbic acid) of 2:1, while Br^- and I^-, which are easily oxidized, interfered at a mole ratio of 0.18 : 1. Sontag and Kainz (1978) found that citric acid, tartaric acid, sucrose, glucose, fructose, sulphite and quinine did not interfere with the determination of ascorbic acid in fruit juice and lemonade by differential pulse polarography. Sulphite is oxidized at high potentials and thus it is possible to determine the concentration of ascorbic acid and sulphite in a mixture (Lindquist, 1975). Reductones (those tested were reductic acid and dihydroxyfumaric acid) interfere (Lindquist, 1975), but can be removed from the sample by the addition of formaldehyde (Strohecker and Henning, 1966). In practice, the standard addition calibration should be used in voltammetry to reduce matrix interference effects. Electrochemical methods have been developed which involve a prior separation of sample components by HPLC (see Chapter 6).

5.3 SPECTROPHOTOMETRIC DETERMINATION OF VITAMIN C

5.3.1 PRINCIPLE OF UV/VISIBLE ABSORPTION SPECTROSCOPY

A molecule with a characteristic structure will absorb radiation in the UV or visible region of the electromagnetic spectrum and undergo a transition to a higher electronic state. If the intensity of the incident radiation is I_0 and that of the transmitted radiation is I_t, then the fraction transmitted is:

$$I_t/I_o = T \text{ (transmittance)}$$

The percentage transmittance is:

$$\%T = 100I_t/I_0$$

Mathematically, absorbance is related to percentage transmittance by the expression

$$A = \log (I_o/I_t) = \log (100/\%T)$$

The Beer–Lambert law states that there is a linear relationship between absorbance and concentration at every wavelength over a limited concentration range. The law is only true for monochromatic radiation, i.e. radiation of a single wavelength or narrow band of wavelengths.

$$A = kcl$$

where l is the optical path length through the sample solution, c is the concentration of absorbing compound in the path l, and k is the absorptivity (or extinction coefficient), which is a constant for a particular compound in a particular solvent at a given wavelength.

The absorbance (A) is a dimensionless number and an absorbance of 1 is usually expressed as 1 absorption unit (AU).

The absorptivity (k) must have units used for the concentration and path length of the sample. It is usually expressed as ε (epsilon), the molar absorptivity or molar absorption (extinction) coefficient, which is the absorbance of a sample concentration of 1 g molecule/litre in a 1-cm path at a given wavelength.

If the molecular weight of the compound is not known, it is usual to calculate $A_{1\,\mathrm{cm}}^{1\%}$, which is the absorbance of a 1% w/v sample concentration in a 1-cm path at a given wavelength.

The relationship between ε and $A_{1\,\mathrm{cm}}^{1\%}$ is

$$\varepsilon = A_{1\,\mathrm{cm}}^{1\%} \times \text{molecular weight}/10$$

Absorbance and quantity are related by the equation:

$$\mathrm{mg} = A \times D \times V \times 10/A_{1\,\mathrm{cm}}^{1\%}$$

where A is the absorbance, D is the dilution factor, and V is the total volume of sample (ml).

A spectrophotometer provides monochromatic radiation of a selected wavelength and measures the ratio of the transmitted radiation (I) to the incident radiation (I_0). For quantitative analysis one usually selects radiation of a wavelength at which k is a maximum, i.e. at the peak (λ_{max}) of the absorption spectrum. A solution of the sample is placed in an optical cell of known path length, and the solvent or suitable blank solution is placed in a similar reference cell. The radiation intensity transmitted by the sample is compared to that transmitted by the reference solution. The spectrophotometer is designed to provide an output in absorbance.

To determine the concentration of an analyte in solution, one constructs a calibration graph of absorbance versus concentration using standard solutions of known concentration of the analyte. The absorbance of the 'unknown' is measured and the concentration is interpolated from the calibration graph. If the absorbance falls outside the linear part of the graph, the sample must be diluted and remeasured.

5.3.2 APPLICABILITY

The application of direct spectrophotometry to the determination of water-soluble vitamins in food extracts is subject to spectral interference from many substances. The extent of the interference depends upon the intensity of the absorbance of the vitamin relative to the absorbances of accompanying substances at the selected wavelength. Direct spectrophotometry has not found widespread routine application in the determination of the water-soluble vitamins in foods, owing to the rigorous sample preparation that would be required to obtain a sufficiently pure solution for assay. Furthermore, for certain vitamins, fluorimetric assay offers superior sensitivity and selectivity.

Direct spectrophotometry has been applied to the determination of ascorbic acid in soft drinks, fruit juices and cordials after correction for background absorption in the UV region (Lau, Luk and Wong, 1986). The method of background correction was to measure the absorbance of the sample solution before and after the catalytic oxidation of ascorbic acid with copper (II) sulphate, and then to calculate the concentration of ascorbic acid from the difference. The sample blank was prepared by adding copper (II) sulphate to an aliquot of diluted sample and heating at 50 °C for 15 min. The heating step was necessary to overcome the inhibitory effect of citrate upon the copper-catalysed oxidation. To correct for the absorption due to copper (II), EDTA was added after the oxidation. Samples and standard solutions were prepared to contain the same concentration of the copper (II)–EDTA complex, which does not catalyse the oxidation of ascorbic acid at room temperature. The absorption due to the copper (II)–EDTA complex constituted part of the reagent blank against which the ascorbic acid standard solutions were read. Absorbance measurements were made at 267 nm and pH 6. The calibration graph was linear within the range 0–20 μg/ml of ascorbic acid. The precision was 0.1–0.5% for ascorbic acid in the concentration range 5–13 μg/ml. The recoveries of ascorbic acid added to lime cordial, orange drink and lemon tea were within 99.8–100.4%: the result for blackcurrant drink was 98.5%.

5.4 COLORIMETRIC METHODS FOR NIACIN AND VITAMIN C

5.4.1 DETERMINATION OF NIACIN BY THE KÖNIG REACTION

The AOAC colorimetric method for the determination of niacin in foods and feeds (AOAC, 1990b) is based on the König reaction, in which pyridine derivatives are reacted with cyanogen bromide and an aromatic amine, sulphanilic acid. The pyridine ring is opened up, and the intermediate product is coupled with the amine to form a yellow dye, whose absorbance can be measured photometrically. Food samples are hydrolysed to liberate niacin from its coenzyme forms, whilst also converting nicotinamide to nicotinic acid. The assay therefore accounts for the total niacin content of the food sample.

The AOAC (1990b) method employs two different procedures: one for non-cereal foods and feeds, and the other for cereal products. Non-cereal foods and feeds are autoclaved with 1 N H_2SO_4 for 30 min at 15 lb (104 kPa) pressure in order to liberate nicotinamide from its coenzyme forms and hydrolyse it to nicotinic acid. The reaction with cyanogen bromide is carried out at room temperature in the presence of sulphanilic acid, and the resulting colour is measured at 450 nm. Cereal products are autoclaved with $Ca(OH)_2$ solution for 2 h at 15 lb pressure to liberate the nicotinic acid from its chemically bound forms. The reaction with cyanogen bromide and sulphanilic acid is carried out in the cold under somewhat different conditions, and the colour is measured at 470 nm. This modified procedure (Pelletier and Campbell, 1959) leads to better recoveries of added niacin and better agreement with microbiological results (Campbell and Pelletier, 1961). An obvious disadvantage of the König reaction is the use of cyanogen bromide, which is toxic and difficult to handle.

5.4.2 DETERMINATION OF VITAMIN C AS THE 2,4-DINITROPHENYLHYDRAZINE DERIVATIVE

The method of Roe and Kuether (1943) involves the oxidation of ascorbic acid to dehydroascorbic acid and subsequent reaction with 2,4-dinitrophenylhydrazine (DNPH) to form the osazone of diketogulonic acid. Treatment with 85% H_2SO_4 yields a stable brownish-red colour with an absorption maximum at 500–550 nm. The absorbance of this colour is measured photometrically at 540 nm, and is proportional to the quantity of ascorbic acid (plus dehydroascorbic acid) present in the solution before oxidation (Roe, 1967).

The method is applicable to foods where a proportion of the vitamin C activity is contributed by dehydroascorbic acid. It is not applicable to food containing erythorbic acid, which participates in the reaction (Tuan, Wyatt and Anglemier, 1987) and would yield a false vitamin C value. Unlike with the DCPIP titrimetric method, metal reducing ions do not interfere, but sugars such as glucose, fructose and glucuronic acid react with DNPH to form yellow osazones. Although the absorption maxima of the latter lie toward shorter wavelengths, they nevertheless absorb sufficient light in the region 520–525 nm to constitute serious interferences in samples containing high levels of sugars or sugar degradation products (Roe, 1954). The interference from any diketogulonic acid that might have been present in the original sample and from reductones cannot be avoided without recourse to chromatographic purification. Pigments do not interfere, owing to their removal by adsorption on the active carbon used in the oxidation reaction.

The assay procedure comprises four main steps: extraction, oxidation, condensation reaction and colour formation. Acetic, trichloroacetic or oxalic acid must be present in the extract to prevent adsorption of the vitamin C upon the active carbon used in the oxidation step (Roe, 1967). Oxalic acid also stabilizes the ascorbic acid (Strohecker and Henning, 1966) and for these reasons is the preferred extractant. Acid-washed charcoal is the recommended oxidizing agent, as it also clarifies sample extracts and removes interfering substances that other oxidants do not remove (Roe, 1967). The condensation reaction between dehydroascorbic acid and DNPH is carried out at 37 °C and takes 3 h to complete. The reaction rate would obviously be increased by raising the temperature, but above 37 °C sugars and glucuronic acid also react to a noticeable extent, leading to falsely high results. With the reaction at 37 °C, Roe (1961) found no interference from glucose or fructose with concentrations up to 0.5% and 0.3%, respectively, while glucuronic acid began to interfere at a concentration of 0.025%. In the analysis of sugar-rich foods (e.g. syrups and fruit juices), the extracts must be diluted so that the concentrations of sugars are below the levels which would cause interference. The addition of thiourea to the solution provides a weakly reducing medium and prevents discoloration of the DNPH solution by any oxidation products that might form (Roe and Kuether, 1943).

The procedure described by Roe (1967) is as follows.

A 0.05% w/v stock solution of ascorbic acid is prepared by dissolving 50 mg of pure L-ascorbic acid in 100 ml of 0.5% oxalic acid. A working standard solution is prepared by diluting 2 ml of stock solution to 100 ml with 4% TCA, or 5% metaphosphoric acid plus 10% acetic acid, the acid being that to be used in the analysis. The solution is oxidized by shaking with acid-washed charcoal (1 g/50 ml of solution) and then filtering. The concentration of dehydroascorbic acid in this working standard solution is 10 μg/ml.

Food samples are homogenized in 4% TCA solution or in 5% metaphosphoric acid plus 10% acetic acid solution. A volume of extract is prepared that is estimated to yield a concentration of 1–10 μg ascorbic acid/ml. The extract is shaken with acid-washed charcoal (1 g/50 ml) and then filtered. Into each of two colorimeter tubes is placed 4 ml of sample filtrate, and into a third tube is placed 4 ml of the standard filtrate containing 10 μg dehydroascorbic acid/ml. To one of the tubes containing the sample filtrate and to the standard tube is added 1 ml of DNPH reagent containing thiourea. The second tube containing the sample filtrate serves as the blank. The three tubes are placed in a water bath at 37 °C for 3 h, after which they are transferred to an ice-water bath. To each of the three tubes is added 5 ml of 85% H_2SO_4, dropwise and slowly. Finally, 1 ml of DNPH reagent is added to the blank tube. Each tube is shaken under the ice water, and then removed to a rack and allowed to stand for 30 min. The absorbances of the coloured solutions are measured at 540 nm.

The concentration of ascorbic acid in the sample is calculated thus:

$$\text{mg ascorbic acid per 100-g sample} = D_U \times S \times \text{ml extract} \times 100/D_S \times 1000 \times 4 \times \text{sample weight (g)}$$

where
D_U = optical density of unknown
D_S = optical density of standard
S = μg ascorbic acid/4 ml standard solution

Pelletier and Brassard (1977) proposed manual and automated discrete sample analytical methods for total vitamin C in food based on the method described above. The interference from high concentrations of sugars was rendered negligible by incubating at 15 °C for 17 h, and by measuring the absorbance 75 min after the addition of sulphuric acid instead of 30 min.

5.4.3 DETERMINATION OF VITAMIN C BY REDUCTION OF TETRAZOLIUM DYE

Beutler and Beinstingl (1980) described a colorimetric method based upon the reduction of the tetrazolium dye 3-(4,5-dimethylthiazolyl-2)-2,5-diphenyltetrazolium bromide by ascorbic acid in the presence of the electron carrier 5-methylphenazinium methyl sulphate at pH 3.5 to form a formazan that absorbs visible light at 578 nm. The effect of interferences is reduced by carrying out a parallel blank determination in which the ascorbic acid is destroyed by the action of ascorbate oxidase. Total vitamin C determinations require reduction of dehydroascorbic acid to ascorbic acid with homocysteine. Interference from sulphur dioxide is eliminated by treatment with formaldehyde, and colour interference from dark juices is prevented by decolorization with 1% polyvinylpolypyrrolidone before filtering. The reagents for this assay are available in kit form from Boehringer Mannheim Biochemicals. The assay has been evaluated for determination of ascorbic acid in beer (Kelley and Siebert, 1989).

5.5 FLUORIMETRIC METHODS FOR THIAMIN, RIBOFLAVIN, VITAMIN B_6 AND VITAMIN C

5.5.1 PRINCIPLE OF FLUORESCENCE SPECTROSCOPY

Fluorescence is a form of luminescence, and refers to the long-wave radiation energy emitted from certain compounds when excited by UV irradiation. When a molecule of a fluorescent compound absorbs a photon of UV radiation the molecule is excited to a higher energy state. The fluorescence is produced when the molecule returns to an intermediate energy level by re-emitting a photon. Since some of the energy of the incident photon is retained in the molecule or is lost by a nonradiative process, the emitted photon has less energy and hence a longer wavelength than the absorbed photon. The fluorescence efficiency or quantum yield of a compound is defined as the fraction of the incident radiation which is re-emitted as fluorescence.

$$\text{Fluorescense intensity } (F) = \phi_f(I_0 - I_t)$$

where I_0 and I_t are the intensities of the incident and transmitted radiation

$$\phi_f = \text{quantum yield}$$

By substituting the exponential form of the Beer–Lambert law in this equation, a relationship between the fluorescence intensity and solute concentration (c) can be obtained. At low solute concentration, where the curve of F plotted against c is almost linear, the relationship can be approximated to

$$F = 2.303\phi_f K I_0 \varepsilon c l$$

where K = efficiency of collection of fluorescence
ε = molar absorptivity of the fluorescent compound
l = optical path length through the sample solution
c = concentration of the fluorescent compound in the path l

As ϕ_f, K, I_0 and ε can be held constant, it can be seen that the fluorescence intensity is proportional to the concentration.

Any fluorescent molecule has two characteristic spectra, namely the excitation spectrum and the emission spectrum. The excitation spectrum is obtained by plotting the intensity of the fluorescence as the wavelength of the exciting radiation is changed: it shows the relative efficiency of different wavelengths of exciting radiation in causing fluorescence. The emission spectrum is obtained by irradiating the sample at the wavelength of maximum absorption and observing the emitted fluorescence. In theory, the excitation spectrum of a given compound is identical to the compound's UV absorption spectrum obtained using a spectrophotometer. In practice, however, excitation spectra are distorted as a result of instrumental artifacts. A characteristic feature of fluorescent molecules is the difference between the wavelengths of the excitation and emission maxima. This physical constant is called the Stoke's shift and indicates the energy dissipated during the lifetime of the excited state before return to the ground state (Guilbault, 1973). Maximum sensitivity in analysis is obtained by selecting the wavelengths of the excitation and emission maxima. Other wavelengths may provide the advantage of greater analytical selectivity, and the sensitivity, although reduced, may still be adequate. Fluorescence spectroscopy is more selective than UV/visible absorption spectroscopy because the former uses two wavelengths in the measurement, and the structural features required in a molecule for fluorescence to occur are more limited. A rigid planar ring system and conjugated double bonds, as found in riboflavin, are favourable for fluorescence.

In a typical fluorescence spectrometer the sample is excited by radiation from a high-intensity lamp at a wavelength determined by a monochromator or narrow band-pass interference filter. The emitted radiation is detected at right-angles to the incident beam through a second monochromator or filter. The sample solution is placed in a cell, of which all four sides are polished. A 150-W high-pressure xenon arc lamp fulfils the requirements of constant output and the emission of radiation over a wide range of wavelengths. Instruments are classified according to the types of wavelength selector. The most versatile instrument is the dual monochromator spectrofluorimeter, which allows any wavelength to be selected for both excitation and emission, and can be used to record both the excitation and emission spectra of a sample. The band-pass of a grating monochromator can be increased by increasing the slit width. An instrument with a single monochromator and a band-pass filter provides a less expensive option while, for quantitative analysis at predetermined wavelengths, a fluorimeter with two band-pass filters is quite adequate.

Quantification in fluorimetric analysis is based upon the dependency of the intensity of fluorescence upon the amount of radiation absorbed, which in turn depends upon the concentration of the fluorescent analyte. At low concentrations a linear calibration graph of fluorescence intensity versus concentration is obtained. At higher concentration, where the absorbance of the sample solution exceeds 0.02, the graph becomes curved. Additional curvature takes place at absorbance values above 0.03 due to the inner filter effect. This phenomenon refers to the absorption of incident radiation by molecules in the sample before it can excite the molecules of the fluorescent species. Self-absorption is another type of inner filter effect, which involves a loss of the emitted radiation by absorption before it leaves the cell. Inner filter effects occur when the sample solution contains a strongly absorbing compound whose absorption band overlaps either the excitation or the emission band of the fluorescent analyte.

The minimum detection limit with fluorescence spectroscopy, given a pure sample and optimal instrumental settings, is at the 1-pg level, compared with 1 ng obtained with UV absorption spectroscopy. Factors that affect the method sensitivity include light scattering, quenching and the presence of fluorescent impurities. The light scatter that occurs at the wavelength of excitation is composed of Rayleigh scattering from the solvent, Tyndall scattering from suspended particles, and scatter from the surface of the cell. Raman scatter is another property of the pure solvent, and occurs at wavelengths longer than the exciting radiation. The provision of an auxiliary cut-off filter helps to reduce stray light by transmitting only the radiation above a specified wavelength. Quenching refers to the loss of energy from excited analyte molecules before they can emit radiation. The energy is transferred directly to other molecules, especially molecules of dissolved oxygen, and, at high concentration, to molecules of the analyte itself. Fluorescent impurities may originate from the sample itself or from the solvent and reagents introduced during the analysis. The isolation and measurement of the fluorescent analyte can be more effectively achieved using HPLC with fluorimetric detection.

Fluorescence spectroscopy generally has enhanced sensitivity, dynamic range and selectivity compared with UV/visible absorption spectroscopy, but reduced precision.

5.5.2 FLUORIMETRIC DETERMINATION OF THIAMIN

The AOAC fluorimetric method is based on the conversion of thiamin to its fluorescent oxidation product, thiochrome, by reaction with alkaline potassium hexacyanoferrate (III) (potassium ferricyanide, $K_3Fe(CN)_6$). Under standardized conditions the method is sensitive and specific, with a reproducibility of ±5–10%, according to the nature of the sample (Strohecker and Henning, 1966). The specificity is achieved by the use of chromatography and extraction into isobutanol, both of which act as purification steps. The latter step also contributes to the sensitivity, since thiochrome is more fluorescent in isobutanol than in aqueous solution.

The AOAC fluorimetric method has been applied to the determination of thiamin in foods, grain products, bread and milk-based infant formula (AOAC, 1990c,d,e,f). In the procedure described for foods containing TPP (AOAC, 1990c), the food sample(s) and a standard solution of thiamin hydrochloride are taken through the following steps: acid digestion, enzymatic hydrolysis, purification by open-column chromatography, oxidation of thiamin to thiochrome and extraction of the thiochrome into isobutanol, and measurement of the fluorescence. Some workers prefer to run an internal standard by adding a known amount of thiamin to a second sample. The methodology has been studied by Conner and Straub (1941) and each step is briefly discussed below.

Acid digestion

The purpose of the acid digestion is to release the thiamin or thiamin phosphate esters that may be bound to protein, and thus effect the complete solution of the various forms of thiamin present in the sample. Thiamin is quite stable under the heating and acidic conditions employed (McRoberts, 1954). A collaborative study of the determination of thiamin in enriched flour (McRoberts, 1954) has shown that there is no apparent difference in the use of hydrochloric or sulphuric acids. However, Deutsch, Schiaffino and Pillsbury (1960) reported signs of thiamin destruction and the possible loss of thiamin by adsorption on precipitated sulphates when sulphuric acid was used in the analysis of a cornmeal enrichment mixture. Consequently, hydrochloric acid is used in AOAC procedures as recommended by McRoberts (1960). For the analysis of yeast and animal tissues, treatment of the acid digest with cysteine has been recommended (Association of Vitamin Chemists, Inc., 1966; Strohecker and Henning, 1966) to reduce any thiamin disulphide that might be present back to thiamin. However, the presence of thiamin disulphide in tissues has not been unequivocally demonstrated (Pearson, 1967a) and the reduction step is not included in any of the AOAC fluorimetric procedures (AOAC, 1990c,d,e,f).

Enzymatic hydrolysis

The phosphate esters of thiamin are converted to thiochrome phosphates by alkaline oxidation, but these derivatized esters are insoluble in isobutanol and therefore not assayed. Phosphorylated thiamin compounds must therefore be hydrolysed to thiamin prior to oxidation, and this hydrolysis can only proceed by the use of phosphatases. Enzyme preparations that have been used for this purpose include Mylase, Takadiastase and α-amylase, which are of fungal origin. The commercial availability of some of these enzymes has been a problem, and Defibaugh (1987) has evaluated suitable alternatives. The acid digest is buffered to pH 4.0–4.5, and then incubated with the enzyme for 3 h at 45–50 °C. The phosphatase treatment is actually not required for the analysis of plant material, because the thiamin is present largely in the free form. However, the enzyme treatment is beneficial for such material because the enzyme preparations used as a source of phosphatase also contain diastase, which breaks down starch into soluble sugars, thereby aiding subsequent filtration (Pearson, 1967a). For highly proteinaceous samples, such as meat and meat products, it has been recommended to add a proteolytic enzyme to the phosphatase/diastase preparation in order to prevent the occlusion of thiamin in the undissolved denatured protein that remains after acid digestion. Papain is suitable for this purpose, as it is active at the pH used for the phosphatase treatment (Strohecker and Henning, 1966).

Open-column chromatography

Purification of the acid digest or enzyme hydrolysate is essential in order to remove (1) substances that produce extraneous fluorescence and (2) reducing compounds that consume the oxidizing agent with the resulting danger of there being insufficient oxidizing agent to convert thiamin quantitatively into thiochrome. The purification is readily effected by means of open-column chromatography using a cation exchanger. The positively charged thiamin, together with other cations, is retained on the column, while unretained anions and non-ionized solutes are washed off with hot distilled water. The thiamin is exchanged for potassium ions and eluted using hot acidified potassium chloride solution. The ion exchanger used for many years was an activated aluminosilicate (Decalso). The purification of sample extracts on Decalso columns, as usually carried out, were reported to give low (about 90%) and inconsistent recoveries of thiamin, but recoveries could be improved (to 97.5%) by increasing the eluent volume from 25 to 50 ml (Pippen and Potter, 1975). This problem is now historical, as Decalso is no longer commercially available (Ellefson *et al.*, 1981) and has been replaced in the AOAC (1990c,d,e,f) procedures by Bio-Rex 70, hydrogen form (Bio-Rad Laboratories). This material is a weakly acidic cation exchange resin containing carboxylic acid exchange groups on a macroreticular acrylic polymer support.

Oxidation and extraction

Thiamin is oxidized by $K_3Fe(CN)_6$ in the presence of strong alkali to yield thiochrome, which is extracted into isobutanol. The yield of thiochrome is not quantitative (Pearson, 1967a), but it is very constant under standard conditions. Thus the oxidation and extraction steps for standards and samples should be performed in a standardized manner.

Measurement

The fluorescence intensity is linear in the range 0–2 μg thiamin. Since thiochrome is gradually destroyed by UV radiation, solutions undergoing measurement should not be exposed to the fluorimeter beam for longer than 15 s (Strohecker and Henning, 1966).

It is necessary to prepare a blank for each of the samples and for the standard in order to correct for the presence of other fluorescent substances. This is usually done by taking a second aliquot of the acidified potassium chloride eluate and treating it identically to the sample or standard, except that 15% NaOH is added instead of alkaline $K_3Fe(CN)_6$. This type of blank assumes that nonthiamin fluorescent substances are not affected differently by alkaline $K_3Fe(CN)_6$ solution and NaOH solution; however, this is not always the case. An alternative blank procedure that has been established for cereal products (McRoberts, 1960) relies upon the quenching of the fluorescence by strong acids. One simply adds a drop of concentrated hydrochloric acid to the cuvette containing the isobutanol solution of thiochrome whose fluorescence has been measured, and measures the fluorescence again.

The AOAC (1990c) procedure for dry or semi-dry foods containing TPP is as follows.

The sample is mixed with 0.1 N HCl at a volume in millilitres equal to at least 10 times the dry weight of sample in grams. The mixture is digested by heating for 30 min at 95–100 °C on a steam bath or by autoclaving for 30 min at 121–123 °C. The cooled digest is diluted to a measured volume containing 0.2–5.0 μg thiamin/ml. An aliquot of the digest containing *c.* 10–25 μg thiamin is diluted to *c.* 65 ml with 0.1 N HCl, and the pH is adjusted to 4.0–4.5 with 2 N sodium acetate. The buffered digest is incubated with enzyme for 3 h at 45–50 °C, followed by cooling and pH adjustment to 3.5. The solution is diluted to 100 ml with water, and filtered. An aliquot of the filtrate containing *c.* 5 μg of thiamin is passed through a suitably prepared Bio-Rex column, and the column is washed with 3 × 5-ml portions of almost boiling water. The thiamin is eluted from the resin with 5 × 4.0–4.5-ml portions of almost boiling acidified KCl solution. The eluate is cooled and then diluted to 25 ml with acidified KCl to give the 'assay sample solution'.

A working standard solution containing 1 μg thiamin hydrochloride/ml is prepared by heating (steam bath) or autoclaving 10 ml of an intermediate 10 μg/ml solution and *c.* 50 ml of 0.1 N HCl, and then diluting the cooled solution to 100 ml with the 0.1 N HCl. A 20-ml aliquot of the working standard solution is subjected to the enzyme hydrolysis and purification steps. The final 25 ml of eluate containing (theoretically) 5 μg of thiamin hydrochloride is designated as 'assay standard solution'.

Into a series of tubes or reaction vessels are placed *c.* 1.5 g of NaCl (or KCl) and 5 ml of assay sample solution or assay standard solution. Within 1–2 s, 3 ml of alkaline $K_3Fe(CN)_6$ reagent is added to the swirled tube contents, followed immediately by 13 ml of isobutanol. Each tube is stoppered and shaken vigorously directly after the addition of isobutanol. After isobutanol has been added to all tubes, the tubes are shaken again for *c.* 2 min, and then centrifuged. The isobutanol extract (upper layer) is taken for thiochrome fluorescence measurement. Sample blanks and a standard blank are prepared in a similar manner, except that the alkaline $K_3Fe(CN)_6$ reagent is replaced by an equal volume of 15% NaOH solution.

A fluorimeter equipped with narrow transmittance range filters with input filter max. at *c.* 365 nm and output filter max. at *c.* 435 nm is satisfactory.

The concentration of thiamin in the original food sample is calculated from the measured fluorescence response of the assay solution relative to that of the oxidized thiamin standard solution after subtraction of blank readings. Thus:

$$\mu g\ \text{thiamin/g} = (U - U_B) \times 25 \times 100/(S - S_B) \times 5 \times V \times M$$

where U and U_B are the fluorescence readings of the unknown (sample) and its blank

S and S_B are the fluorescence readings of the standard and its blank (the factor 1/5 converts the reading to μg/ml instead of μg/5 ml aliquot)

V = volume of solution applied to the chromatography column (the factor $25/V$ corrects for volume changes during chromatographic purification and elution; the eluate is made up to a final volume of 25 ml)

The factor $100/M$ accounts for the weight of sample in g (M) that when extracted yields 100 ml of assay solution

For the analysis of grain products (e.g. wheat flour, macaroni, and noodle products, which do not contain significant amounts of phosphorylated or protein-bound thiamin) the enzymatic hydrolysis and chromatographic purification steps have beem omitted (AOAC, 1990d). The autoclaving conditions prescribed for grain products are 20 min at 108–109 °C; the higher temperature of 121–123 °C employed for 'foods' (AOAC, 1990c) resulted in a loss of thiamin using this rapid procedure (McRoberts, 1954). The enzymatic hydrolysis step (but not the chromatography) is essential for bread and wheat germ (AOAC, 1990e), which both contain phosphorylated thiamin (Bechtel and Hollenbeck, 1958).

5.5.3 FLUORIMETRIC DETERMINATION OF RIBOFLAVIN

This discussion is confined to the determination of total vitamin B_2; the simultaneous determination of riboflavin, FMN and FAD is more appropriate to biological, chemical and clinical applications. Early chromatographic methods for determining individual flavins involved long and tedious procedures, and have been superseded by HPLC separations (Russell and Vanderslice, 1990).

Direct fluorescence method

The native fluorescence exhibited by riboflavin enables this vitamin to be assayed fluorimetrically without the need for chemical derivatization. This technique has been applied successfully to the analysis of milk and milk products, eggs, meats and grain products. Quantification is based on a comparison of the fluorescence intensity of the sample assay solution with that of a sample assay solution to which a known amount of riboflavin has been added (internal standard). It is assumed that interfering substances will affect both standard and sample fluorescence to a similar extent. The use of an internal standard does not, however, assure an absolutely correct determination, since the synthetic riboflavin added to the sample extract may behave in a slightly different manner than native flavins. The error caused by this phenomenon will be greater the higher the concentration of interfering substances in the assay solution (Koziol, 1971). The method is not applicable to many low-potency materials or to samples in which interfering colours, like caramel, develop on heating (Pearson, 1967b).

The direct fluorescence method has been adopted as Final Action for the determination of riboflavin in foods, including ready-to-feed milk-based infant formula, by the AOAC. The general procedure (AOAC, 1990g) involves the following steps: acid digestion, precipitation of proteinaceous material, oxidation, and measurement of the fluorescence. Each of these steps will be discussed in turn.

Acid digestion

The purpose of the acid digestion is to release noncovalently bound flavins from their association with proteins, and to completely convert FAD to FMN and riboflavin, whilst also denaturing the proteins and inactivating any enzymes that might be present. The food sample is mixed with 0.1 N HCl and autoclaved for 30 min at 121–123 °C. Alternatively, the extraction may be carried out using a boiling water bath (1 h with frequent shaking) or by refluxing for 45 min (Pearson, 1967b).

Precipitation of proteinaceous material

The proteinaceous material is precipitated by pH adjustment to 4.5 (the isoelectric point of many proteins) and removed by filtration.

Oxidation

Most of the interfering fluorescent substances and pigments are irreversibly oxidized by brief (2 min) treatment of the extract with 4% potassium permanganate solution, the excess of which is then rapidly destroyed by the addition of 3% hydrogen peroxide solution. This oxidation step, as applied to food extracts, does not affect the riboflavin present in the assay solution, provided that the fluorescent measurement is carried out immediately afterwards.

Measurement

The total fluorescence of the sample assay solution is measured, after which powdered sodium hydrosulphite (sodium dithionite, $Na_2S_2O_4$) is added to the tube or cuvette, and the solution is measured again to give the residual fluorescence (blank reading). The $Na_2S_2O_4$ reduces the riboflavin to its nonfluorescent leuco base, and therefore the difference in the two readings corrects for the presence of nonreducible interfering pigments and fluorescent substances in the sample assay solution. This technique is not always specific for riboflavin, since some fluorescent compounds may behave like riboflavin, whereas other compounds may become fluorescent after reduction. Such phenomena have been observed for extracts from plant tissues (Koziol, 1971).

The AOAC (1990g) procedure for dry or semi-dry foods is as follows.

The sample is mixed with 0.1 N HCl at a volume in millilitres equal to at least 10 times the dry weight of sample in grams, and then autoclaved for 30 min at 121–123 °C. The cooled digest is adjusted to pH 6.0–6.5 with NaOH solution, followed immediately by the addition of dilute HCl until no further precipitation occurs. The mixture is diluted to a measured volume containing >0.1 μg riboflavin/ml, filtered, and then checked for the absence of dissolved protein by the dropwise addition of HCl. If further precipitation occurs, the pH must be readjusted to the point of maximum precipitation. If no further precipitation occurs, the pH is adjusted with NaOH to 6.8, and the solution is diluted to a final measured volume containing *c.* 0.1 μg riboflavin/ml.

Into a tube or reaction vessel is placed 10 ml of the sample solution, 1 ml of water and 1 ml of acetic acid. The tube contents are mixed, and then 0.5 ml of 4% potassium permanganate solution is added with mixing. After standing for 2 min, 0.5 ml of 3% hydrogen peroxide is added (the permanganate colour must be destroyed within 10 s). The internal standard is prepared in a similar manner, except that the 1 ml of water is replaced by 1 ml of standard riboflavin working solution (1 μg/ml). The fluorescence of the sample and internal standard solutions are measured, after which 20 mg of powdered $Na_2S_2O_4$ is added with mixing, and the solutions are read again within 5 s to give the corresponding blank readings.

The concentration of riboflavin in the original food sample is calculated from the measured fluorescence response of the assay solution relative to that of the internal standard solution.

$$\mu g \text{ riboflavin} = (A - B) \times R \times \text{dilution factor}/(C - A) \times V \times W$$

where A = fluorescence of the sample solution
B = fluorescence of the sample solution after addition of $Na_2S_2O_4$ (sample blank)
C = fluorescence of the sample solution containing added riboflavin (internal standard)
R = riboflavin added (1 μg)
V = volume of sample aliquot (10 ml)
W = sample weight (g)

As a means of eliminating the troublesome generation of oxygen gas, Jacobson (1977) substituted hydroxylamine hydrochloride for the hydrogen peroxide used to destroy the excess permanganate after the oxidation step.

In a rapid procedure for determining added riboflavin in dried milk products (Woodrow, Torrie and Henderson, 1969), samples were acidified to pH 4.2–4.8 and the precipitated proteins were removed by filtration. Fluorescence readings of the filtrates were obtained without further purification. The recoveries of riboflavin added at different levels to skimmed milk powder were 90.7–98.8%. Rashid and Potts (1980) removed the protein from milk and milk products by a single filtration step after treatment with acidified lead acetate solution. The addition of ethanol to 2% partially skimmed chocolate milk and nonfat dry milk improved recoveries.

Lumiflavin fluorescence method

Lumiflavin, obtained from riboflavin by photolysis in alkaline medium, is soluble in chloroform and barely soluble in water. This property enables lumiflavin to be separated from many potentially interfering substances, and hence imparts a high specificity for its fluorimetric measurement. The method based upon this principle is also more sensitive than measurement of the native fluorescence of riboflavin. In a procedure described by Strohecker and Henning (1966) food samples are extracted by autoclaving for 30 min. with 0.1 N HCl, after which the digest is buffered to pH 4.5 and treated with diastase. It is then cooled to room temperature, diluted with water and filtered. The filtrate is shaken with chloroform to remove any chloroform-soluble impurities that may be present, and the mixture is centrifuged. Concentrated NaOH solution is added to the clear aqueous layer and the alkaline solution (of pH 10–12) is diluted so that a range of aliquots contains 2 to 20 μg of riboflavin. The solutions are irradiated, then immediately acidified with glacial acetic acid and extracted with chloroform. The chloroform extracts are dried over anhydrous sodium sulphate and measured fluorimetrically.

5.5.4 FLUORIMETRIC DETERMINATION OF VITAMIN B_6

Vitamin B_6 constitutes pyridoxine (PN), pyridoxal (PL), pyridoxamine (PM) and their corresponding phosphorylated analogues PNP, PLP and PMP. Open-column chromatographic techniques using ion exchange resins have been developed for the separation of some or all of the six B_6 vitamers extracted from biological tissues with deproteinizing agents (e.g. TCA, metaphosphoric acid and perchloric acid) that do not hydrolyse the phosphorylated vitamers (Sauberlich, 1967; Loo and Cort, 1972). With the exception of PLP, all of the B_6 vitamers exhibit measurable fluorescence and can be estimated by direct fluorimetry. PLP can be oxidized by the catalytic action of cyanide to 4-pyridoxic acid 5′-phosphate, which also exhibits measurable fluorescence (Ohishi and Fukui, 1968). The methodology involved in this approach is somewhat laborious and the information provided is more applicable to clinical analysis than to food analysis.

The general strategy in food analysis is to hydrolyse the phosphorylated vitamin B_6 compounds by autoclaving with strong acid, and then to separate the PL, PN and PM vitamers chromatographically. The earlier work discussed in this section utilizes ion exchange resins packed into open columns, but HPLC permits the use of alternative column packings. Fluorimetric measurement of each vitamer can then be performed directly, or indirectly by forming a fluorophore such as 4-pyridoxic acid lactone (Figure 5.6). This compound exhibits a fluorescence intensity approximately 1000 times that of PN, PL or PM under defined measurement conditions (Toepfer and Polansky, 1964). In the anion form at pH 8–13, 4-pyridoxic acid lactone displays excitation and emission maxima at 360 nm and 430 nm, respectively (Bridges, Davies and Williams, 1966).

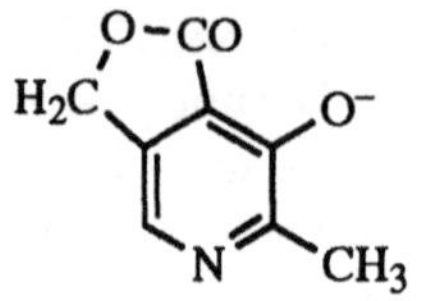

Figure 5.6 Structure of 4-pyridoxic acid lactone (anion form).

4-Pyridoxic acid lactone fluorescence method

The first published methods for the fluorimetric determination of vitamin B_6 in foods (Fujita, Fujita and Fujino, 1955a,b; Fujita, Matsuura and Fujino, 1955) involved acid hydrolysis of the food samples, chromatographic purification, chemical conversion of the eluted vitamers to 4-pyridoxic acid, and acid treatment of this intermediate to form the lactone derivative. Different pretreatment procedures were necessary to selectively determine each of the vitamers. PN was eluted from an activated Decalso ion exchange column and oxidized with potassium permanganate to 4-pyridoxic acid. PM was converted to PN by deamination with nitrous acid before Declaso chromatography, and calculated by subtracting the PN value of the unconverted fraction from that of the converted fraction. PL was eluted from an Amberlite IR-112 ion exchange column and oxidized with ammoniacal silver to 4-pyridoxic acid.

The procedure described by Fujita, Matsuura and Fujino (1955) for determining PN was adapted by Hennessy *et al.* (1960) to the analysis of white flour enriched by the addition of PN.HCl, as well as bread made from this flour. Modifications included an additional enzymatic (Mylase) digestion step after acid hydrolysis. A simplified modification of the Hennessy method was applied to PN.HCl-enriched foods in general (Strohecker and Henning, 1966). Ion exchange purification of the extract was not always adequate, and in these cases the alternative use of thin-layer chromatography was suggested.

In the fluorimetric procedures of Fujita, Fujita and Fujino (1955a,b) and Fujita, Matsuura and Fujino (1955), column chromatography was used to remove interfering substances, and not to separate the B_6 vitamers. However, MacArthur and Lehmann (1959) obtained variable results using the Fujita procedures if any B_6 vitamers, other than the one specifically being determined, were present during the oxidation reaction. These researchers developed a new chromatographic procedure using a strong acid cation exchanger (Dowex AG 50W-X8 resin) to obtain the complete separation and quantitative recovery of PN, PM and PL, which permitted their individual fluorimetric determination after conversion to 4-pyridoxic acid lactone. The average conversion of PN to the lactone was 26% and that of PL was 67%. These yields were consistent within a set and were fairly reproducible from day to day. When the Fujita fluorimetric procedures using Dowex chromatography were applied to extracts of food samples, the fluorescence of substances other than B_6 vitamers in the eluted fractions interfered with the assay (Toepfer, MacArthur and Lehmann, 1960).

Toepfer and Polansky (1964) proposed alternative methods for converting B_6 vitamers to the 4-pyridoxic acid lactone fluorophore based on the cyanide-catalysed oxidation of PL to the lactone first reported by Bonavita (1960) and elucidated by Ohishi and Fukui (1968). Hydrolysed food extracts were fractionated on Dowex AG 50W-X8 ion exchange columns as described by Toepfer and Lehmann (1961). The resin, prepared in the potassium form, was rinsed with hot 0.01 M potassium acetate at pH 4.5 before addition of the extract. The B_6 vitamers were retained on the column, which was washed with hot 0.02 M potassium acetate at pH 5.5. The PL, PN and PM vitamers were eluted separately, in that order, with two 50-ml portions of the following solutions: boiling 0.04 M potassium acetate at pH 6.0 (PL), boiling 0.1 M potassium acetate at pH 7.0 (PN), and boiling 1.0 M potassium chloride/0.1 M K_2HPO_4 at pH 8.0 (PM). This chromatographic technique was adopted as Final Action in 1975 by the AOAC for the microbiological determination of PN, PL and PM in food extracts (Toepfer and Polansky, 1970; AOAC, 1990h). PM was determined by Al^{3+}-catalysed transamination to PL with sodium glyoxylate, and calculated by subtracting the PL (unconverted) value from the converted value. The transamination step was rapid, but the subsequent oxidation of the PL product to the lactone required 2 h to reach completion (Toepfer, Polansky and Hewston, 1961). The third vitamer, PN, was determined in a similar indirect manner after oxidation to PL with manganese dioxide (Polansky, Camarra and Toepfer, 1964). The above procedure was successfully applied to the determination of PL in dried milk; recoveries of PL added to powdered whole milk ranged between 99.0 and 101.4% (Fiedlerová and Davídek, 1974).

Gregory and Kirk (1977) reported that certain Maillard browning pigments, which were formed during the standard autoclave extraction procedure, reacted with cyanide during lactone formation to form highly fluorescent products. These pigments appeared in the PL fraction obtained from the Dowex column by the procedure of Toepfer and Lehmann (1961) and caused erroneously high PL values. Alternative chromatographic elution procedures using Dowex AG 50W-X8 columns were developed to eliminate these interfering compounds from the PL fraction. PL was eluted with 0.15 M phosphate buffer at pH 6.3 from one column, while PN and PM were eluted in a single fraction from a second column with 0.5 M potassium acetate at pH 8.0. All separations were performed at room temperature. The effectiveness of the improved chromatographic procedure was demonstrated on selected food samples (corn flakes, dried infant formula and cured ham).

Direct fluorescence method

The determination of PN in enriched foodstuffs has been carried out by measuring its natural fluorescence (Söderhjelm, 1975). Hydrolysed sample extracts were purified on suitably prepared Dowex AG 50W-X8 ion exchange columns, and the PN fraction (also containing PL and PM) was eluted with 0.2 M ammonia buffer, pH 9.2. The eluate (100 ml) was divided into two equal portions, and the fluorescence of one portion was measured to give the uncorrected PN reading. The blank reading was obtained after addition of solid sodium tetraborate to the second portion of eluate (excess borate quenches the fluorescence of PN). The interference of PL and PM was less than 5% for each when they were present in equimolar amounts to PN. Riboflavin, which is the only other water-soluble vitamin that interferes, was removed by the ion exchange chromatography. The practical working range for the method was 0.1–20 μg PN/ml, which was sensitive enough to assay PN in the samples tested (enriched wheat flours, macaroni and an infant feeding formula). The overall recovery of PN added to wheat flour was 97 ± 6%. The PN values obtained were lower than those obtained with the microbiological assay using *Saccharomyces carlsbergensis*. This was attributed to the latter assay giving an approximately equal response to PN, PL and PM, as opposed to the specific response to PN with the fluorimetric method.

5.5.5 FLUORIMETRIC DETERMINATION OF VITAMIN C

A fluorimetric method for determining microgram quantities of total vitamin C (ascorbic acid plus dehydroascorbic acid) in pharmaceutical preparations, beverages and special dietary foods has been described by Deutsch and Weeks (1965). The method involves the oxidation of ascorbic acid to dehydroascorbic acid with active charcoal, and subsequent reaction with *o*-phenylenediamine (OPDA) to form a fluorescent quinoxaline derivative. The blank reveals any fluorescence due to interfering substances, and is prepared by complexing the oxidized vitamin with boric acid to prevent the formation of the quinoxaline derivative.

The method shows a high degree of specificity. Deutsch and Weeks (1965) ascertained that a substance will only interfere in the assay if all of the following conditions are satisfied. (1) The substance must have α-diketo groups, which react with the OPDA under the assay conditions. (2) The excitation and emission wavelengths of the quinoxaline derivative must be within the regions prescribed for the assay. (3) It must contain adjacent *cis* hydroxyl groups, which react with the boric acid solution to form a complex. Additionally, the substance must be present in the sample assay solution in sufficient quantity to have an effect. Of a large number of possibly interfering substances tested (Deutsch and Weeks, 1965; Deutsch, 1967), no individual compound was found which satisfied all of the above criteria. The procedure was therefore judged to be suitable for samples containing large amounts of reducing substances. An additional advantage is its ability to cope with highly coloured materials. Christie (1975) reported from the Laboratory of the Government Chemist in the UK that the method could be applied successfully to a wide range of foodstuffs, including liver, milk, fresh and canned fruit, raw and cooked vegetables and potato powder. However, Augustin, Beck and Marousek (1981) obtained unrealistically high vitamin C values with the fluorimetric method in the analysis of processed potato products.

The Deutsch and Weeks (1965) method has been tested collaboratively using a modified DCPIP titrimetric procedure and the 2,4-dinitrophenylhydrazine (DNPH) colorimetric method as comparative assays (Deutsch, 1967). It was concluded that the fluorimetric method is suitable for the determination of vitamin C activity of foods and pharmaceutical preparations, and that the method is less susceptible to interference than are the other two assays. The fluorimetric method showed less variability than the analogous DNPH method, besides being less time-consuming and less tedious. Consequently, the fluorimetric method has been adopted as Final Action by the AOAC (AOAC, 1990i) for vitamin preparations.

The AOAC (1990i) procedure is as follows.

A 10 mg/100 ml standard solution of ascorbic acid is prepared immediately before use by dissolving 50 mg of pure L-ascorbic acid in 50 ml of extracting solution (8% v/v acetic acid and 3% w/v metaphosphoric acid in water) and then diluting 10 ml to 100 ml with extracting solution. Solid food samples are blended with extracting solution, and then diluted with extracting solution to give an estimated ascorbic acid concentration of about 100 μg/ml. Liquid samples are diluted with extracting solution to give a similar concentration of ascorbic acid. The final volume of this sample assay solution is designated as *V* ml. One hundred millilitre volumes of the standard and sample assay solutions are shaken with 2 g of acid-washed charcoal, and then filtered. Five-millilitre aliquots of each filtrate are transferred to separate 100-ml volumetric flasks containing 5 ml of freshly prepared boric acid/sodium acetate solution (3 g of boric acid dissolved in 100 ml of 50% w/v sodium acetate). The solutions, which are designated as standard blank or sample blank solutions, are allowed to stand for

15 min with occasional swirling. (Note: Christie (1975) reported that at least 30 min standing was required for the complexing reaction between dehydroascorbic acid and boric acid to be practically complete.) During the standing period, 5 ml of each filtrate is transferred to a 100-ml volumetric flask containing 5 ml of 50% w/v sodium acetate and about 75 ml of water, and then diluted to volume with water. Two-millilitre aliquots of each solution are transferred to each of three test tubes, which are designated as standard or sample tubes. After the 15-min standing, the blank solutions are diluted to volume with water. Two-millilitre aliquots of each solution are transferred to each of three test tubes, which are designated as standard blank or sample blank tubes. To all of the tubes is added 5 ml of freshly prepared OPDA reagent (0.02% w/v OPDA hydrochloride in water). The tube contents are mixed and allowed to stand for 35 min at room temperature, protected from light. The fluorescence of each tube is measured using a spectrophotofluorimeter set at the wavelength maxima of 350 nm excitation and 430 nm emission. Alternatively, a fluorimeter fitted with the appropriate filters can be used. The readings from each triplicate set of tubes are averaged.

The concentration of total vitamin C (ascorbic acid plus dehydroascorbic acid) in the sample is calculated thus:

$$\text{mg vitamin C per g (or per ml) of sample} = (C - D) \times S \times V/(A - B) \times 100 \times E$$

where A = fluorescence of standard tube
B = fluorescence of standard blank tube
C = fluorescence of sample tube
D = fluorescence of sample blank tube
$S/100$ = standard (10 mg ascorbic acid standard per 100 ml)
V = volume (ml) of initial sample assay solution
E = sample weight (g) or sample volume (ml)

The AOAC fluorimetric method has been extended and modified by Weeks and Deutsch (1967) to permit the independent determination of ascorbic acid and erythorbic acid. Sample extracts and standards are subjected to chromatography on silicic acid-impregnated glass fibre paper developed with water-saturated methyl ethyl ketone. The isomers are separated in 25 min, with R_f values of 0.52 for ascorbic acid and 0.63 for erythorbic acid. The spots are visualized by spraying with DCPIP solution, and then cut out of the chromatogram in the form of discs. The acids are eluted from the discs by immersion in the acetic acid/metaphosphoric acid extracting solution. The oxidation step is performed using DCPIP solution rather than active carbon, and the excess DCPIP is extracted with xylene. The OPDA reagent (0.01% w/v) is added to the aqueous extract, and the fluorescence is measured after the 35-min development period.

5.6 CONTINUOUS-FLOW ANALYSIS FOR THE DETERMINATION OF THIAMIN, RIBOFLAVIN, NIACIN AND VITAMIN C

5.6.1 PRINCIPLES OF CONTINUOUS-FLOW ANALYSIS

Continuous-flow analysis has been used to automate the chemical stages of the AOAC fluorimetric methods for thiamin, riboflavin and vitamin C, and the AOAC colorimetric method for niacin. The modified AOAC procedures reviewed by Roy and Conetta (1976) and Roy (1979) utilize the Technicon AutoAnalyzer II modular system, which was introduced commercially in 1957 for use in clinical analysis. Within this system, the chemical reactions take place in a continuously flowing stream segmented by air bubbles to limit sample dispersion and to promote mixing of sample with diluent or reagent by so-called bolus flow. The mixing is enhanced by arrangement of the tubing as a horizontally orientated helical coil. For some applications, a dialyser is incorporated into the system. A peristaltic proportioning pump moves sample (or standard) and reagents through the system to the photometric or fluorimetric detector. The concentration of reaction product corresponding to a state of chemical equilibrium is recorded as a flat-topped profile, the height of which can be compared with that of a standard to give the analyte concentration (Snyder *et al.*, 1976). Segmented-flow methods are usually operated at sampling rates of 30–60/h.

A more recent innovation is flow-injection analysis, in which there is no air segmentation and it is not necessary for a state of chemical equilibrium to be reached. In flow-injection analysis, the sample is introduced into the carrier stream as a discrete plug, and the presence of a sample–carrier interface allows diffusion-controlled dispersion of the sample as it is swept through narrow-bore tubing to create a concentration gradient. The flow-through detector monitors the change in concentration of the reaction product, which is displayed as a well-defined peak. Quantification of analyte concentration can be achieved by comparing the peak height of the sample with that of a standard. In practice, the area of the peak is measured by integration, since the peak width will not vary significantly. Flow-injection systems permit faster sampling rates and consume less reagent than comparable segmented-flow methods. The technique depends on precise sample injection, reproducible timing and controlled sample dispersion. These features preclude the requirement for reaching the state of chemical equilibrium, since the residence time of the sample in the analytical system is constant. Optimization of a flow-injection system for a given application is achieved by empirical selection of manifold design (tubing bore size and length), sample and reagent volume, and flow rate (Betteridge,

1978; Ranger, 1981). Application of flow-injection analysis to vitamin assays in foods has so far been limited to the determination of ascorbic acid.

5.6.2 APPLICATIONS

Because the extraction of the vitamins from foods must be performed manually, the modified AOAC methods can only be truly described as semi-automated procedures. Comparison of results obtained by semi-automated and corresponding manual procedures show overall good agreement. As well as reducing the labour requirement, the automation significantly improves the precision of reactions in which timing and reagent volume are critical, such as the chemical oxidation of thiamin to thiochrome. Osborne and Tyson (1988) have reviewed the principles, instrumentation and techniques of flow-injection analysis, and considered the scope of its actual and potential applications in food and beverage analysis.

Thiamin

Segmented-flow analysis has been used to automate the oxidation reaction and subsequent steps of the AOAC fluorimetric procedure at a sampling rate of 30/h (Kirk, 1974, 1977; Ribbron, Stevenson and Kirk, 1977; Pelletier and Madère, 1975). Partial separation of thiamin from extraneous substances was achieved by on-line dialysis (Roy and Conetta, 1976), and interferences from the remaining impurities were corrected by measuring the blank of the sample solution. Examination of the manual extraction stage (Pelletier and Madère, 1977) revealed that acid digestion before enzymatic hydrolysis can cause lower yields of thiamin from fish and from certain non-processed meat such as beefsteak. Losses of thiamin incurred during the separation of insoluble matter from certain fruits was prevented by addition of ethylene glycol monomethyl ether (Pelletier and Madère, 1977). Kirk (1974) observed that the chromatographic purification step, normally used for sample clean-up, was not required for most samples. When high blank values interfered with the assay results, interference was eliminated by extracting the sample with water-saturated isobutanol before automated analysis. Only sample extracts containing chocolate were found to require the use of column chromatography (Kirk, 1977). Pelletier and Madère (1975) included the chromatographic purification step in the extraction procedure, although they observed that with certain foods it appeared to be unnecessary. Soliman (1981) used neither column chromatography nor isobutanol washing to clean up sample extracts. Instead, extracts were analysed before and after the addition of benzenesulphonyl chloride, which inhibited thiochrome formation and provided a more representative blank based on the fluorescence of all the reactants except thiochrome.

Riboflavin

The AOAC fluorimetric method for determining riboflavin has been semi-automated using segmented-flow analysis to perform in-line dialysis, and permanganate oxidative clean-up after manual acid digestion of food samples (Egberg and Potter, 1975). Excess permanganate was reduced with sodium bisulphite, and metaphosphoric acid was added as a manganese-sequestering ligand to prevent the precipitation and build-up of manganese dioxide in the reagent lines. A collaborative study (Egberg, 1979a) led to the adoption of the method by the AOAC as Final Action in 1982 (AOAC, 1990j). Roy, Salpeter and Dunmire (1976) evaluated a urea–acid system as an extraction medium for riboflavin from a wide variety of food products. Riboflavin present in hamburger and pork was extracted by autoclaving with urea and 1 N HCl for 30 min at 121 °C; fruits and all other food samples tested required urea in the presence of 0.1 N H_2SO_4 and 0.2 N H_2SO_4, respectively. Dunbar and Stevenson (1979) reported the simultaneous determination of thiamin and riboflavin in infant formula products using segmented-flow analysis and a common extraction procedure involving both acid and enzymatic hydrolysis.

Russell and Vanderslice (1992) applied flow-injection analysis to the standard AOAC fluorimetric method (AOAC, 1990g) using $Na_2S_2O_4$ dissolved in 0.4% sodium acetate as the blank determination, as specified in the AOAC semi-automated method for total riboflavin (AOAC, 1990j).

Niacin

The AOAC colorimetric method using cyanogen bromide (König reaction) has been semi-automated using segmented-flow analysis with on-line dialysis for the determination of nicotinic acid (representing total niacin) released from food samples by autoclaving with calcium hydroxide solution (Egberg, Potter and Honold, 1974). A reference flow cell was employed to eliminate blank colour interference. The semi-automated procedure was shown to compare favourably with a specific microbiological assay for 63 different food products (r = 0.9937). The method has been adopted as Final Action by the AOAC for the determination of niacin in cereal products (Gross, 1975; AOAC, 1990k) and foods and feeds (Egberg, 1979b; AOAC, 1990l). Roy and Merten

(1983) extracted cereals and other selected food products by autoclaving with 1 N HCl in the presence of urea for 30 min at 121 °C.

van Gend (1973) utilized segmented-flow analysis with on-line dialysis to determine free (added) nicotinic acid extracted from minced meat with water. The nicotinic acid was reacted with cyanogen chloride generated *in situ* using potassium cyanide and chloramine-T. The colorimetric reaction took place in an acetone/water medium in which, at the detection wavelength of 470 nm, there was no significant interference from nicotinamide. The on-line generation of cyanogen chloride using the Technicon AutoAnalyzer II system has been investigated by Ge, Oman and Ebert (1986) and shown to represent a definite improvement in the safe handling of the reagents used for niacin determination.

Vitamin C

Segmented-flow analysis has been utilized for modifying the AOAC microfluorimetric procedure for total vitamin C using DCPIP (Kirk and Ting, 1975) or *N*-bromosuccinimide (Roy, Conetta and Salpeter, 1976) as the oxidizing agent instead of activated charcoal. Roy, Conetta and Salpeter (1976) reported that cocoa and chocolate, known to contain significant amounts of reductic acids, reductones and alkaloids, required prior filtration through charcoal to remove interfering fluorescent compounds. On the basis of this observation, Egberg, Potter and Heroff (1977) proposed a semi-automated method involving simultaneous oxidation and clean-up with charcoal prior to automated analysis. Dunmire *et al.* (1979) compared the methods of Roy, Conetta and Salpeter (1976) and Egberg, Potter and Heroff (1977) and concluded that the latter method, with its potential for sample clean-up, was more appropriate for the majority of food commodities analysed. Following a collaborative study (DeVries, 1983), the semi-automated microfluorimetric procedure was adopted as Final Action by the AOAC in 1985 (AOAC, 1990m).

Lázaro, Luque de Castro and Valcárcel (1987) proposed a flow-injection method for the simultaneous determination of ascorbic acid and sulphite in soft drinks based on the reaction with chloramine-T. The sample, dissolved in an acidic medium, is injected into the chloramine-T stream after merging with a starch–iodide stream. Iodide forms HI in an acidic medium, and this subsequently reacts with chloramine-T to liberate iodine. The iodine oxidizes ascorbic acid and sulphite and, as soon as these reducing analytes have disappeared, the remaining iodine binds to starch to form the starch–iodine complex, whose absorbance is monitored at 581 nm. Maximum absorbance is obtained with the blank sample because no iodide is consumed when the reducing analytes are absent; thus the difference in absorbance between the blank and sample solutions is related to the concentration of analyte. The absorbance due to sulphite alone is determined by simultaneously injecting a sample previously mixed with NaOH to destroy the ascorbic acid. The ascorbic acid content can then be calculated by subtracting the result of the NaOH-treated sample from the untreated sample.

Using simple flow-injection apparatus, Elgilany Elbashier and Greenway (1990) determined ascorbic acid in beverages by monitoring fluorimetrically the reduction of cerium (IV) to cerium (III) by the action of ascorbic acid in acidic conditions. Vanderslice and Higgs (1989) combined a flow-injection system with a robotic extraction procedure to automate the determination of total vitamin C in fruits, juices and vegetables from after sample weighing to final quantification. The procedure was based on the AOAC microfluorimetric method, except that mercuric chloride was used as the oxidizing agent.

Greenway and Ongomo (1990) devised a flow-injection system for determining ascorbic acid in fruit and vegetable juices using an amperometric detector and an on-line column containing ascorbate oxidase immobilized on activated Sepharose 4B. On passage through the immobilized enzyme, a fraction of the ascorbic acid was converted into the electrochemically inactive dehydroascorbic acid, and the decrease in signal compared with that obtained using a blank (no enzyme) column was measured. The signal from the blank column represented total oxidizable material, while the signal from the enzyme column represented total oxidizable material less ascorbic acid. The difference between the two signals therefore gave the ascorbic acid content, with the enzyme reaction providing the selectivity. Glucose, oxalic acid, citric acid and tartaric acid did not seriously interfere, even in great excess, while interference from copper was eliminated by addition of EDTA. The immobilized enzyme was used continuously each day for a period of 3 weeks without significant loss in activity.

5.7 GAS CHROMATOGRAPHIC METHODS FOR THIAMIN, NIACIN, VITAMIN B_6, PANTOTHENIC ACID AND VITAMIN C

5.7.1 PRINCIPLE OF GAS–LIQUID CHROMATOGRAPHY (GLC)

GLC is a technique for separating volatile substances by passing a stream of inert gas (mobile phase) over a film of nonvolatile organic liquid (stationary phase) contained within a heated column. The stationary phase is either coated onto a porous support material (packed-bed column) or onto the wall of a capillary column (wall-coated open tubular column). The sample extract is introduced at the column inlet, and the volatile components are retained as a result of selective molecular interactions between the components and the stationary phase. Separation is effected as a consequence of the numerous sorption–desorption cycles that take place as the volatile sample material passes through the column. Detection of the separated components is carried out by continuous monitoring of the gaseous column effluent.

5.7.2 COLUMN TECHNOLOGY

The published GLC applications for those water-soluble vitamins discussed in this text have utilized packed columns in which the support material is diatomaceous earth. The surfaces of untreated diatomaceous earth are covered with silanol (≡Si–OH) groups, which function as active sites in promoting severe peak tailing of polar compounds. The diatomaceous earth is therefore deactivated before coating with stationary phases of low or intermediate polarity by treatment with dimethyldichlorosilane (DMCS) or similar silylating reagent. Typical packed column dimensions are 2–4 mm internal diameter (i.d.) and 1.5 m up to 3 m or 4 m length. The chief advantages of packed columns over capillary columns are high sample capacity, sample ruggedness, ease of preparation and low cost.

The stationary phases employed in water-soluble vitamin assays are either polysiloxanes or polyethylene glycol. The backbone of a polysiloxane is –Si–O–Si–, with the other two valencies (not shown) of the silicon atom satisfied by different R groups, which impart different polarities to the liquid phase. Of the nonpolar dimethyl polysiloxanes, SE-30 and OV-1 are high molecular weight ($>10^6$) gums, and SP-2100 and OV-101 are oils of lower molecular weight. OV-17 is a phenylmethyl (50% phenyl) oil of intermediate polarity, while Carbowax 20M is a polyethylene glycol gum of higher polarity. The terminal silanol groups of the polysiloxane phases are end-capped with a silylating reagent to maximize thermal stability.

Open-tubular capillary columns provide superior separating efficiencies compared with packed columns, and the sharper peaks facilitate a more accurate integration, as well as a greatly improved detectability. The stationary liquid phase is coated as a film upon the inner deactivated surface of a fused silica capillary column, leaving a lumen extending throughout the length of the column. The efficiency is therefore governed solely by the rate of mass transfer in the stationary phase, and the absence of a support material leads to an improved inertness. Another feature is a low stationary phase bleed, which is an advantage in temperature-programmed separations. The column is coated on the outside with a protective layer of polyimide resin to impart mechanical strength and flexibility. The standard capillary columns are of 0.25 or 0.32 mm i.d. and 10 m up to 50 m or even 100 m in length, with a film thickness of up to 1 μm (typically 0.25 μm). Such columns require special injection systems to cope with the limited sample capacity.

Since 1983, wide-bore, thick-film capillary columns have become available which bridge the gap between capillary and packed column gas chromatography. The combination of increased i.d. and increased film thickness permits a significant increase in the sample capacity, allowing the use of a simple on-column injector (as used for packed columns) with its inherent ease of operation and quantitative assay. The column i.d. is most commonly 0.53 mm, and cross-linked nonpolar polysiloxane phases can be coated in thicknesses of 1–8 μm in 1-μm increments. The immobilized stationary phase is non-extractable, which allows the column to be flushed with pure solvents to remove contaminants, nonvolatiles and pyrolysis products. A 10-m wide-bore capillary column approximates the sample capacity and separation efficiency of a 1.8 m × 2 mm i.d. packed column with a 3–5% phase loading at the same operating conditions (Wiedemer, McKinley and Rendl, 1986). However, when the carrier gas flow rate is optimized for the capillary tubing, the wide-bore column produces far superior separations, with an increased speed of analysis. The low pressure drop across the column offers a very practical way to increase the efficiency several-fold, simply by increasing the column length.

5.7.3 DETECTORS

The detector monitors the gaseous column effluent and measures compositional variations attributable to eluted components. The output signal is produced in response to the mass or concentration of the eluted compound passing through the detector. The linear range refers to the range of solute concentration over which the detector response is linear, from the minimum detectable level (two or three times the noise level) to the upper concentration, which produces a departure from linearity of about 5%. Different compounds can produce signals of varying magnitude for a given concentration, so the signal observed needs to be corrected by applying a response factor to obtain accurate ratios of components in a mixture. For a mass-sensitive detector, such as the flame ionization detector, the response factor is expressed as the ratio of the peak area to the mass of solute injected. Response factors are frequently determined using an internal standard as a marker. A known amount of the internal standard is added to a standard mixture of all the components of interest, and the response factors relative to the internal standard are calculated. The same amount of internal standard is added to each sample, and the peak areas are corrected by dividing the areas by the response factors.

Three types of detector employed for water-soluble vitamin determinations are ionization detectors; they are the flame ionization detector (FID), the nitrogen–phosphorus detector (NPD) and the electron capture detector (ECD). A flame photometric detector (FPD) has also been employed. Interfacing a gas chromatograph with a mass spectrometer (GC-MS) provides information on the molecular weight and structure of the compound, in addition to its quantitative detection.

The flame ionization detector

In the FID the carrier gas emerging from the column outlet is mixed with hydrogen. This mixture is then combined with air and burned at a small metal jet that is insulated from the body of the detector. Organic compounds eluted from the column are ionized in the flame. A collector electrode situated a few millimetres above the flame is maintained at a negative potential with respect to the jet. The current produced by the accelerated movement of ions to the collector electrode is proportional to the mass of ions present in the flame and this, in turn, is proportional to the number of carbon atoms present. The current is converted to a voltage, which is amplified for output to a chart recorder or a data-handling system.

The FID is a rugged detector which has a high sensitivity and shows similar response factors for all compounds which contain carbon–hydrogen bonds. It is stable to small changes in operational parameters (temperature, carrier gas flow rate and pressure) and has little or no response to the common carrier gas impurities (water and CO_2). The detector has an exceptional linear response range of up to seven orders of magnitude of solute concentration.

The nitrogen–phosphorus detector

This detector is a modified FID in which a stable population of alkali metal ions generated by flameless thermionic ionization interacts with pyrolysis products of nitrogen- and phosphorus-containing compounds to produce electrons. The collection of electrons creates a current; hence the selective response.

When compared with a standard FID, the NPD is approximately 50 times more sensitive for nitrogen-containing compounds and 500 times more sensitive for phosphorus compounds. The linear response range is four or five orders of magnitude of solute concentration.

The electron capture detector

In the ECD a stream of beta-particles from a radioactive source (usually ^{63}Ni) is used to bombard the neutral molecules of carrier gas passing through the detector cell. The secondary electrons produced by these collisions are collected by applying an electric potential between the source and a collector electrode, thereby establishing a standing current. When an electrophilic compound enters the cell it captures an electron to produce a negative ion. These negative ions take longer to migrate to the collector electrode than do the electrons, and therefore have a higher probability of recombining with positive ions before reaching the electrode. As a result, the standing current of the detector is decreased during the elution of the electrophilic compound, and it is this change which is displayed as a peak on the recorder or integrator.

The ECD is selective for the detection of electrophilic compounds such as alkyl halides, conjugated carbonyls, nitriles and nitrates, and has a high sensitivity in the order of 10^{-12} g/s. The linear response range for an ECD with a modified pulsed-sampling technique for measuring the thermal electron concentration in the detector cell is four or five orders of magnitude of solute concentration (Poole and Schuette, 1984). As the response factors cover a wide range for electrophilic compounds, each compound to be quantified must have an individual calibration curve.

Gas chromatography–mass spectrometry

The eluted compounds are bombarded with high-energy electrons in an ionization chamber under vacuum, which causes the molecules to fragment. The fragments are directed to a mass analyser, where they are separated on the basis of their mass/charge ratio. The mass spectrum is presented as a bar diagram in the normalized form, i.e. with the intensity of the most abundant ion taken as 100.

The flame photometric detector

The FPD offers selectivity for sulphur and phosphorus compounds, and has been applied to the determination of thiamin in foods. Excited sulphur- and phosphorus-containing species generated by the combustion of eluted organic compounds containing these elements exhibit characteristic emission spectra on return to the electronic ground state. The emitted radiation is reflected through an appropriate band-pass filter (392 nm for sulphur and 526 nm for phosphorus) to a photomultiplier tube, which detects and amplifies the emission. Dual-channel FPDs are available which can detect both sulphur and phosphorus simultaneously, although it is necessary to separate the sulphur-containing compounds from the phosphorus compounds. At optimum carrier gas flow rates, the minimum detectable level for phosphorus is given as 0.1–2 pg/s, and for sulphur as 2–50 pg/s. Phosphorus compounds generally give a linear response over four orders of magnitude, but the sulphur signal is often nonlinear (Ravindranath, 1989).

5.7.4 DERIVATIZATION TECHNIQUES

A prerequisite for a sample to be analysed by GLC is that the components are sufficiently volatile without decomposing under the conditions of separation. For the water-soluble vitamins the required volatility and stability are achieved either by making a suitable degradation product or preparing a chemical derivative by reaction with a suitable reagent. The most widely used derivatization technique is silylation, whereby a trimethylsilyl (TMS) group is introduced into a wide variety of organic compounds containing −OH, −COOH, −SH, $-NH_2$ and =NH groups. The replacement of active hydrogen by the silyl group reduces the polarity of the compound and decreases the possibility of hydrogen bonding, with the resultant increase in volatility. Furthermore, stability is enhanced by reduction in the number of reactive sites. The trifluoroacetate (TFA) derivative offers the advantage of compatibility with the highly sensitive ECD (Ahuja, 1976).

5.7.5 APPLICATIONS

The chromatographic operating conditions for determining some of the water-soluble vitamins in foods are summarized in Table 5.1.

Thiamin

Attempts to chromatograph TMS and other derivatives of thiamin have been unsuccessful because the derivatives are not sufficiently volatile at normal gas chromatographic operating temperatures, whereas they pyrolyse above 250 °C (Velíšek and Davídek, 1986). The ability of sulphite treatment to quantitatively split the thiamin molecule into substituted pyrimidine and thiazole moieties has been exploited in GLC methods for determining thiamin in food samples (Echols *et al.*, 1983; Echols, Miller and Thompson, 1985; Echols, Miller and Foster, 1986; Velíšek *et al.*, 1986). The thiazole compound 4-methyl-5-(β-hydroxyethyl)-thiazole possesses the necessary attributes of being soluble in organic solvents and sufficiently volatile to permit its direct determination by GLC. The general procedure entails acid and enzyme hydrolysis of the sample, cleavage of thiamin by bisulphite, extraction of the thiazole compound by chloroform, and GLC. The FID provides adequate sensitivity for the analysis of food samples containing relatively large concentrations of thiamin: the NPD is about 1000 times more sensitive and is more selective.

Table 5.1 GLC methods used for the determination of water-soluble vitamins

Compound	Food	Internal standard	Column/ temperature	Stationary phase/ support	Detector	Reference
Thiamin (as thiazole compound)	Pork chops, cornflakes, milk	3-(3-pyridyl)-1-propanol	Glass 1.8 m × 2 mm i.d. 190 °C	5% OV-1 or 5% OV-17 on Chromosorb W-DMCS	NPD	Echols, Miller and Thompson (1985); Echols, Miller and Foster (1986)
Thiamin (as thiazole compound)	Liver, lean pork, skim milk, egg yolk, whole-grain wheat flour, white beans	Not used	Glass 2.4 m × 2 mm i.d. 220 °C	10% Carbowax 20M on Inerton AW	FPD	Velíšek *et al.* (1986) (Figure 5.8)
Nicotinamide (as 3-cyanopyridine)	Meats and meat products	1,2,4-Trichloro-benzene	Glass 2 m × 3 mm i.d. 130 °C	5% OV-17 on Chromosorb W-AW-DMCS	FID	Tanaka *et al.* (1989) (Figure 5.9)
Vitamin B_6 (PN, PM and PL as TFA derivatives)	Enriched white bread, non-fat dry milk, peas	Deoxypyridoxine	Glass 1.54 m × 2 mm i.d. 125 °C	10% SP-1200 on Supelcoport	ECD (^{63}Ni)	Lim *et al.* (1982) (Figure 5.10)
Pantothenic acid (as lactone)	Liver, egg yolk, soybean flour, whole-grain wheat flour, bakers' yeast	Ethyl laurate	Glass 2.4 m × 2 mm i.d. 120–220 °C at 5 °/min	10% Carbowax 20M on Chromaton N-AW-DMCS	FID	Davídek *et al.* (1985) (Figure 5.12)
Ascorbic acid (as TMS ether)	Fortified food products, including instant potatoes, breakfast cereal, infant milk	Glutaric acid	Glass 1.5 m × 2 mm i.d. 60–210 °C at 6 °/min	3% SE-30 on Varaport 30	FID	Schlack (1974) (Figure 5.13)
Ascorbic acid (as TMS ether)	Foods and feed-stuffs	Not used	Glass 1.75 m × 4 mm i.d. 155 °C	3% SE-30 on GasChrom Q	FID	Gerstl and Ranfft (1974)
Ascorbic acid (as TMS ether)	Instant orange powder	Triphenylethylene	Glass 1.5 m × 6 mm i.d. 160 °C	1.5% SE-30 on Chromosorb W-DMCS	FID	Koeppen (1973)

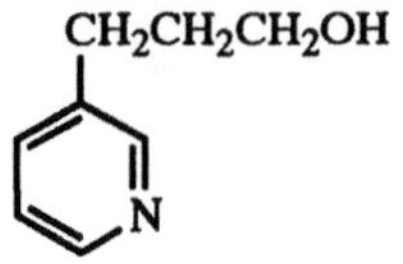

Figure 5.7 Structure of 3-(3-pyridyl)-1-propanol.

Echols, Miller and Thompson (1985) used a pre-extraction internal standard, 3-(3-pyridyl)-1-propanol (Figure 5.7), in a method to determine the thiamin content of hydrolysed extracts of meat (pork chops) and cereals (corn flakes). Meat samples were blended with 0.3 N HCl and internal standard, and then heated to liberate thiamin pyrophosphate from its protein-bound forms. After cooling, adjustment to pH 5 and centrifugation, the enzymes Mylase and papain were added and the resulting mixture was allowed to stand overnight at room temperature. The liberated thiamin was then cleaved by reaction with sodium bisulphite at 100 °C, followed by addition of TCA, additional heating and filtration. The filtrate was extracted with chloroform, and the chloroform extract was evaporated to dryness. The residue was taken up with methanol for analysis by GLC using an NPD and a stationary phase of either 5% OV-1 (nonpolar) or 5% OV-17 (polar). A similar sample pretreatment was adopted for cereals, except that the enzyme treatment was unnecessary, as the nonphosphorylated thiamin predominates. The authors accounted for the different extractabilities of the internal standard and the thiazole compound into chloroform by determining the extraction ratio of each compound from a standard solution. This predetermined ratio, together with the molecular weight ratio of thiamin to thiazole compound, was used in the equation to calculate the thiamin concentration in food samples.

Echols, Miller and Foster (1986) modified the above procedure to determine free (nonphosphorylated) thiamin and total thiamin in milk. Free thiamin was determined by treatment of the milk sample with bisulphite to form the thiazole compound, followed by additional heating with hydrochloric and trichloroacetic acid. This acid treatment served to decompose the bisulphite into sulphur dioxide and water, whilst also precipitating soluble proteins that interfered with the extraction. (A proteinase such as papain was not used in this determination.) Extraction with chloroform was carried out at high pH (>10.5) in order to convert the thiamin phosphates into their anion salts, which cannot be extracted with chloroform. Total thiamin was determined by treatment with Mylase to convert phosphorylated thiamin to free thiamin, followed by bisulphite treatment. The rest of the procedure followed that for quantifying free thiamin.

Velísěk *et al.* (1986) used an FPD to determine thiamin in foods after acid and enzymatic hydrolysis of the sample, and bisulphite treatment to form the thiazole compound. A chromatogram of a lean pork extract is shown in Figure 5.8. The sensitivity of the determination was comparable with that achieved by the AOAC fluorimetric method. The results obtained by the two methods did not significantly differ at a probability level of 99%, the correlation coefficient being $r = 0.992$.

Niacin

No GLC applications have been reported for determining naturally occurring niacin in foods. Nicotinamide, added to meats and meat products to stabilize the red colour (this practice is not permitted in the UK and in certain other countries), has been determined as 3-cyanopyridine after dehydration by heptafluorobutyric anhydride (HFB) (Tanaka *et al.*, 1989). Although nicotinamide can be chromatographed as such, 3-cyanopyridine was found to be over six times more sensitive

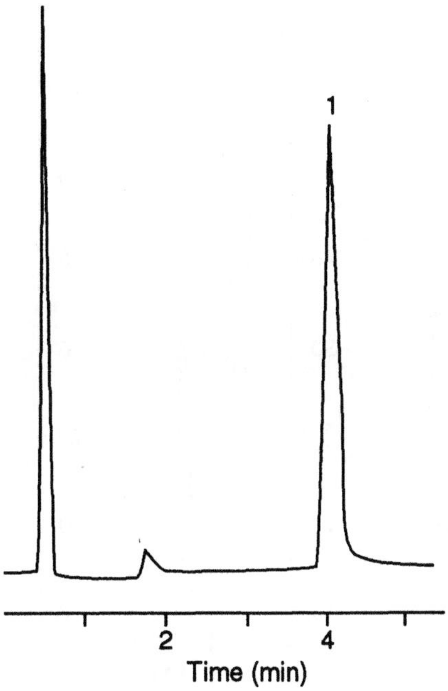

Figure 5.8 GLC determination of thiamin in lean pork after release of the free thiamin by acid and enzyme hydrolysis and bisulphite treatment to form the thiazole compound (peak 1). Glass column, 2.4 m × 2 mm i.d.; column packing, 10% Carbowax 20M on Inerton AW; column temp., 220 °C; FPD (from Velísek *et al.*, 1986).

towards GLC. The procedure involved extraction of the nicotinamide with acetonitrile, evaporation to dryness, and addition to the residue of an internal standard (1,2,4-trichlorobenzene) and HFB. The reaction was completed within 5 min at room temperature. GLC was performed using a stationary phase of 5% OV-17 and an FID (Figure 5.9). The minimum detection limit was 5 ppm and the recovery ranged from 93.4 to 104.6% (average 98.0%).

Vitamin B_6

TMS derivatives are not ideal for the analysis of vitamin B_6-fortified foods, as PN-TMS generally yields two peaks whose relative areas are dependent on the silylation reaction conditions (Korytnyk, Fricke and Paul, 1966). Of the numerous other derivatives that have been

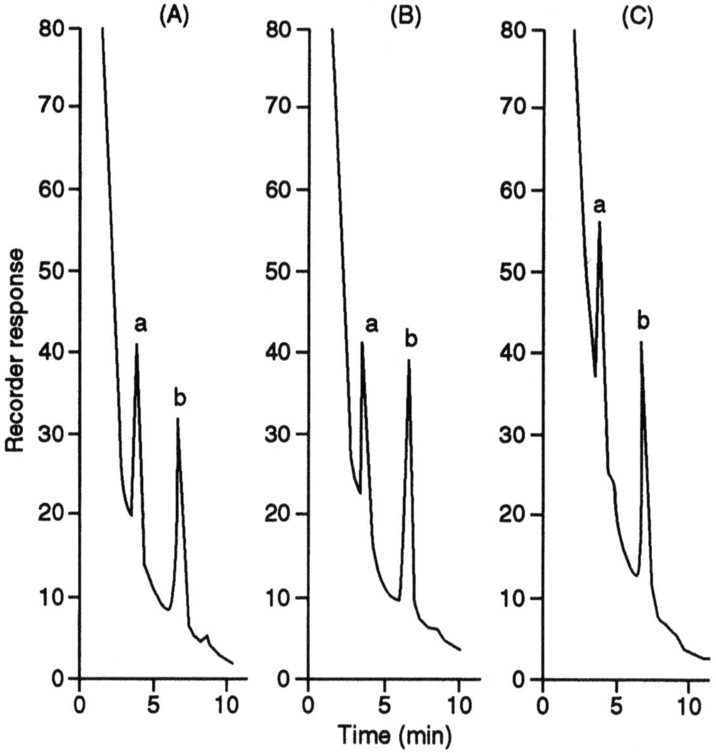

Figure 5.9 GLC determination of nicotinamide in (A) a standard reaction mixture, (B) chicken meat and (C) tuna meat after conversion to 3-cyanopyridine. Peaks: (a) 3-cyanopyridine; (b) 1,2,4-trichlorobenzene (internal standard). Glass column, 2 m × 3 mm i.d.; column packing, 5% OV-17 on Chromosorb W-AW-DMCS 80–100 mesh; column temp., 130 °C; FID (from Tanaka *et al.*, 1989).

investigated (Velíšek and Davídek, 1986), the TFA offers advantages of greater volatility, as well as compatibility with the ECD. A suitable internal standard for chromatographing the TFA derivatives of B_6 vitamers is desoxypyridoxine (Patzer and Hilker, 1977). The derivatizing agent employed is *N*-methyl-bis-trifluoroacetamide (MBTFA), which reacts with primary and secondary amines, and hydroxyl and thiol groups under mild acidic conditions. Lim *et al.* (1982) used this reagent to determine the TFA derivatives of PN, PM and PL in hydrolysed extracts of enriched white bread, non-fat dry milk and peas. The procedure entailed release of the free B_6 vitamers by acid digestion, and enzymatic treatment using α-amylase, pepsin and papain. The filtered solution was passed through an ion exchange column, and then reacted with MBTFA to form the TFA derivatives. Absolute ethanol was then added to convert PL-TFA to its hemiacetal in order to distinguish it from PN-TFA. Analysis was performed using a stationary phase of 10% SP-2100 and a ^{63}Ni ECD. Trifluoroacetylation of PL and PM gave rise to single peaks, whereas the corresponding PN derivative gave rise to two peaks – a major peak closely preceded by a minor peak (Figure 5.10).

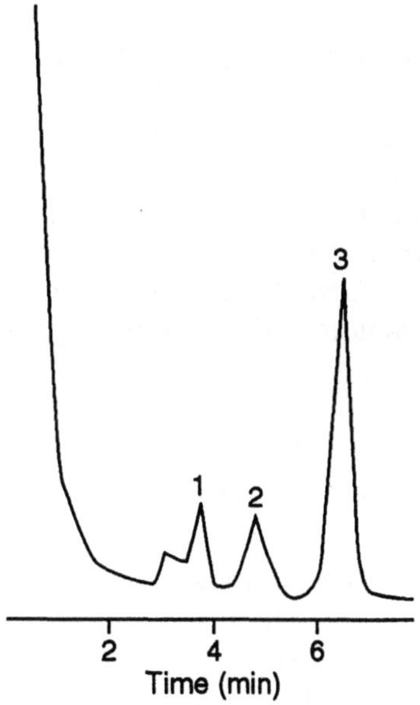

Figure 5.10 GLC determination of vitamin B_6 in non-fat dry milk after release of the free vitamers by acid and enzyme hydrolysis and conversion to their trifluoroacetate (TFA) derivatives. Peaks: (1) PN-TFA; (2) PL-TFA (hemiacetal form); (3) PM-TFA. Glass column, 1.54 m × 2 mm i.d.; column packing, 10% SP-2100 on Supelcoport 80–100 mesh; column temp., 125 °C; ECD (from Lim *et al.*, 1982).

The calibration curve for PN was plotted using the sum of the peak heights. The minimum detectable quantity of all three vitamers was 0.01 ng on-column. Relative standard deviations (duplicate analyses) for total vitamin B_6 in enriched white bread, nonfat dry milk and peas were, respectively, 22.9%, 15.3% and 14.9%.

Pantothenic acid

Salts of pantothenic acid have been analysed by GLC after conversion to volatile acetate, TFA or TMS derivatives (Prosser and Sheppard, 1969, 1971), but such methods are only applicable to relatively pure samples such as pharmaceutical preparations. An alternative approach, which does not involve derivatization, is to chromatograph the pantoyl lactone formed from pantothenic acid by acid hydrolysis (Tarli, Benocci and Neri, 1971; Figure 5.11). This approach is applicable to foodstuffs, because the hydrolysis reaction liberates the lactone from the free and bound pantothenic acid in the food matrix with a recovery of >95% (Velíšek and Davídek, 1986). For the analysis of fresh beef liver, spray-dried egg yolk, soybean flour, whole-grain wheat flour and dried bakers' yeast (Davídek *et al.*, 1985), samples were hydrolysed in dilute hydrochloric acid and the neutralized hydrolysate, after filtration, was extracted with dichloromethane. The combined extracts, to which 50 μg of ethyl laurate was added as an internal standard, were concentrated by rotary evaporation, and then analysed by GLC using a polar stationary phase of 10% Carbowax 20M and an FID. Gas chromatograms of hydrolysed fresh beef liver and whole-grain wheat flour are depicted in Figure 5.12. On comparison of the gas chromatographic results with results obtained by the currently accepted microbiological method, no significant difference was found at the 95% probability level, and the

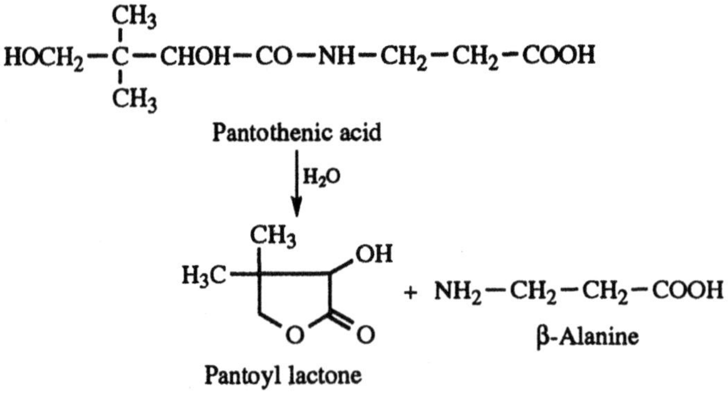

Figure 5.11 Hydrolysis of pantothenic acid.

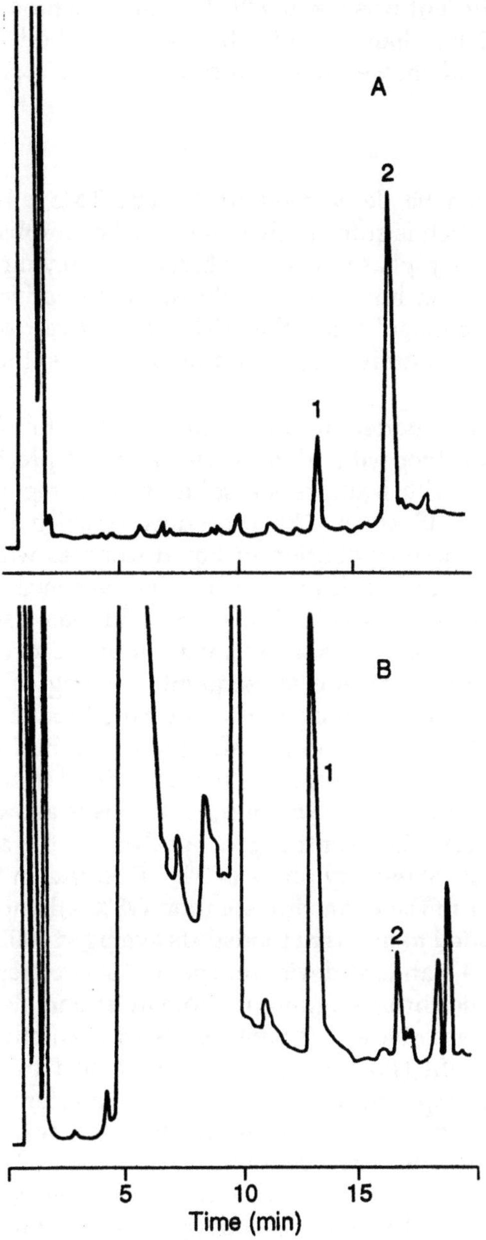

Figure 5.12 GLC determination of pantothenic acid in (A) fresh beef liver and (B) whole-grain wheat flour after formation of the pantoyl lactone by acid hydrolysis. Peaks: (1) ethyl laurate (internal standard); (2) pantoyl lactone. Glass column, 2.4 m × 2 mm i.d.; column packing, 10% Carbowax 20M on Chromaton N-AW-DMCS; column temp., 120–220 °C at 5 °/min; FID (from Davídek *et al.*, 1985).

correlation coefficient was $r = 0.975$. The GLC method was considered to be more reliable than the microbiological method, as it was more rapid, simpler and showed higher reproducibility.

Vitamin C

Ascorbic acid can be derivatized to its tetra-TMS ether (Vecchi and Kaiser, 1967), which is sufficiently volatile to be chromatographed on a nonpolar stationary phase. The feasibility of applying GLC to a food product depends on how successfully the TMS derivative of ascorbic acid can be separated from the TMS derivatives of all the other hydroxylated compounds (sugars and organic acids) that are present in the final extract.

Schlack (1974) reported a procedure suitable for foods in which ascorbic acid, together with other organic acids, is precipitated from an ethanolic extract with lead acetate solution, and regenerated from its lead salt as its TMS ether. The procedure entailed extraction of the homogenized sample or dilution of liquid samples with 95% ethanol, and precipitation of the lead salts in the presence of glutaric acid (internal standard) and Celite 545. Citric acid was also added at this stage (where necessary) to aid precipitation and prevent formation of colloidal suspensions during subsequent washing of the precipitate. After centrifugation, the precipitate was washed sequentially with 95% ethanol and diethyl ether, and the precipitate was broken up and dried for 1 h at 100 °C. The silylating reagent was added to the dried powder plus a drying agent, and the reaction mixture was allowed to digest for 1 h at 55–60 °C and then centrifuged. Analysis of the supernatant was performed using a stationary phase of 3% SE-30 and an FID. Despite the lack of stabilizer in the extracting solution (95% ethanol), recoveries of ascorbic acid added to different foodstuffs averaged 100.1% (range 99.1–103.0%) and the standard deviation (pooled sets of replicate analyses) was ±0.23%. The chromatogram of a tomato extract depicted in Figure 5.13 shows that ascorbic acid is well separated from other organic acids.

Gerstl and Ranfft (1974) extracted ascorbic acid from food samples with 5% metaphosphoric acid, and removed interfering substances by open-column liquid chromatography on cellulose. The fraction containing ascorbic acid was dried by evaporation, and then silylated. The TMS ether of ascorbic acid was determined using a stationary phase of 3% SE-30 and an FID. Total vitamin C activity was determined by reducing dehydroascorbic acid to ascorbic acid with hydrogen sulphide before clean-up by column chromatography.

For the determination of ascorbic acid in instant orange powder, Koeppen (1973) extracted the sample with hot ethanol, and silylated the dried residue in the presence of an internal standard, triphenylethylene

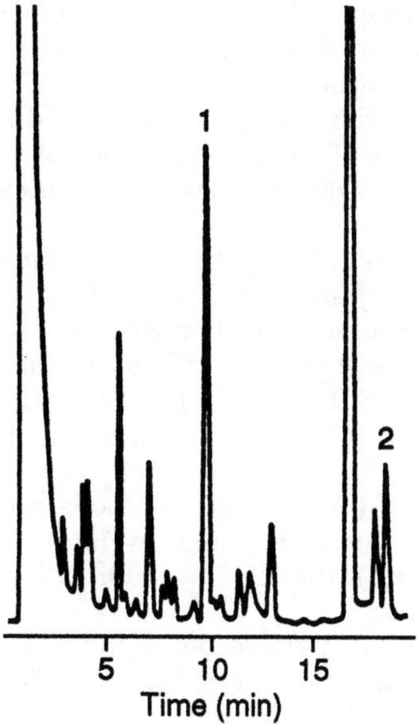

Figure 5.13 GLC determination of ascorbic acid in a tomato extract after regeneration from its lead salt as its trimethylsilyl (TMS) ether. Peaks: (1) glutaric acid-TMS (internal standard); (2) ascorbic acid-TMS. Glass column, 1.5 m × 2 mm i.d.; column packing, 3% SE-30 on Varaport 30 60–80 mesh; column temp., 60–210 °C at 6 °/min; FID. From Schlack, 1974. Reprinted from the *Journal of the AOAC*, Vol. 57, No. 06, pp. 1346–8, 1974. Copyright 1974 by AOAC International.

(TPE). Analysis was carried out using a stationary phase of 1.5% SE-30 and an FID. TMS-ascorbic acid and the internal standard were well separated from the other extract constituents, the order of elution being citric acid, D-fructose, α-D-glucose, ascorbic acid, β-D-glucose, TPE and sucrose. The result obtained for the orange powder (310.4 mg ascorbic acid/100 g) was in good agreement with that obtained by titration with DCPIP (313.8 mg/100 g).

REFERENCES

Ahuja, S. (1976) Derivatization in gas chromatography. *J. Pharm. Sci.*, **65**, 163–82.

AOAC (1990a) Vitamin C (ascorbic acid) in vitamin preparations and juices. 2,6-Dichloroindophenol titrimetric method. Final action 1968. In *AOAC Official Methods of Analysis*, 15th edn (ed. K. Helrich), Association of Official Analytical Chemists, Inc., Arlington, VA, 967.21.

AOAC (1990b) Niacin and niacinamide in drugs, foods and feeds. Colorimetric method. Final action 1962. In *AOAC Official Methods of Analysis*, 15th edn (ed. K. Helrich), Association of Official Analytical Chemists, Inc., Arlington, VA, 961.14.

AOAC (1990c) Thiamin (vitamin B_1) in foods. Fluorometric method. Final action. In *AOAC Official Methods of Analysis*, 15th edn (ed. K. Helrich), Association of Official Analytical Chemists, Inc., Arlington, VA, 942.23.

AOAC (1990d) Thiamine (vitamin B_1) in grain products. Fluorometric (rapid) method. Final action. In *AOAC Official Methods of Analysis*, 15th edn (ed. K. Helrich), Association of Official Analytical Chemists, Inc., Arlington, VA, 953.17.

AOAC (1990e) Thiamine (vitamin B_1) in bread. Fluorometric method. Final action 1960. In *AOAC Official Methods of Analysis*, 15th edn (ed. K. Helrich), Association of Official Analytical Chemists, Inc., Arlington, VA, 957.17.

AOAC (1990f) Thiamine (vitamin B_1) in milk-based infant formula. Fluorometric method. Final action 1988. In *AOAC Official Methods of Analysis*, 15th edn (ed. K. Helrich), Association of Official Analytical Chemists, Inc., Arlington, VA, 986.27.

AOAC (1990g) Riboflavin (vitamin B_2) in foods and vitamin preparations. Fluorometric method. Final action 1971. In *AOAC Official Methods of Analysis*, 15th edn (ed. K. Helrich), Association of Official Analytical Chemists, Inc., Arlington, VA, 970.65.

AOAC (1990h) Vitamin B_6 (pyridoxine, pyridoxal, pyridoxamine) in food extracts. Microbiological method. Final action 1975. In *AOAC Official Methods of Analysis*, 15th edn (ed. K. Helrich), Association of Official Analytical Chemists, Inc., Arlington, VA, 961.15.

AOAC (1990i) Vitamin C (ascorbic acid) in vitamin preparations. Microfluorometric method. Final action 1968. In *AOAC Official Methods of Analysis*, 15th edn (ed. K. Helrich), Association of Official Analytical Chemists, Inc., Arlington, VA, 967.22.

AOAC (1990j) Riboflavin in foods and vitamin preparations. Automated method. Final action 1982. In *AOAC Official Methods of Analysis*, 15th edn (ed. K. Helrich), Association of Official Analytical Chemists, Inc., Arlington, VA, 981.15.

AOAC (1990k) Niacin and niacinamide in cereal products. Automated method. Final action 1976. In *AOAC Official Methods of Analysis*, 15th edn (ed. K. Helrich), Association of Official Analytical Chemists, Inc., Arlington, VA, 975.41.

AOAC (1990l) Niacin and niacinamide in foods, drugs and feeds. Automated method. Final action 1982. In *AOAC Official Methods of Analysis*, 15th edn (ed. K. Helrich), Association of Official Analytical Chemists, Inc., Arlington, VA, 981.16.

AOAC (1990m) Vitamin C (total) in food. Semiautomated fluorometric method. Final action 1985. In *AOAC Official Methods of Analysis*, 15th edn (ed. K. Helrich), Association of Official Analytical Chemists, Inc., Arlington, VA, 984.26.

Association of Vitamin Chemists, Inc. (1966) *Methods of Vitamin Assay*, 3rd edn, Interscience Publishers, New York.

Augustin, J., Beck, C. and Marousek, G.I. (1981) Quantitative determination of ascorbic acid in potatoes and potato products by high performance liquid chromatography. *J. Fd Sci.*, **46**, 312–3, 316.

Ballantine, J. and Woolfson, A.D. (1980) The application of differential pulse voltammetry at the glassy carbon electrode to multivitamin analysis. *J. Pharm. Pharmac.*, **32**, 353–6.

Barakat, M.Z., El-Wahab, M.F.A. and El-Sadr, M.M. (1955) Action of *N*-bromosuccinimide on ascorbic acid. New titrimetric method for estimation of vitamin C. *Analyt. Chem.*, 27, 536–40.

Bechtel, W.G. and Hollenbeck, C.M. (1958) A revised thiochrome procedure for the determination of thiamine in cereal products. *Cereal Chem.*, **35**, 1–14.

Betteridge, D. (1978) Flow injection analysis. *Analyt. Chem.*, **50**, 832A–3A, 835A–6A, 839A–40A, 842A–4A, 846A.

Beutler, H.O. and Beinstingl, G. (1980) Determination of L-ascorbic acid in foods. *Dtsch. Lebensmitt. Rundschau*, **76**, 69–75 (in German).

Bonavita, V. (1960) The reaction of pyridoxal 5-phosphate with cyanide and its analytical use. *Arch. Biochem. Biophys.*, **88**, 366–72.

Bond, A.M. (1980) *Modern Polarographic Methods in Analytical Chemistry*, Marcel Dekker, Inc., New York.

Bridges, J.W., Davies, D.S. and Williams, R.T. (1966) Fluorescence studies on some hydroxypyridines including compounds of the vitamin B_6 group. *Biochem. J.*, **98**, 451–68.

Campbell, J.A. and Pelletier, O. (1961) Determination of niacin in cereals. *J. Ass. Off. Analyt. Chem.*, **44**, 431–6.

Christie, A.A. (1975) Analysis for selected vitamins in a nutritional labelling programme. *Inst. Fd Sci. Technol. Proc.*, **8**, 163–8.

Conner, R.T. and Straub, G.J. (1941) Determination of thiamin by the thiochrome reaction. *Ind. Engng Chem. Analyt. Edn*, **13**, 380–4.

Davídek, J., Velíšek, J., Černá, J. and Davídek, T. (1985) Gas chromatographic determination of pantothenic acid in foodstuffs. *J. Micronutr. Anal.*, **1**, 39–46.

Defibaugh, P.W. (1987) Evaluation of selected enzymes for thiamine determination. *J. Ass. Off. Analyt. Chem.*, **70**, 514–17.

Deutsch, M.J. (1967) Assay for vitamin C: a collaborative study. *J. Ass. Off. Analyt. Chem.*, **50**, 798–806.

Deutsch, M.J., Schiaffino, S.S. and Pillsbury, H.C. (1960) Stability and determination of thiamine in a cornmeal enrichment mixture. *J. Ass. Off. Analyt. Chem.*, **43**, 45–6.

Deutsch, M.J. and Weeks, C.E. (1965) Microfluorometric assay for vitamin C. *J. Ass. Off. Analyt. Chem.*, **48**, 1248–56.

DeVries, J.W. (1983) Semiautomated fluorometric method for determination of vitamin C in foods: collaborative study. *J. Ass. Off. Analyt. Chem.*, **66**, 1371–6.

Dunbar, W.E. and Stevenson, K.E. (1979) Automated fluorometric determination of thiamine and riboflavin in infant formulas. *J. Ass. Off. Analyt. Chem.*, **62**, 642–7.

Dunmire, D.L., Reese, J.D., Bryan, R. and Seegers, M. (1979) Automated fluorometric determination of vitamin C in foods. *J. Ass. Off. Analyt. Chem.*, **62**, 648–52.

Echols, R.E., Miller, R.H. and Foster, W. (1986) Analysis of thiamine in milk by gas chromatography and the nitrogen-phosphorus detector. *J. Dairy Sci.*, **69**, 1246–9.

Echols, R.E., Miller, R.H. and Thompson, L. (1985) Evaluation of internal standards and extraction solvents in the gas chromatographic determination of thiamine. *J. Chromat.*, **347**, 89–97.

Echols, R.E. Miller, R.H., Winzer, W., Carmen, J. and Ireland, Y.R. (1983) Gas chromatographic determination of thiamine in meats, vegetables and cereals with a nitrogen-phosphorus detector. *J. Chromat.*, **262**, 257–63.

Egberg, D.C. (1979a) Semiautomated method for riboflavin in food products: collaborative study. *J. Ass. Off. Analyt. Chem.*, **62**, 1041–4.

Egberg, D.C. (1979b) Semiautomated method for niacin and niacinamide in food products: collaborative study. *J. Ass. Off. Analyt. Chem.*, **62**, 1027–30.

Egberg, D.C. and Potter, R.H. (1975) An improved automated determination of riboflavin in food products. *J. Agric. Fd Chem.*, **23**, 815–20.

Egberg, D.C., Potter, R.H. and Heroff, J.C. (1977) Semiautomated method for the fluorometric determination of total vitamin C in food products. *J. Ass. Off. Analyt. Chem.*, **60**, 126–31.

Egberg, D.C., Potter, R.H. and Honold, G.R. (1974) The semiautomated determination of niacin and niacinamide in food products. *J. Agric. Fd. Chem.*, **22**, 323–6.

Elgilany Elbashier, E. and Greenway, G.M. (1990) Determination of vitamin C in karkady using flow injection analysis. *J. Micronutr. Anal.*, **8**, 311–16.

Ellefson, W.C., Richter, E., Adams, M. and Baillies, N.T. (1981) Evaluation of ion exchange resins and various enzymes in thiamine analysis. *J. Ass. Off. Analyt. Chem.*, **64**, 1336–8.

Evered, D.F. (1960) Determination of ascorbic acid in highly coloured solutions with *N*-bromosuccinimide. *Analyst, Lond.*, **85**, 515–17.

Fiedlerová, V. and Davídek, J. (1974) Fluorimetric determination of pyridoxal in dried milk. *Z. Lebensmittelunters. u.-Forsch.*, **155**, 277–81.

Flato, J.B. (1972) The renaissance in polarographic and voltammetric analysis. *Analyt. Chem.*, **44**(11), 75A–87A.

Fleet, B. and Fouzder, N.B. (1979) Unit processes in organic voltammetric analysis – II. Determination. In *Polarography of Molecules of Biological Significance* (ed. W. Franklin Smyth), Academic Press, London, pp. 37–76.

Fujita, A., Fujita, D. and Fujino, K. (1955a) Fluorometric determination of vitamin B_6. 2. Determination of pyridoxamine. *J. Vitam.*, **1**, 275–8.

Fujita, A., Fujita, D. and Fujino, K. (1955b) Fluorometric determination of vitamin B_6. 3. Fractional determination of pyridoxal and 4-pyridoxic acid. *J. Vitam.*, **1**, 279–89.

Fujita, A., Matsuura, K. and Fujino, K. (1955) Fluorometric determination of vitamin B_6. 1. Determination of pyridoxine. *J. Vitam.*, **1**, 267–74.

Ge, H., Oman, G.N. and Ebert, F.J. (1986) On-line generation of cyanogen chloride in semiautomated determination of niacin and niacinamide in food products. *J. Ass. Off. Analyt. Chem.*, **69**, 560–2.

Gerstl, R. and Ranfft, K. (1974) A gas chromatographic method for determination of vitamin C. *Z. Lebensmittelunters. u.-Forsch.*, **154**, 12–17 (in German).

Greenway, G.M. and Ongomo, P. (1990) Determination of L-ascorbic acid in fruit and vegetable juices by flow injection with immobilised ascorbate oxidase. *Analyst, Lond.*, **115**, 1297–9.

Gregory, J.F. and Kirk, J.R. (1977) Improved chromatographic separation and fluorometric determination of vitamin B_6 compounds in foods. *J. Fd Sci.*, **42**, 1073–6.

Gross, A.F. (1975) Automated method for the determination of niacin and niacinamide in cereal products: collaborative study. *J. Ass. Off. Analyt. Chem.*, **58**, 799–803.

Guilbault, G.G. (1973) *Practical Fluorescence. Theory, Methods, and Techniques*, Marcel Dekker, Inc., New York.

Hart, J.P. (1984) Polarography and its application to the determination of low levels of vitamins and coenzymes. In *Investigative Microtechniques in Medicine and Biology*, Vol. 1 (eds J. Chayen and L. Bitensky), Marcel Dekker, Inc., New York, pp. 199–250.

Hart, J.P. (1986) Polarographic and voltammetric techniques and their application to the determination of vitamins and coenzymes. *Trends Analyt. Chem.*, **5**, 20–5.

Hennessy, D.J., Steinberg, A.M., Wilson, G.S. and Keaveney, W.P. (1960) Fluorometric determination of added pyridoxine in enriched white flour and in bread baked from it. *J. Ass. Off. Analyt. Chem.*, **43**, 765–8.

Henshall, J.D. (1981) Ascorbic acid in fruit juices and beverages. In *Vitamin C (Ascorbic Acid)* (eds J.N. Counsell and D.H. Hornig), Applied Science Publishers, London, pp. 123–37.

Jacobson, B.S. (1977) Hydroxylamine hydrochloride in automated and manual methods for riboflavin determination. *J. Ass. Off. Analyt. Chem.*, **60**, 147–50.

Karayannis, M.I. and Farasoglou, D.I. (1987) Kinetic-spectrophotometric method for the determination of ascorbic acid in orange juice, parsley and potatoes. *Analyst, Lond.*, **112**, 767–70.

Kelley, J.J. and Siebert, K.J. (1989) Evaluation of a colorimetric method for determination of ascorbates in beer. *J. Am. Soc. Brewing Chem.*, **47**, 57–61.

Kirk, J.R. (1974) Automated method for the analysis of thiamine in milk, with application to other selected foods. *J. Ass. Off. Analyt. Chem.*, **57**, 1081–4.

Kirk, J.R. (1977) Automated analysis of thiamine, ascorbic acid, and vitamin A. *J. Ass. Off. Analyt. Chem.*, **60**, 1234–7.

Kirk, J.R. and Ting, N. (1975) Fluorometric assay for total vitamin C using continuous flow analysis. *J. Fd Sci.*, **40**, 463–6.

Koeppen, B.H. (1973) Determination of ascorbic acid by gas-liquid chromatography. *S. Afr. J. Sci.*, **69**, 376–7.

Korytnyk, W., Fricke, G. and Paul, B. (1966) Pyridoxine chemistry. XII. Gas chromatography of compounds in the vitamin B_6 group. *Analyt. Biochem.*, **17**, 66–75.

Koziol, J. (1971) Fluorometric analyses of riboflavin and its coenzymes. *Methods Enzymol.*, **18B**, 253–85.

Lau, O.-W., Luk, S.-F. and Wong, K.-S. (1986) Background correction method for the determination of ascorbic acid in soft drinks, fruit juices and cordials using direct ultraviolet spectrophotometry. *Analyst, Lond.*, **111**, 665–70.

Lau, O.-W., Shiu, K.-K. and Chang, S.-T. (1985) Determination of ascorbic acid in vegetables and fruits by differential pulse polarography. *J. Sci. Fd Agric.*, **36**, 733–9.

Lázaro, F., Luque de Castro, M.D. and Valcárcel, M. (1987) Simultaneous determination of ascorbic acid and sulphite in soft drinks by flow injection analysis. *Analysis*, **15**, 183–7.

Lechien, A., Valenta, P., Nürnberg, H.W. and Patriarche, G.J. (1982) Determination of ascorbic acid by differential pulse voltammetry. *Z. Analyt. Chem.*, **311**, 105–8.

Lim, K.L., Young, R.W., Palmer, J.K. and Driskell, J.A. (1982) Quantitative separation of B_6 vitamers in selected foods by a gas-liquid chromatographic system equipped with an electron-capture detector. *J. Chromat.*, **250**, 86–9.

Lindquist, J. (1975) Voltammetric determination of ascorbic acid by use of a carbon paste electrode. *Analyst, Lond.*, **100**, 339–48.

Loo, Y.H. and Cort, W.M. (1972) Assay of pyridoxal and its derivatives. *Methods Neurochem.*, **2**, 169–204.

MacArthur, M.J. and Lehmann, J. (1959) Chromatographic separation and fluorometric measurement of vitamin B_6 components in aqueous solutions. *J. Ass. Off. Analyt. Chem.*, **42**, 619–22.

McRoberts, L.H. (1954) Report on the determination of thiamine in enriched flour. Comparison of fluorometric methods, *J. Ass. Off. Agric. Chem.*, **37**, 757–70.

McRoberts, L.H. (1960) Determination of thiamine in enriched cereal and bakery products. *J. Ass. Off. Analyt. Chem.*, **43**, 47–54.

Mapson, L.W. (1943) Vitamin methods. VI. The estimation of ascorbic acid in the presence of reductones and allied substances. *J. Soc. Chem. Ind., Lond.*, **62**, 223–32.

Ohishi, N. and Fukui, S. (1968) Further study on the reaction products of pyridoxal and pyridoxal 5′-phosphate with cyanide. *Arch. Biochem. Biophys.*, **128**, 606–10.

Olliver, M. (1967) Ascorbic acid. IV. Estimation. In *The Vitamins. Chemistry, Physiology, Pathology, Methods*, 2nd edn, Vol. 1 (eds W.H. Sebrell, Jr and R.S. Harris), Academic Press, New York, pp. 338–59.

Osborne, B.G. and Tyson, J.F. (1988) Review: flow injection analysis – a new technique for food and beverage analysis. *Int. J. Fd. Sci. Technol.*, **23**, 541–54.

Owen, R.S. and Franklin Smyth, W. (1975) The determination of ascorbic acid in foods by reverse sweep cathode ray polarography. *J. Fd Technol.*, **10**, 263–72.

Pachla, L.A. and Kissinger, P.T. (1976) Determination of ascorbic acid in foodstuffs, pharmaceuticals, and body fluids by liquid chromatography with electrochemical detection. *Analyt. Chem.*, **48**, 364–7.

Patzer, E.M. and Hilker, D.M. (1977) New reagent for vitamin B_6 derivative formation in gas chromatography. *J. Chromat.*, **135**, 489–92.

Pearson, W.N. (1967a) Thiamine. In *The Vitamins. Chemistry, Physiology, Pathology, Methods*, 2nd edn, Vol. VII (eds P. György and W.N. Pearson), Academic Press, New York, pp. 53–94.

Pearson, W.N. (1967b) Riboflavin. In *The Vitamins. Chemistry, Physiology, Pathology, Methods*, 2nd edn, Vol. VII (eds. P. György and W.N. Pearson), Academic Press, New York, pp. 99–134.

Pelletier, O. and Brassard, R. (1977) Determination of vitamin C (L-ascorbic acid and dehydroascorbic acid) in food by manual and automated photometric methods. *J. Fd. Sci.*, **42**, 1471–7.

Pelletier, O. and Campbell, J.A. (1959) A modified procedure for the determination of niacin in cereal products. *J. Ass. Off. Analyt. Chem.*, **42**, 625–30.

Pelletier, O. and Madère, R. (1975) Comparison of automated and manual procedures for determining thiamine and riboflavin in foods. *J. Fd Sci.*, **40**, 374–9.

Pelletier, O. and Madère, R. (1977) Automated determination of thiamin and riboflavin in various foods. *J. Ass. Off. Analyt. Chem.*, **60**, 140–6.

Pelletier, O. and Morrison, A.B. (1966) Determination of ascorbic acid in the presence of ferrous and stannous salts. *J. Ass. Off. Analyt. Chem.*, **49**, 800–3.

Perone, S.P. and Kretlow, W.J. (1966) Application of controlled potential techniques to study of rapid succeeding chemical reaction coupled to electro-oxidation of ascorbic acid. *Analyt. Chem.*, **38**, 1760–3.

Pippen, E.L. and Potter, A.L. (1975) Quantitating the recovery of thiamine (vitamin B_1) from Decalso in the thiochrome method for the determination of thiamine. *J. Agric. Fd Chem.*, **23**, 523–6.

Polansky, M.M., Camarra, R.T. and Toepfer, E.W. (1964) Pyridoxine determined fluorometrically as pyridoxal cyanide compound. *J. Ass. Off. Analyt. Chem.*, **47**, 827–8.

Poole, C.F. and Schuette, S.A. (1984) *Contemporary Practice of Chromatography*, Elsevier, Amsterdam, Oxford, New York and Tokyo.

Prosser, A.R. and Sheppard, A.J. (1969) Gas–liquid chromatographic determination of pantothenates and panthenol. *J. Pharm. Sci.*, **58**, 718–21.

Prosser, A.R. and Sheppard, A.J. (1971) GLC of trimethylsilyl derivatives of pantothenyl alcohol and pantothenates. *J. Pharm. Sci.*, **60**, 909–12.

Ranger, C.B. (1981) Flow injection analysis. Principles, techniques, application, design. *Analyt. Chem.*, **53**, 20A–22A, 24A, 26A, 28A, 30A, 32A.

Rashid, I. and Potts, D. (1980) Riboflavin determination in milk. *J. Fd Sci.*, **45**, 744–5.

Ratzkowski, C. and Korol, J. (1977) The quantitative, differential determination of ascorbic acid and erythorbic acid in foods by polarography. *J. Inst. Can. Sci. Technol. Aliment.*, **10**, 215–18.

Ravindranath, B. (1989) *Principles and Practice of Chromatography*, Ellis Horwood Ltd, Chichester.

Ribbron, W.M., Stevenson, K.E. and Kirk, J.R. (1977) Comparison of semi-automated and manual methods for the determination of thiamine in baby cereals and infant and dietary formulas. *J. Ass. Off. Analyt. Chem.*, **60**, 737–8.

Riley, T. and Watson, A. (1987) *Polarography and other Voltammetric Methods*, John Wiley & Sons, Chichester.

Roe, J.H. (1954) Chemical determination of ascorbic, dehydroascorbic, and diketogulonic acids. In *Methods of Biochemical Analysis*, Vol. I (ed. D. Glick), Interscience Publishers, Inc., New York, pp. 115–39.

Roe, J.H. (1961) Appraisal of methods for the determination of L-ascorbic acid. *Ann. N.Y. Acad. Sci.*, **92**, 277–83.

Roe, J.H. (1967) Ascorbic acid. In *The Vitamins. Chemistry, Physiology, Pathology, Methods*, 2nd edn, Vol. VII (eds P. György and W.N. Pearson), Academic Press, New York, pp. 27–51.

Roe, J.H. and Kuether, C.A. (1943) The determination of ascorbic acid in whole blood and urine through the 2,4-dinitrophenylhydrazine derivative of dehydroascorbic acid. *J. Biol. Chem.*, **147**, 399–407.

Roy, R.B. (1979) Application of Technicon AutoAnalyzer II to the analysis of water-soluble vitamins in foodstuffs. In *Topics in Automatic Chemical Analysis*, Vol. I, Technicon Ind. Systems, Tarrytown, New York, pp. 138–62.

Roy, R.B. and Conetta, A. (1976) Automated analysis of water-soluble vitamins in food. *Fd Technol.*, **30**(10), 94, 95, 98, 100, 103, 104.

Roy, R.B., Conetta, A. and Salpeter, J. (1976) Automated fluorometric method for the determination of total vitamin C in food products. *J. Ass. Off. Analyt. Chem.*, **59**, 1244–50.

Roy, R.B. and Merten, J.J. (1983) Evaluation of urea–acid system as medium of extraction for the B-group vitamins. Part II. Simplified semi-automated chemical analysis for niacin and niacinamide in cereal products. *J. Ass. Off. Analyt. Chem.*, **66**, 291–6.

Roy, R.B., Salpeter, J. and Dunmire, D.L. (1976) Evaluation of urea–acid system as a medium of extraction for B-group vitamins. Simplified automated analysis of riboflavin in food products. *J. Fd Sci.*, **41**, 996–1000.

Russell, L.F. and Vanderslice, J.T. (1990) A comprehensive review of vitamin B_2 analytical methodology. *J. Micronutr. Anal.*, **8**, 257–310.

Russell, L.F. and Vanderslice, J.T. (1992) Comments on the standard fluorometric determination of riboflavin in foods and biological tissues. *Fd Chem.*, **43**, 79–82.

Santhanam, K.S.V. and Krishnan, V.R. (1961) Estimation of ascorbic acid by controlled potential coulometry. *Analyt. Chem.*, **33**, 1493–5.

Sarwar, M., Iqbal, Z. and Zaidi, S. (1975) Modified method for the estimation of ascorbic acid from preserved juices and squashes. *Mikrochim. Acta*, **II**, 699–704.

Sauberlich, H.E. (1967) Vitamin B_6. In *The Vitamins. Chemistry, Physiology, Pathology, Methods*, 2nd edn, Vol. VII (eds P. György and W.N. Pearson), Academic Press, New York, pp. 169–205.

Schlack, J.E. (1974) Quantitative determination of L-ascorbic acid by gas–liquid chromatography. *J. Ass. Off. Analyt. Chem.*, **57**, 1346–8.

Snyder, L., Levine, J., Stoy, R. and Conetta, A. (1976) Automated chemical analysis: update on continuous-flow approach. *Analyt. Chem.*, **48**, 942A–944A, 946A, 948A, 950A, 952A, 954A, 956A.

Söderhjelm, P. (1975) The determination of pyridoxine in enriched foodstuffs by direct spectrofluorometric measurement. *J. Sci. Fd Agric.*, **26**, 1469–72.

Söderhjelm, P. and Lindquist, J. (1976) Electrochemical assay of thiamine, riboflavin, pyridoxine, nicotinamide and ascorbic acid in pharmaceutical preparations. *Acta Pharm. Suec.*, **13**, 201–12.

Soliman, A.-G.M. (1981) Comparison of manual and benzenesulphonyl chloride-semiautomated thiochrome methods for determination of thiamine in foods. *J. Ass. Off. Analyt. Chem.*, **64**, 616–22.

Sontag, G. and Kainz, G. (1978) Determination of ascorbic acid in fruit juices and lemonades by differential-pulse polarography. *Mikrochim. Acta*, **I**, 175–84 (in German).

Spaeth, E.E., Baptist, V.H. and Roberts, M. (1962) Rapid potentiometric determination of ascorbic acid. *Analyt. Chem.*, **34**, 1342.

Strohecker, R. and Henning, H.M. (1966) *Vitamin Assay – Tested Methods*, Verlag Chemie, Weinheim.

Tanaka, A., Iijima, M., Kikuchi, Y., Hoshino, Y, and Nose, N. (1989) Gas chromatographic determination of nicotinamide in meats and meat products as 3-cyanopyridine. *J. Chromat.*, **466**, 307–17.

Tarli, P., Benocci, S. and Neri, P. (1971) Gas-chromatographic determination of pantothenates and panthenol in pharmaceutical preparations by pantoyl lactone. *Analyt. Biochem.*, **42**, 8–13.

Toepfer, E.W. and Lehmann, J. (1961) Procedure for chromatographic separation and microbiological assay of pyridoxine, pyridoxal and pyridoxamine in food extracts. *J. Ass. Off. Analyt. Chem.*, **44**, 426–30.

Toepfer, E.W., MacArthur, M.J. and Lehmann, J. (1960) Chromatographic separation of vitamin B_6 components in food extracts. *J. Ass. Off. Analyt. Chem.*, **43**, 57–9.

Toepfer, E.W. and Polansky, M.M. (1964) Recent developments in the analysis for vitamin B_6 in foods. *Vitams Horm.*, **22**, 825–32.

Toepfer, E.W. and Polansky, M.M. (1970) Microbiological assay of vitamin B_6 and its components. *J. Ass. Off. Analyt. Chem.*, **53**, 546–50.

Toepfer, E.W., Polansky, M.M. and Hewston, E.M. (1961) Fluorometric determination of pyridoxamine by conversion to pyridoxal cyanide compound. *Analyt. Biochem.*, **2**, 463–9.

Tuan, S., Wyatt, J. and Anglemier, A.F. (1987) The effect of erythorbic acid on the determination of ascorbic acid levels in selected foods by HPLC and spectrophotometry. *J. Micronutr. Anal.*, **3**, 211–28.

Vanderslice, J.T. and Higgs, D.J. (1989) Automated analysis of total vitamin C in food. *J. Micronutr. Anal.*, **6**, 109–17.

van Gend, H.W. (1973) An automated colorimetric method for the determination of free nicotinic acid in minced meat. *Z. Lebensmittelunters. u.-Forsch.*, **153**, 73–7.

Vecchi, M. and Kaiser, K. (1967) The gas chromatographic determination of ascorbic acid in the form of its trimethylsilyl ether derivative. *J. Chromat.*, **26**, 22–9.

Velíšek, J. and Davídek, J. (1986) Gas–liquid chromatography of vitamins in foods: the water-soluble vitamins. *J. Micronutr. Anal.*, **2**, 25–42.

Velíšek, J., Davídek, J., Mňuková, J. and Pištěk, T. (1986) Gas chromatographic determination of thiamin in foods. *J. Micronutr. Anal.*, **2**, 73–80.

Weeks, C.E. and Deutsch, M.J. (1967) *l*-Ascorbic and *d*-isoascorbic acids: quantitative separation and assay. *J. Ass. Off. Analyt. Chem.*, **50**, 793–8.

Wiedemer, R.T., McKinley, S.L. and Rendl, T.W. (1986) Advantages of wide-bore capillary columns. *Int. Lab.*, **16**, May, 68, 70, 72, 74, 76, 77.

Woodrow, I.L., Torrie, K.M. and Henderson, G.A. (1969) A rapid method for the determination of riboflavin in dried milk products. *J. Inst. Can. Technol. Aliment.*, **2**, 120–2.

High-performance liquid chromatographic methods for the determination of thiamin, riboflavin, niacin, vitamin B_6, folate and vitamin C

6

6.1 GENERAL ASPECTS OF HPLC

6.1.1 PRINCIPLE OF HPLC

In HPLC, a small volume (typically 10–100 μl) of the suitably prepared sample extract is applied to a column packed with 5- or 10-μm particles, whose surfaces constitute the stationary phase, and eluted with a liquid mobile phase. The microparticulate column packings permit rapid solute distributions between the mobile and stationary phases. To overcome the very low permeability of such packings, a high-pressure pump provides a controlled flow of mobile phase, and a precise sample loading is achieved using either manual syringe injection or automatic injection. Detection of the separated components is achieved by continuous monitoring of the column effluent. HPLC allows hundreds of individual separations to be carried out on a given column with high speed, efficiency and reproducibility.

The separation of sample components in HPLC is the result of specific interactions between component molecules and the stationary and mobile phases, so many experimentally variable parameters are available for optimizing a separation. Detection relies mainly on the UV absorption or fluorescence spectral characteristics of the analyte, and therefore provides a marked selectivity in addition to the column separation.

6.1.2 THE COLUMN

The majority of published vitamin assays involving HPLC have utilized stainless steel columns of 25 or 30 cm length and standard internal diameter (i.d.) 4.6 mm. Cartridge columns of shorter length, which can be readily connected to the system by means of finger-tight end-fittings, have also found application. The insertion of a short guard column between the injector and analytical column protects the latter against loss of efficiency from strongly retained sample components. The guard column is usually packed with the same material as the analytical column, and should not increase band spreading by more than 5–10%.

6.1.3 THE MOBILE PHASE

Selection of the mobile phase (also referred to as the eluent) is made on the basis of solvent strength and solvent selectivity. The general strategy in optimizing a separation is first to adjust the solvent strength to maintain solute capacity factors (*k* values) in the range 1–10 and then, while holding the solvent strength constant, to alter the selectivity of the mobile phase. Compounds having *k* values in the optimum range of 1–10 can be separated using isocratic elution, i.e. using a mobile phase whose solvent strength remains constant throughout the separation. Compounds having widely different *k* values can often be separated by gradient elution, in which the solvent strength is increased continuously throughout the separation.

6.1.4 COLUMN SWITCHING

Column switching is a technique whereby selective fractions of the effluent from one chromatographic column are transferred to the inlet of another column. Automatic on-line column switching is achieved via one or more high-pressure switching valves actuated by time-programmable events from a microprocessor chromatograph. A particularly useful application of column switching is sample clean-up, which, in its simplest form, uses two columns containing identical packing material and one mobile phase. The initial separation takes place on a short column such that unwanted early-eluting components are routed to waste, and the fraction containing the components of interest is diverted onto the analytical column. The valve is then switched back to its initial position so that, while the components of interest are undergoing analysis, the more highly retained components are eluted from the short column directly to waste. A more complicated configuration is on-line multidimensional HPLC (Majors, 1980a), where fractions from one column are transferred to another column of different chromatographic mode. This configuration is used for better resolution of complex samples as well as for sample clean-up.

6.1.5 THE DETECTOR

Three types of in-line detector have been routinely employed to monitor the column effluent in HPLC systems for the determination of water-soluble vitamins in food samples. These are the photometric detector, the fluorescence detector, and the electrochemical detector. Absorption monitoring provides a convenient means of detecting niacin, folate compounds and ascorbic acid; fluorimetric detection provides a greater selectivity and sensitivity for detecting thiamin (as thiochrome), riboflavin, vitamin B_6 and pterin breakdown products of folic acid, DHF and THF; and electrochemical detection provides high selectivity and sensitivity for ascorbic acid.

6.1.6 DERIVATIZATION

The derivatization of some vitamins may be necessary to facilitate the use of a more suitable means of detection (usually fluorimetric) and/or a more suitable chromatographic mode. Either pre-column or post-column derivatization may be employed, depending upon whether one wishes to chromatograph the derivatized vitamer or the underivatized vitamer. In pre-column derivatization the reaction is carried out before HPLC, so it is the derivatized compounds that are actually chromatographed. In post-column derivatization the sample extract is injected onto the HPLC column, and the separated vitamers in the effluent are reacted with the derivatizing agent in a reaction coil located between a mixing tee and the detector (Froehlich and Wehry, 1981).

A post-column derivatization system requires a second pump to introduce the derivatizing agent but, once set up, the system provides an automatic and standardized means of preparing the derivatives. There will inevitably be some degree of peak broadening due to the increased distance between the HPLC column and the detector. Another disadvantage is that there is no opportunity to remove or separate excess reagent or impurities within the reagent that might impair the sensitivity of detection. Pre-column derivatization requires manual manipulations, and hence more skill and non-standardized reaction conditions, unless rigorously controlled. Advantages are the opportunity to clean up the reaction mixture before HPLC, and the operation of a simpler and more efficient chromatographic system.

6.1.7 QUANTIFICATION

Peak height or peak area?

Quantitative analysis utilizes the peak height or the peak area in the chromatogram to determine the concentration of a specific solute in the sample. In order to decide between height and area measurement as a means of obtaining optimum precision, a number of factors relating to system performance must be considered (Bakalyar and Henry, 1976). The key point to remember is that chromatographic development is based on elution volume, not time. If the mobile phase flow rate should slow down or stop when a solute band is passing through the flow cell of a concentration-sensitive detector, the peak height will be unaltered, but the area will continue to increase as it is accrued on a time basis.

Hence area measurement is quite sensitive to deficiencies in the pumping system, and to possible changes in the viscosity and compressibility of solvents that could affect flow rate during gradient elution. Minor changes in mobile phase composition or slight changes in the column temperature will affect retention times, with a consequent effect on peak width and hence peak height. Peak area will remain constant because the height decreases as the width increases. Possible causes of variation in mobile phase composition are evaporation of the organic solvent component and poor reproducibility of gradient programmes. It follows that, if the mobile phase composition and column temperature can be maintained precisely, but the flow rate is variable, peak height measurement yields greater precision than peak area measurement. Conversely, if the mobile phase composition and/or temperature cannot be maintained precisely, but flow rate is constant, peak area measurement is preferred. The use of peak area also relies on the accurate electronic assignment of the beginning and end of the solute peak. The errors will be greater for the narrow peaks at the beginning of a chromatogram, and hence in practice it is sometimes found that peak height measurement is more precise for early-eluting peaks, while peak area is more reproducible for later peaks.

Internal standardization

HPLC assays should, if possible, include an internal standard for calibration purposes, especially when uncontrolled losses of analyte occur during the course of the sample work-up. Internal standardization is a technique designed to compensate for analyte (vitamin) losses incurred during the sample work-up and final chromatographic analysis. The technique involves adding a known amount of a suitable compound (internal standard) to the sample at the earliest possible point in the analytical procedure, and measuring the peak heights or areas of the analyte and internal standard in the chromatogram. The quantification is based upon the comparison of the ratio of the internal standard peak size to analyte peak size in the sample with that ratio in a standard solution containing known amounts of the analyte and internal standard. As the calculation involves ratios of peak size, and not the absolute peak size, the injection volumes need not be constant. The concentrations of the analyte and internal standard must, however, remain within the linear range of the detector.

The ideal internal standard conforms to the following requirements:

1. It must resemble the analyte as closely as possible in terms of chemical and physical properties (including stability), and behave in a similar manner to the analyte during all steps in the analytical procedure (extraction, derivatization, etc.).

2. It must be commercially available in high purity.
3. It must never occur naturally in the original sample.
4. It should not react with any components of the sample or with the column packing.
5. It must elute near to the analyte, whilst being completely resolved from the analyte and from other neighbouring components.

The internal standardization technique actually increases the precision error by a factor of 1.4 ($\sqrt{2}$), as two peaks (analyte and internal standard) are measured (Snyder and Kirkland, 1979). The inherent errors will be minimized if the analyte and internal standard yield peaks of similar size, since errors in measuring peaks of about the same size will tend to cancel out. The effect of changing the peak size ratios can be ascertained by chromatographing a series of standard solutions containing different concentrations of analyte and a fixed concentration of internal standard. A calibration plot is then constructed in which the analyte to internal standard peak height (or peak area) ratios are plotted against the concentration of analyte. A linear calibration plot which intercepts the origin is evidence that the relative response factor is constant at all concentration ratios of internal standard and analyte over the concentration range of analyte to be used.

External standardization

For HPLC methods that require a less stringent sample work-up, the external standardization (direct calibration) method is more applicable. An external standard is a standard analyte solution of known concentration that has been carried through all operations in parallel with the sample. This technique obviates the problem of finding a suitable internal standard, and only one standard needs to be prepared for a series of samples. The quantification is based upon the ratio of analyte peak size (height or area) in the sample to analyte peak size in the standard. The technique involves absolute measurements of peak size, and hence is dependent upon the precise control of injection volume. As peak measurements in external calibration are compared from separate chromatograms, it is advisable to inject the standard solution at frequent intervals during the analysis in order to minimize errors arising from changes in the chromatographic conditions (e.g. temperature, flow rate, mobile phase composition).

Standard additions

A third calibration method that is advantageous in the analysis of complex mixtures, such as food extracts, is the method of standard additions. This technique compensates for matrix interferences, whereby

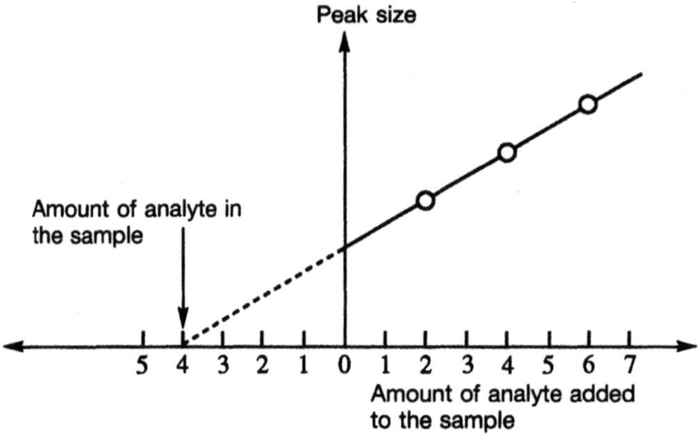

Figure 6.1 Standard additions calibration plot.

the presence of other compounds in the sample may affect the retention and/or the peak size of the analyte. In this procedure, three or four identical aliquots of the sample extract are spiked with increasing known amounts of the pure analyte (aliquots from a standard solution), and each solution is chromatographed. The peak areas or heights are measured and plotted as a function of the added amounts of analyte. The amount of analyte in the original sample can then be determined by extrapolating the standard additions calibration plot to the point of intersection of the concentration axis as shown in Figure 6.1.

Calibration plots

In practice, quantification of the water-soluble vitamins is usually carried out by reference to calibration plots (standard curves) of the vitamin in the free form, and not by use of internal or external standards. If the linearity of the calibration plot has been established, a one-point calibration can be performed. In this procedure, chromatograms are obtained of the sample extract *per se* and of the sample extract which has been spiked with a known amount of analyte. The concentration of the analyte can be determined using the calibration factor, R, defined by the following equation:

$$R = h'_A - h_A/W_A$$

Where h'_A is the height of the analyte (A) in the spiked sample, h_A is the height of A in the unspiked sample, and W_A is the weight of analyte added. The weight of analyte in the original sample is given by:

$$W_A = \frac{h_A}{R}$$

If a sample can be obtained that is known to be free of the analyte (e.g. a nonfortified sample of a foodstuff that is normally fortified), this sample blank can be used as a matrix for preparing standards for normal calibration. That is, several identical sample blanks are separately spiked with graded amounts of the analyte, and a calibration plot is constructed.

6.2 CHROMATOGRAPHIC MODES

The principal chromatographic modes that have been utilized in the analysis of water-soluble vitamins are ion exchange, ion exclusion partition, normal-phase, reversed-phase and ion interaction chromatography.

6.2.1 ION EXCHANGE CHROMATOGRAPHY

An ion exchange material comprises a porous support matrix bearing fixed ionogenic groups which, when ionized, function as the ion exchange sites. Depending on their function, ion exchange materials are either anion exchangers or cation exchangers, bearing positively charged and negatively charged functional groups, respectively. The positive charges of anion exchangers result from the protonation of basic groups, while the negative charges of cation exchangers are produced by the protolysis of acidic groups (Table 6.1). The functional groups are located mainly within the extensive pore structure of the matrix. To preserve electrical neutrality, each fixed ion is paired with an exchangeable counterion of opposite charge. The type of counterion specifies the 'form' of the ion exchanger; for example, a strong anion exchanger is usually supplied in the chloride form, i.e. the counterion is Cl^-.

Theoretical concepts

The concept of the Donnan membrane potential, which governs the diffusion of electrolytes across biological membranes, is fundamental in understanding ion exchange processes. When an anion exchanger is

Table 6.1 Characterization of ion exchangers

Type	Functional group	Usable pH range
Strong cation exchanger (SCX)	Sulphonic acid $-SO_3^-$	Above pH 1
Strong anion exchanger (SAX)	Quaternary amine $-NR_3^+$	Below pH 11
Weak cation exchanger (WCX)	Carboxylic acid $-CO_2^-$	Above pH 6
Weak anion exchanger (WAX)	Primary amine $-NH_3^+$	Below pH 8

immersed in a dilute solution of an electrolyte containing the same type of counterion (C^-), there is a higher concentration of C^- in the exchanger than in the surrounding solution. The C^- ion will therefore begin to diffuse out of the exchanger, following the concentration gradient. The diffusion occurs to only a minute degree, though, owing to the uncompensated fixed positive charge on the matrix, which makes it more difficult for further counterions to escape. Those which do diffuse into the external solution remain near to the surface of the exchanger, and the separation of positive and negative charges within the double layer so formed creates an electrical potential across the exchanger–solution interface. This Donnan potential tends to return the counterions of the double layer to their matrix sites against the concentration gradient, and thus the counterions of the double layer are in dynamic equilibrium with those of the exchanger. The migration of just a few counterions is sufficient to build up the Donnan potential, and so the conditions of electrical neutrality within the exchanger and the external solution are, for all practical purposes, maintained. Introducing foreign counterions into the external solution results in these mixing with and displacing the original counterions of the double layer, allowing them to enter and occupy sites within the exchanger. The same principle applies to a cation exchanger, except that the electrical charges have the opposite sign.

In ion exchange chromatography, the separation of sample ions depends upon the selectivity at the numerous sorption–desorption cycles that take place as the sample material passes through the column. Ions having a strong affinity for the functional groups will be retained on the column, whilst ions that interact only weakly will be easily displaced by competing ions, and eluted early.

The true ion exchange process represents the interaction of ionogenic (coulombic) forces, whereby the different sample anions or cations compete with each other and with the counterions to pair with the functional groups on the matrix (Mx).

Ion exchange processes may be represented thus:

Anion exchange. $Mx\text{-}\overset{+}{N}R_3C^- + X^+ + A^- \rightleftharpoons Mx\text{-}\overset{+}{N}R_3A^- + X^+ + C^-$

Cation exchange. $Mx\text{-}SO_3^-C^+ + X^- + A^+ \rightleftharpoons Mx\text{-}SO_3^-A^+ + X^- + C^+$

For anion exchange, the cation X^+, which accompanies the sample anion A^- in the above case, is referred to as the co-ion. Similarly, for cation exchange the anion X^- is the co-ion. Co-ions are not exchangeable, owing to their exclusion by the Donnan potential, but they play an important role in the mechanism of ion exchange chromatography in competing with the functional groups to attract counterions. Because electrical neutrality between the exchanger and the solution must be maintained, the ion exchange process is strictly stoichiometric.

Ion exchangers are further classified as strong or weak according to the ionization properties of the basic or acidic functional groups (Table 6.1). The degree of ionization depends upon the pK_a of the functional group and on the pH of the mobile phase, and is directly proportional to the ion exchange capacity. The capacity is maximal when all of the functional groups are ionized. The exchange capacity as a function of pH for the different types of ion exchanger is illustrated in Figure 6.2. It is seen that for strong anion and cation exchangers the maximum exchange capacity is maintained over a wide pH range, whereas for weak exchangers the usable pH range is limited (Table 6.1).

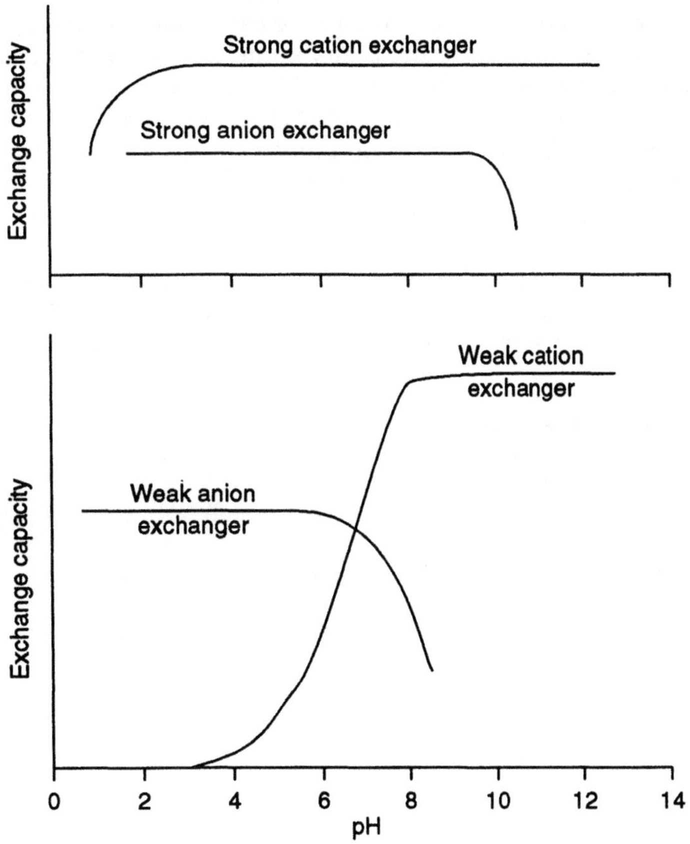

Figure 6.2 Exchange capacity of various ion exchangers as a function of pH. From Snyder, L.R. and Kirkland, J.J. (1979) *Introduction to Modern Liquid Chromatography*, Copyright © 1979, by John Wiley & Sons, Inc. Reprinted by permission of John Wiley & Sons, Inc.

Column packing materials

Totally porous resins

Most classical ion exchange resins are polystyrene–divinylbenzene (PS-DVB) copolymers to which the ionogenic functional groups are attached (Figure 6.3). The resins are available as uniformly sized spherical microparticles of about 10 μm diameter. During the polymerization reaction, the linear chains of polystyrene become cross-linked at fixed distances by the divinylbenzene to form a three-dimensional network. The hydration of the functional groups in an aqueous medium sets up an osmotic pressure inside the network, which causes the resin to swell considerably. The degree of cross-linking determines the extent to which a resin is free to swell or shrink. Highly cross-linked resins will have a relatively small swollen volume for essentially the same number of exchange sites, and thus the wet volume ion exchange capacity is increased accordingly. The relative swelling of the particle determines its porosity; that is, the percentage of DVB is inversely proportional to the average pore size. A decrease in porosity is accompanied by slower ion exchange kinetics, due mainly to small diffusion coefficients; conversely, an increase in porosity permits faster ion exchange kinetics, but the resin structure is less rigid and is highly compressible under HPLC conditions. In practice, an 8% (by weight) DVB cross-linked resin is a good compromise between pore size and mechanical strength. The PS-DVB resins are remarkably stable, being insoluble in concentrated

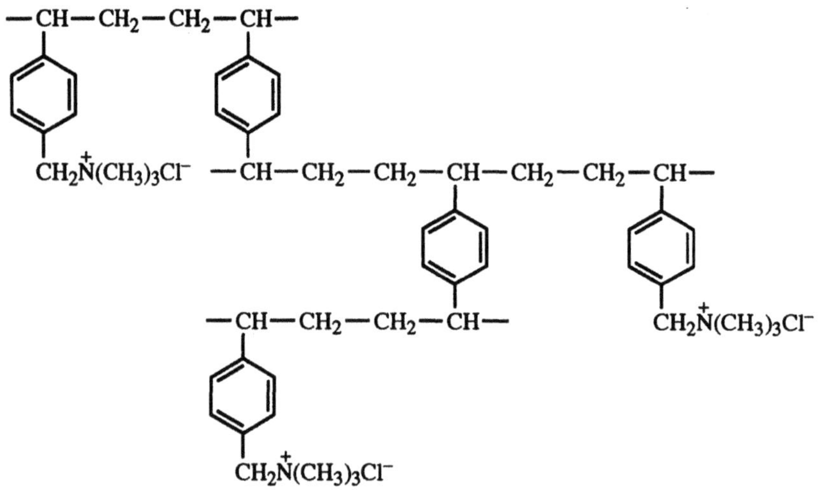

Figure 6.3 Structure of a typical polystyrene–divinylbenzene strong anion exchange resin.

acids, bases and salts, and resistant to oxidation, reduction and radiation (Khym, 1974). However, such resins exhibit a relatively slow diffusion of solutes within the deep pores containing stagnant mobile phase, and this leads to major band broadening. For this reason, such resins were often operated at elevated temperatures to speed mass transfer through a decrease in mobile phase viscosity.

Pellicular particles

One way of minimizing the diffusion path and improving the efficiency of the separation is to use pellicular particles, which have a non-porous impervious solid core surrounded by a thin coating of active stationary phase. The first pellicular particles were prepared by polymerizing a film of PS-DVB on glass beads of 50 μm diameter, and then introducing the functional groups (Horvath, Preiss and Lipsky, 1967). These novel packings were rapidly superseded by a wide range of superficially porous siliceous supports, typified by Zipax, which comprises glass beads of 25–37 μm diameter coated with a 1-μm porous layer of 0.2 μm diameter alumina-modified silica particles (Locke, 1973). The larger pore diameters of porous silica result in a higher column efficiency compared with the efficiencies obtained with PS-DVB-based coatings.

The stationary phases in the original Zipax type of exchanger were mechanically coated; that of Zipax-SAX, for example, was a methylacrylate polymer bearing quaternary ammonium functional groups (Majors, 1975). Such packings are limited in that they cannot be used in the presence of organic solvents or at temperatures exceeding 50 °C (Williams, Baker and Schmit, 1973). Bonded phase pellicular packings such as Permaphase-AAX were then introduced in which the stationary phase is covalently attached to the silica surface of the particle by thermally and hydrolytically stable siloxane bonds (Henry, Schmit and Williams, 1973).

The pellicular particles are much more efficient than totally porous particles of the same size, due to the improved mass transfer of solutes within the short pores of the superficial stationary phase. Furthermore, their structure allows high mobile phase flow rates to be used, while still maintaining near-equilibrium exchange conditions. The lower ion exchange capacity of pellicular packings compared with totally porous resins results in less retention of solutes, which can be overcome by the use of low ionic strength mobile phrases.

Microparticulate packings

Another way of minimizing band broadening is to use a column packing with a much smaller particle diameter. This concept has promoted the development of totally porous microparticulate silica-based packings, which can be tightly and uniformly packed into a column using a balanced density slurry technique (Majors, 1972). The short pore lengths and small interparticle channels facilitate fast exchange rates, leading to a dramatic improvement in efficiency and speed compared with the resins and pellicular types of column packing. A particle size in the range of 5–10 μm diameter represents a good compromise among column efficiency, packing ability and permeability (Majors, 1975). The greater efficiency of microparticulate particles allows shorter columns to be used, thus providing fast separations at lower column inlet pressures. Owing to the large specific surface area of the totally porous silica particles, the ion exchange capacity is much higher than that of pellicular packings, and this allows a higher sample loading. In contrast to the soft polystyrene-based resins, microparticulate (and pellicular) materials do not swell or shrink if the pH or ionic strength of the mobile phase alters, so pH or concentration gradients are possible in HPLC systems. Silica-based packings are stable at temperatures up to 80 °C, but strongly acidic (pH <2) or mildly basic (pH >7.5) conditions destroy the silicon structure, leading to drastic increase in column resistance and loss of efficiency. This problem has prompted investigation into new supports for a second generation of microparticulate bonded phases.

Mobile phase parameters

The chief mobile phase parameters that control sample retention and separation selectivity are ionic strength and pH. The role of the buffer component is to maintain the pH at the selected value and to provide the desired solvent strength in terms of the appropriate type of counterion at the right concentration. The aim is to achieve a satisfactory resolution of sample components within a short analysis time, preferably using isocratic elution. A gradient elution programme, in which either the ionic strength or the pH is increased during a run, may be required to promote faster elution or to control selectivity. A disadvantage of gradient elution is the need to regenerate the column after each run.

In optimizing the elution conditions, the parameters that can be adjusted are ionic strength, pH, temperature, flow rate, type of counterion and organic modifier. The effects of varying each of these parameters will be discussed in turn.

Ionic strength

The ionic strength of the mobile phase can be regarded as a measure of the number of counterions present, and is the most important parameter controlling the ion exchange equilibria. The sample ions and mobile phase counterions of the same charge compete for the ion exchange sites, and hence an increase in ionic strength will proportionately decrease solute retention, and vice versa. In other words, the solvent strength increases with increasing ionic strength, accompanied by a minimal change in solute selectivity. The ionic strength of the mobile phase can be increased by either increasing the molarity of the buffer solution while holding the pH constant, or adding a non-buffer salt such as sodium nitrate when it is undesirable to increase the buffer concentration. The molarity of the buffer or neutral salt in the mobile phase should be adjusted to suit the exchange capacity of the column packing used, and is usually between 1 and 100 mM for totally porous microparticulate silica-based packings. Within this range of concentrations, the aim is to adjust the ionic strength until the solute capacity factors (k values) are between 2 and 10. Samples containing solutes of similar charge can usually be eluted isocratically, but if charges vary from weak to strong, it may be necessary to employ a gradient elution programme. This entails commencing with a mobile phase of low ionic strength to encourage sorption of weakly charged solutes, and then gradually increasing the ionic strength to elute the most strongly retained solutes.

pH

The retention of weak acids and bases can also be controlled through variation of the mobile phase pH. The primary effect of pH is to control the ionization of organic acids and bases in the sample as shown below.

$$HA \rightleftharpoons H^+ + A^-$$
$$B + H^+ \rightleftharpoons BH^+$$

Increasing the pH leads to an increased ionization of acids and decreased ionization of bases, and vice versa for a decrease in pH. An increase in ionization in each case leads to increased solute retention.

The operating pH range for a separation can be estimated from the pK_a values of the sample components. Solute pK_a and mobile phase pH values are related by the Henderson–Hasselbalch equation which, for an acid, is:

$$\mathrm{pH} = \mathrm{p}K_a + \log \frac{[A^-]}{[HA]}$$

The pH of an equimolar (1 : 1) solution of undissociated acid (HA) and conjugate base (A^-) is equal to the pK_a of the acid involved, since the logarithm of 1 is zero. Thus the pK_a can be defined as the pH at which the acid is half ionized. The degree of ionization of ascorbic acid (with a pK_a value of 4.2) as a function of pH is shown in Figure 6.4. At a pH of

1 unit above the pK_a of the weak acid, the ratio of A^- (ionized acid) to HA (nonionized acid) is 10 : 1, and at 2 pH units above, the ratio will be 100 : 1. It is evident that large changes in selectivity can occur through changing the pH if the various solutes present possess different pK_a values. The initial pH is selected on the basis of the solute pK_a, and then further adjusted in increments of 0.1 pH units in the direction which appears to give further improvement in resolution. A pH gradient of a narrow range may be used to control selectivity. A good starting pH for an organic acid is 1.5 pH units above the pK_a of the acid involved. There does not appear to be a corresponding generalization for bases, except that they are usually chromatographed within the range of pH 3–6 (Johnson and Stevenson, 1978).

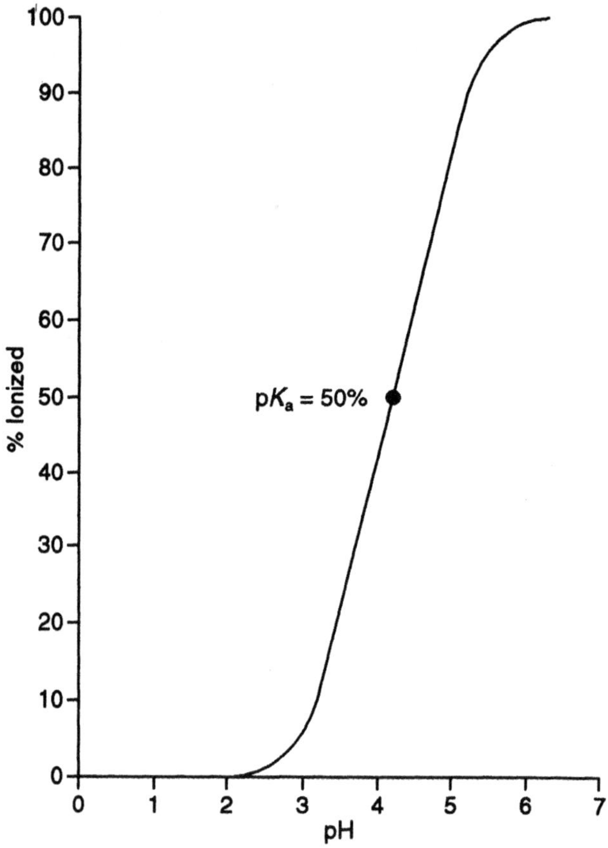

Figure 6.4 Degree of ionization of ascorbic acid (pK_a of 4.2) as a function of pH. From Bidlingmeyer (1980). Reproduced from the *Journal of Chromatographic Science* by permission of Preston Publications, a Division of Preston Industries, Inc.

The influence of mobile phase pH on the retention of weak acidic and basic solutes depends upon whether a strong or a weak ion exchanger is employed. For strong anion and cation exchangers, retention is solely dependent upon solute pK_a value. For weak exchangers the situation is somewhat different, because the ion exchange capacity also depends on the pH; however, the dominant effect of changes in pH is usually on the sample.

Temperature

Although silica-based pellicular and microparticulate packings are designed to reach equilibrium quickly at ambient temperature, elevated temperatures up to at least 60 °C will further increase efficiency, and may also cause selectivity changes. Biologically active samples such as vitamins are commonly chromatographed at ambient temperature to avoid possible degradation and interactions.

Flow rate

The solutes need a finite time to reach equilibrium with as many exchange sites as possible, so a mobile phase flow rate that is too fast will result in a low column efficiency. The flow rates used in practice should be a compromise between maximum efficiency and minimum elution time.

Type of counterion

The retention of sample ions also depends on the competition from counterions in the mobile phase for the ion exchange sites. Counterions having a strong affinity for the exchanger will permit the earlier elution of sample ions than those having a weak affinity, and thus solute selectivity can be altered by changing the counterion. In general, the ion exchanger shows the greatest affinity for ions with a higher electrical charge (valence), a smaller solvated volume and a greater polarizability. The relative affinities for cations and anions on strong cation and anion exchangers have been established and a selection is shown below:

For strong cation exchangers: $Fe^{3+} > Ba^{2+} > Pb^{2+} > Ca^{2+} > Cu^{2+} > Co^{2+} > Zn^{2+} > Mg^{2+} > Ag^{+} > K^{+} > NH_4^{+} > Na^{+} > H^{+} > Li^{+}$

For strong anion exchangers: $\text{citrate}^{3-} > SO_4^{2-} > \text{oxalate}^{2-} > I^{-} > \text{borate}^{2-} > NO_3^{-} > Br^{-} > Cl^{-} > \text{formate}^{-} > \text{acetate}^{-} > OH^{-} > F^{-}$

The above sequences also hold for weak cation and anion exchangers, except that H^+ and OH^- have the highest eluting strength. This is because the dissociation of the respective exchange sites diminishes in an acid or alkaline medium.

Thus, when using a strong cation exchanger, elution of sample ions will be more rapid when a mobile phase buffer is prepared with potassium salt than when prepared with sodium salt at the same molarity. Similarly, when using a strong anion exchanger, elution will be more rapid with a mobile phase containing nitrate ions than one containing chloride ions.

In practice, corrosive anions (e.g. halide ions), reducing anions and highly UV-absorbing anions are avoided, the most common counterions being phosphate, borate, nitrate and perchlorate, with sulphate, acetate and citrate occasionally being considered (Meyer, 1988).

It must be emphasized that ions with a low affinity for the exchanger can replace ions of a greater affinity if the former are present at a higher concentration. This property is utilized in the regeneration of ion exchange resins.

Organic modifiers

Water-miscible organic solvents such as acetonitrile, propan-2-ol and ethanol are frequently added as modifiers to the aqueous mobile phase as a means of lowering the viscosity and improving mass transfer kinetics. Typical amounts of added solvent range between 3% and 10% by volume. The effect of the organic modifier upon the ion exchange equilibria is relatively minor, and any significant changes that result from such additions are mainly attributed to hydrophobic mechanisms. In weak anion exchange chromatography an appreciable proportion of an organic acid solute will exist in the nonionized form, and thus behave differently to the ionized form (anion). The resultant peak tailing caused by the mixed-mode chromatography can be eliminated by use of an organic modifier, which also decreases the retention time. In general, using a modifier can dramatically improve a separation, although the effect is unpredictable and has to be determined empirically. It is obviously important to ascertain beforehand that the column packing material is compatible with the proposed organic solvent.

6.2.2 ION EXCLUSION PARTITION CHROMATOGRAPHY

Ion exclusion partition chromatography is a technique in which an ion exchange resin is employed for separating ionic molecules from nonionic or weakly ionic molecules. Ions having the same charge as the functional groups of the support (i.e. co-ions) are repelled by the Donnan potential and excluded from the aqueous phase within the pore volume of the resin beads. Nonionic or weakly ionic molecules are not excluded and, provided they are small enough, may freely diffuse into the matrix, where they can partition between the aqueous phase within the resin beads and the aqueous phase between the resin beads. Therefore, ionized sample solutes pass quickly through the column, whereas nonionic or weakly ionic solutes pass through more slowly. The retention mechanisms of the nonionic solutes include polar attraction between the solute and the resin functional groups (i.e. adsorption), van der Waal's forces between the solute and the hydrocarbon portion of the resin (primarily the benzene rings) and size exclusion. The overall separation is accomplished without any exchange of ions, so the column does not require regeneration after use.

Ion exclusion partition chromatography using a strong cation exchange resin has been successfully applied to the separation of organic acids, including ascorbic acid. The technique here is to suppress the ionization of the weak organic acid by adding sulphuric acid to the water mobile phase so that the highly ionized sulphate ion is excluded and quickly eluted, while the undissociated organic acid enters the resin pore structure and is retained. The mobile phase pH should be lower than the pK_a of the organic acid to ensure that the acid is undissociated. PS-DVB types of resin, rather than silica-based exchangers, are used because of their swelling properties. The volume of aqueous phase within the resin bead must be sufficient to allow partition of the nonionic solutes to take place and, to achieve optimum separation, must be greater than the sample volume.

6.2.3 NORMAL-PHASE CHROMATOGRAPHY

In normal-phase chromatography the surface of microparticulate silica (or other adsorbent) constitutes the polar stationary phase. The mobile phase is a nonpolar solvent containing a varying percentage of a more polar solvent to deactivate the strong adsorption sites (silanol groups in the case of silica). Separation occurs by competition between the solute and the mobile phase for the remaining adsorption sites, so the more polar the solute is, the more strongly it is retained. Conversely, solutes are eluted more rapidly by increasing the polarity of the mobile phase. Normal-phase chromatography has been applied to the determination of thiamin as thiochrome, and riboflavin as lumiflavin, after extraction of these reaction products into isobutanol and chloroform, respectively (Ang and Moseley, 1980). The analysis of the actual (unmodified) water-soluble vitamins by normal-phase chromatography is precluded by their lack of solubility in the organic mobile phase.

6.2.4 REVERSED-PHASE CHROMATOGRAPHY

Principle

In reversed-phase chromatography a nonpolar stationary phase is used in conjunction with a polar mobile phase. Solute elution is the opposite to that observed in normal-phase chromatography; polar solutes prefer the mobile phase and elute first, while nonpolar solutes prefer the essentially hydrophobic stationary phase and elute later. Reversed-phase chromatography exhibits improved stability and reproducibility compared with normal-phase chromatography. Interactions between solute and nonpolar stationary phases involve weaker forces, so analyses are rapid and re-equilibration times are short. The latter is particularly advantageous following solvent compositional changes during method development, and following gradient elution. The weaker forces also minimize the risk of on-column artifact formation.

Column packing materials

Most published separations involving reversed-phase chromatography have utilized totally porous microparticulate silica-based packings in which the nonpolar stationary phase, usually octadecylsilane (ODS), is chemically bonded to the silica surface through a siloxane bridge. Phenyl-bonded and cyanopropyl-bonded phases have also been used in certain applications.

The bonding chemistry invariably used in microparticulate silica-based packings involves the reaction between the surface silanol (≡Si—OH) groups on the silica matrix with an organosilane reagent to form a siloxane (—Si—O—Si) bonded phase, thus:

$$\equiv \mathrm{Si{-}OH} + \mathrm{Cl{-}}\overset{\displaystyle \mathrm{CH_3} \atop |}{\underset{\displaystyle | \atop \mathrm{CH_3}}{\mathrm{Si}}}\mathrm{{-}R} \rightarrow \equiv \mathrm{Si{-}O{-}}\overset{\displaystyle \mathrm{CH_3} \atop |}{\underset{\displaystyle | \atop \mathrm{CH_3}}{\mathrm{Si}}}\mathrm{{-}R} + \mathrm{HCl}$$

R is the ligand of interest, usually an octadecyl (C_{18}) hydrocarbon. In a monofunctional silanizing agent, only one of the three remaining substituents is a reative group, usually either chloro or alkoxy (methoxy or ethoxy); the other two substituents are usually methyl groups. Silanizing agents containing two and three reactive groups are referred to as di- and trifunctional. A monofunctional agent reacts with the silanol groups on the silica surface to form a monomolecular layer or monomeric phase. The corresponding di- and trifunctional silanizing agents react in a more complicated fashion and, depending on the reaction conditions, can form a monolayer, multilayer or cross-linked polymer of the bonded phase. Monomeric bonded phases exhibit faster diffusion rates in the stationary phase compared with multilayer or cross-linked phases and, hence, in theory, provide greater column efficiencies.

Differences in selectivity and chromatographic performance between ODS columns from different manufacturers are attributable to particle characteristics (size, shape and porosity), the coverage of the bonded phase and the surface configuration, and the percentage of accessible residual silanol groups. Some silica-based reversed-phase packings are 'end-capped', whereby unwanted residual silanol groups trapped by steric hindrance after reaction with the organosilane reagent are reacted with a small monofunctional silane reagent to give a more or less completely hydrophobic surface. In non-endcapped packings, solute retention is complicated by interactions of solute with accessible residual silanol groups on the stationary phase.

The amount of ODS ligate bound to the silica surface is commonly expressed as percentage carbon (weight per weight) or simply carbon load. The percentage of carbon will depend on the surface area of the silica support, which is governed by the mean pore diameter and by other factors (Cooke and Olsen, 1979). The term carbon load has little meaning without taking the surface area into account, and a more informative term of surface coverage is carbon content per unit specific surface area, expressed in $\mu mol/m^2$. Take, for example, LiChrosorb RP-18 and Zorbax ODS, which have similar carbon loads of 17% and 16% respectively. The surface area of the LiChrosorb material (150 m^2/g) is less than one-half of that of the Zorbax (350 m^2/g). Thus, in terms of carbon content per unit specific area, LiChrosorb RP-18 has a surface coverage that is more than double that of Zorbax ODS. High loading phases are highly retentive and facilitate a high solute load capacity. Phases with low carbon loadings are less retentive and therefore allow shorter analysis times.

Microparticulate rigid PS-DVB polymeric packings have been developed in which the neutral nonpolar polystyrene surface will function as a stationary phase for reversed-phase separations with aqueous eluents. One such polymeric packing that has been used successfully for determining ascorbic acid is PLRP-S 100 Å (Polymer Laboratories, UK), which is a 5-μm PS-DVB copolymer that can withstand pressures up to 5000 lb/in^2 (Dawkins, Lloyd and Warner, 1986).

Theoretical concepts

According to the solvophobic theory of solute retention for bonded phases, the very high cohesive density of the mobile phase, arising from the three-dimensional hydrogen bonding network, causes the less polar solutes to be literally 'squeezed' out of the mobile phase, enabling them to bind with the hydrocarbon ligands of the stationary phase (Horvath and Melander, 1977). The selectivity of the separation results, therefore, almost entirely from specific interactions of the solute with the mobile phase. The retention behaviour of solutes using cross-linked polystyrene packings will be somewhat different from that using alkyl-bonded silica packings because of the presence of aromatic groups, and the absence of interactions with residual silanol groups will result in a greatly reduced peak tailing of polar solutes.

Ionic compounds cannot be analysed as such by reversed-phase HPLC, since they elute near the void volumes. Ion suppression is a reversed phase chromatographic technique in which the ionic equilibrium of the sample is controlled by adjusting the pH of the mobile phase to obtain retention and separation of the components according to their pK_a values (Bidlingmeyer, 1980). By buffering of the mobile phase at 1–2 pH units below the pK_a value for a weak acid, and a corresponding amount above the pK_b value for a weak base, the ionization is suppressed and the undissociated compound, having a greater affinity for the stationary phase, is retained. Thus weak acids and weak bases can be retained in the pH regions 2–5 and 7–8, respectively. Strong acids and bases would require extreme pH values (<2 and >8, respectively) for ion suppression. Silica-based reversed-phase packings are unstable outside the pH range 2–7.5, so the ion suppression technique should not be used for strong acids and bases with such phases. Polymeric-based packings have the advantage over silica-based packings in being stable throughout the entire practical pH range (pH 1–13) (Lee, 1982). Reversed-phase chromatography with ion suppression has the advantage over classic ion exchange chromatography in permitting the simultaneous analysis of both ionized and nonionized solutes.

Mobile phase parameters

The polar mobile phase, in the simplest case, is composed of water, to which is added a varying percentage of a miscible organic solvent (usually methanol or acetonitrile) as modifier. The important properties of the solvents commonly used in reversed-phase chromatography are listed in Table 6.2. The surface tension of the eluent plays the major role in governing solute retention in accordance with the solvophobic theory; of secondary importance is the dielectric constant. Solvent viscosity is related to solute diffusivity in the mobile phase, so an increase in temperature, by reducing viscosity, increases column efficiency. Water, having the highest surface tension, is the weakest solvent, while neat methanol or acetonitrile are the strongest solvents employed in reversed-phase chromatography. Methanol and acetonitrile are the most popular organic solvents because they have relatively low UV cut-off points and viscosity, and are commercially available with sufficient purity. Eluents of intermediate strengths are obtained by mixing one of these solvents with water (Horvath and Melander, 1977). Increasing the proportion of water in water/organic mobile phases causes an increased retention of the more hydrophobic solutes relative to the more polar solutes. Increasing the concentration of organic component with time is a convenient way of performing gradient elution in reversed-phase chromatography.

6.2.5 ION INTERACTION CHROMATOGRAPHY

Principle

Ion interaction chromatography is probably better known as ion pair chromatography, but current theory of retention mechanisms favours the use of the former term. The technique employs the same types of column packing and water/organic mobile phases as those used in conventional reversed-phase HPLC. The pH of the mobile phase is adjusted to encourage ionization of the ionogenic solutes, and retention is controlled by adding to the mobile phase an amphiphilic ion interaction agent bearing an opposite charge to that of the analyte. The ion interaction agent should be univalent, aprotic and soluble in the mobile phase. It should ideally give a low UV-absorbing background, although for special applications a reagent with a strong chromophore

Table 6.2 Properties of solvents used in reversed-phase chromatography (from Horvath and Melander, 1977)

Solvent	Surface tension (dyn/cm)	Dielectric constant	Viscosity (cP)	UV cut-off[a] (nm)
Methanol	22	32.7	0.584	205
Acetonitrile	29	38.8	0.358	190
Propan-2-ol	21	19.9	2.39	205
Water	73	78.5	1.00	170

[a] The wavelength at which the optical density of a 1-cm-thick neat sample is unity as measured against air.

Reproduced from the *Journal of Chromatographic Science*, **15**, by permission of Preston Publications, a Division of Preston Industries, Inc.

can be used to enhance the response of an absorbance detector. The retention behaviour of nonionic solutes is not affected by the presence of the ion interaction agent, so both ionized and nonionized solutes may be resolved in the same chromatographic run. Use of ion interaction chromatography for water-soluble vitamin assays is advantageous, as many polar interferences elute in the dead volume, and hydrophobic compounds would be in low concentration in the aqueous extract of the sample.

Theoretical concepts

Research into the phenomena involved in ion interaction chromatography is continuing in an attempt to elucidate the retention mechanisms. Two stoichiometric models representing extreme situations are the ion pair model and the dynamic ion exchange model. The ion pair model postulates that the charged solute forms a neutral ion pair with the amphiphilic 'ion pairing agent' in the mobile phase, followed by sorption of the ion pair onto the nonpolar stationary phase. In the dynamic ion exchange model the lipophilic alkyl tail of the unpaired amphiphile is sorbed onto the stationary phase, with the ionic group orientated towards the more favourable aqueous media. The modified stationary phase then behaves like a dynamically formed ion exchanger.

Stoichiometric models are incapable of explaining a number of phenomena encountered in ion interaction chromatography. Current theory supports the concept of dynamic sorption of the unpaired amphiphile onto the stationary phase, forming, with its counterion, an electrical double layer that creates a surface potential analogous to the Donnan potential of static ion exchange systems. In the ion interaction model proposed by Bidlingmeyer *et al.* (1979), charged sample solutes interact with the electrical double layer, not only by electrostatic forces, but also by absorptive and solvophobic forces, resulting in the selective sorption of solute ions onto the stationary phase. This concept has been expanded by Stranahan and Deming (1982) to include interfacial tension effects.

Applications

For the determination of ascorbic acid (an anionic solute) a great many organic amines have been employed as ion interaction agents, representing primary, secondary, tertiary and quaternary amines. One of the more popular of these is tetrabutylammonium (Bu_4N^+) phosphate, which is commercially available as a prepared 5 mM solution in pH 7.5 buffer (PIC A reagent, Waters Associates). This aprotic quaternary amine interacts with strong and weak acids, and the buffering to pH 7.5

suppresses weak base ions. Tetrabutylammonium phosphate has found application in the determination of nicotinic acid and folic acid, as well as ascorbic acid. A less frequently used anionic ion interaction agent is sodium dodecylsulphate, which has been utilized in nicotinic acid assays.

For the separation of cationic solutes such as protonated amines, a range of alkyl sulphonates having the formula $CH_3(CH_2)_nSO_3^-$ (with n = 4–7) predominates. Selection of the appropriate reagent is based on solute retention time, which increases with an increase in the length of the alkyl chain. Prepared 5 mM solutions of the sodium salts in pH 3.5 buffer are available from Waters Associates; namely, pentane sulphonic acid (PIC B5), hexane sulphonic acid (PIC B6), heptane sulphonic acid (PIC B7) and octane sulphonic acid (PIC B8). These reagents interact with strong and weak bases, and the buffering to pH 3.5 suppresses weak acid ions. The alkyl sulphonates have found application in the determination of thiamin, riboflavin, nicotinamide and vitamin B_6.

Column packing materials

Most ion interaction chromatographic applications reported for vitamin assays up to the present day have utilized conventional 5- or 10-μm silica-based C_{18} bonded phase packings. Monomeric phases yield better-shaped peaks than polymeric phases, and high carbon loadings ensure good retention properties (Majors, 1980b). PS-DVB copolymers developed for HPLC have also been utilized for ion interaction chromatography (Iskandarani and Pietrzyk, 1982).

Mobile phase parameters

Mobile phase parameters that can be adjusted to optimize retention and selectivity in ion interaction chromatography are type and concentration of the ion interaction agent, pH, ionic strength, percentage of organic modifier and temperature. The effects of varying each of these parameters will be discussed in turn.

Type of ion interaction agent

The retention of ionic solutes can be readily increased by choosing a more hydrophobic ion interaction agent of the same class. For example, the use of pentane sulphonic acid resulted in insufficient retention of water-soluble vitamins, but changing to heptane sulphonic acid increased retention, particularly of thiamin, the most strongly ionic compound present (Bidlingmeyer, 1980). It is also possible to mix two reagents having different chain lengths to 'fine tune' a separation.

Selectivity changes can be effected by changing the counterion of the ion interaction agent, for example from tetrabutylammonium phosphate to tetrabutylammonium sulphate. The effect of the added anion in reducing the analyte retention follows the order:

$$Br^- > NO_3^- > Cl^- > citrate^{3-} > formate^- > PO_4^{3-} > SO_4^{2-} > F^-$$

(Iskandarani and Pietrzyk, 1982).

Concentration of ion interaction agent

Variation of the concentration of agent in the mobile phase provides a simple means of controlling solvent strength. The concentrations of the agents used in water-soluble vitamin assays are generally 5 mM or thereabouts, and such low concentrations will have little, if any, effect on the retention of nonionic solutes (Majors, 1980b). Selectivity remains more or less constant if the sample solutes are fully ionized, but if the solutes are not completely ionized or are nonionized, selectivity does vary with a change in concentration of ion interaction agent (Snyder and Kirkland, 1979). As expected, an increase in the concentration of the agent causes an increase in solute retention but, beyond a certain limit, a further increase in concentration causes a decrease in retention. A possible explanation for this reversal effect is that the increased amount of adsorbed surfactant lowers the interfacial tension between the modified stationary phase and the surrounding aqueous medium to a point at which solute retention is decreased (Stranahan and Deming, 1982). This nonionic theory also accounts for the observed decrease in retention of neutral solutes with increasing concentration of ion interaction agent.

pH

The pH of the mobile phase influences solute ionization in accordance with the solute pK_a values, as previously discussed; therefore, altering the pH will have a pronounced effect upon separation selectivity for weak acids and weak bases. Maximal retention is obtained where the solute and ion interaction agent are completely ionized, conditions under which ion interaction is optimal. The reagents, being strong acids or salts of strong bases, remain completely dissociated over a wide pH range, so that the pH can be adjusted to an optimal value for the separation. Weak acid solutes (pK_a >2) are usually separated at a pH of 6–7.4, and weak bases at pH 2–5 (Gloor and Johnson, 1977) using a buffer to hold the pH constant. When PIC reagents (Waters Associates) are used, the mobile phase is buffered to pH 7.5 for the separation of anionic solutes, and 3.5 for cationic solutes. Buffer salts should have poor ion association properties, but good solubilities in the mobile phase. The buffer concentration should be relatively low (*c.* 5 mM) to avoid possible salting-out anomalies (Adams, 1985). Strong acids and bases can be retained throughout the usable pH range. Again, the pH compatibility of silica gel (pH 2–7.4) must be considered.

Ionic strength

An excessive concentration of buffer salt, or the addition of neutral salt to the mobile phase, results in the surplus ions of such salts competing successfully with analyte ions for association with the adsorbed ion interaction agent, thus causing a decrease in retention. Unlike in ion exchange chromatography, ionic strength is not commonly used for controlling solute retention in ion interaction chromatography. In practice, the ionic strength should be kept as low as possible, commensurate with satisfactory retention characteristics and reproducibility.

Percentage of organic modifier

Methanol, rather than acetonitrile, is preferred as the organic modifier because of its superior solubilizing properties for the commonly used ion interaction agents. However, long-chain ($>C_{10}$) detergent-like reagents show better solubility in water/acetonitrile mixtures. Increasing the proportion of organic modifier increases the solvent strength, resulting in an overall lowering of solute retention. Solvent strength does not follow the solvent polarity index described for conventional reversed-phase chromatography. Rather, the concentration of organic modifier affects the surface potential (and hence solute retention) by influencing the sorption of the ion interaction agent onto the stationary phase (Bartha, Vigh and Varga-Puchony, 1990).

Temperature

Solute pK_a values are affected by a change in temperature, so significant changes in selectivity can occur with relatively small changes in column temperature. To ensure reproducible separations, it is thus good practice to maintain a constant column temperature. Ion interaction chromatography is usually carried out at ambient temperature, although operation at 50–60 °C will improve peak resolution (with a slight decrease in retention) by reducing the viscosity of the mobile phase. The combination of elevated temperature and the use of quaternary amines as ion interaction agents may reduce the life of bonded silica-based column packings, and a safe upper limit with such a combination would be 60 °C (Adams, 1985).

Strategy

The general strategy for separating complex mixtures of non-ionic and ionic solutes is firstly to adjust the percentage of organic modifier (usually methanol) to obtain optimum retention and separation of nonionic solutes. One then adds a suitable ion interaction agent in the appropriate buffer to the previously established mobile phase to separate the ionic compounds isocratically. Gradient elution programmes usually involve a decrease in the concentration of ion interaction agent with time as a means of decreasing retention. A gradient involving an increase in the concentration of ion interaction agent is better avoided, owing to problems of insolubility.

Precautions

Ion interaction agents may irreversibly adsorb onto the stationary phase, thereby changing the phase chemistry and reducing the apparent pore volume. Columns used for ion interaction chromatography should therefore be reserved exclusively for this purpose. The practice of ion interaction chromatography has been discussed by Gloor and Johnson (1977).

6.3 DETECTION SYSTEMS

6.3.1 GENERAL PROPERTIES OF DETECTORS

Photometric, fluorescence and electrochemical detectors respond to changes in concentration (mass per unit volume) and are sensitive to changes in the mobile phase flow rate. They are also dependent on solute dilution during chromatography, so the flow cell volume should be as small as possible (typically 8 μl for a photometric detector and 15 μl for a fluorescence detector). The plot of detector output as a function of time is called the chromatogram. The dynamic range of a detector is the concentration range over which a change in the amount of sample induces a measurable change in the detector signal. Quantitative analysis is concerned with the linear part of the dynamic range, over which the detector response is directly proportional to the concentration of solute in the flow cell. This linear dynamic range extends from the minimum detectable concentration (determined from a measurement of the detector noise) to the highest concentration, determined from the linear plot. The term 'limit of detection' refers to the total analytical method, and is affected by factors such as analyte loss incurred during sample preparation. The fundamental principles of absorption spectroscopy, fluorescence spectroscopy and voltammetry (electrochemistry) are discussed in Chapter 5.

6.3.2 ABSORBANCE DETECTION

Absorbance measurement represents the most versatile detection method employed in HPLC, and may be performed using a variety of photometric detectors. The linear dynamic range is over three orders of magnitude, and nanogram quantities of solutes can be detected, depending upon their absorptivity. Fixed single-wavelength photometers emit radiation at 254 nm from a low-pressure mercury source and can achieve a very high signal/noise ratio. Their main limitation is that the analyte must have sufficient absorption at the operating wavelength of 254 nm to be detected. Fixed multi-wavelength photometers are also available that provide several selectable fixed wavelengths (220, 254, 280, 313, 334 and 365 nm) from a medium-pressure mercury lamp and a series of filters. The energy emitted at these other wavelengths is only a fraction of the source energy at 254 nm, so these detectors are less sensitive than the fixed single-wavelength instrument. Continuously variable wavelength spectrophotometers disperse the incident radiation by means of a monochromator, so that the radiation entering the cell is of a given wavelength selected from the UV–visible range of 190–900 nm. These detectors have the versatility and convenience of allowing operation at the absorption maximum of the analyte, or at a wavelength that provides maximum selectivity. Some instruments facilitate stop-flow scanning, in which the absorbance peak can be trapped in the cell and automatically scanned to produce an absorbance spectrum. The chromatographic peak is lost using this technique, and therefore the injection must be repeated for quantitative assay. Rapid-scanning instruments can acquire spectra without interruption of the mobile phase flow. In the photodiode array detector, the 'white light' containing all the wavelengths generated by the source passes through the flow cell, and the transmitted radiation is then dispersed over an array of photodiodes. Each diode detects radiation of a discrete wavelength, so that the entire spectral transmission is monitored simultaneously. Quantitative analysis at a particular selected wavelength can be performed by monitoring the output from a specific diode. In addition, the absorption spectrum of the contents of the flow cell can be obtained by scanning all the diodes. The disadvantage of passing polychromatic radiation through the flow cell (as opposed to monochromatic radiation) is the increased probability of fluorescence, which may result in a distorted absorbance spectrum. The sensitivity of the photodiode array detector is less than that of a conventional photometric detector, due to the dark current noise from the diode array, and to the difference in light-sensitive area between the diode array and photomultiplier (Arai and Hanai, 1988).

A pure compound measured spectrophotometrically at two different wavelengths will exhibit a characteristic absorbance ratio. If the chromatographic peak of the compound in question contains an unresolved contaminant, the absorbance ratio will change. Thus the measure of absorbance ratios provides a means of testing for peak purity. The technique relies upon the impurity having a significantly different spectrum from the compound in question. The principle of the technique is based on the ratio of the absorbances becoming the ratio of the extinction coefficients, the latter ratio being an intrinsic characteristic of a compound (Yost, Stoveken and Maclean, 1977). Either a dual-channel variable-wavelength detector or a photodiode array detector can produce an absorbance ratio plot ('ratiogram') for investigating peak purity. A homogeneous peak in the chromatogram appears as a square wave in the ratiogram with a height proportional to the ratio of absorptivities, whilst a non-homogeneous peak appears as a distorted wave (Drouen, Billiet and De Galan, 1984). Spectra obtained at different points of a peak (say the apex and half-height on either slope) can be normalized and overlaid to give a visual indication of peak purity. If the eluting compound is pure, spectra taken at any point in the peak profile should be superimposable. With a photodiode array detector and computer, a three-dimensional plot displaying wavelength, time and absorbance can be obtained (Jones, 1985). None of the above tests provide absolute proof of peak purity (Schieffer, 1985).

6.3.3 FLUORESCENCE DETECTION

Fluorescence detectors range in complexity from simple filter instruments to dual monochromator spectrofluorimeters. Electronic array instruments have also been employed as fluorescence detectors (Sepaniak and Kettler, 1986). Compared with conventional radiation sources such as the xenon arc, lasers provide a higher power intensity and monochromaticity, and the incident beam has little tendency to diverge. These properties result in an increased fluorescence signal, with reduced spectral interference, provided that photochemical decomposition of the analyte does not occur (Yeung and Sepaniak, 1980).

The dynamic range of fluorescence detectors extends to four orders of magnitude, but the linear dynamic range usually occurs over a concentration range of two to three orders of magnitude. Sensitivity is some 100 times greater than that obtained with an absorbance detector, and detection limits down to 1 pg can be obtained under favourable circumstances.

6.3.4 ELECTROCHEMICAL DETECTION

Instruments used for the detection of electroactive solutes in HPLC operate on the principle of steady-state hydrodynamic chronovoltammetry, in which current is measured as a function of time. In this case, the mass transfer of the solute to the working electrode occurs by forced convection, rather than solely by diffusion, and this results in a thinner diffusion layer at the electrode compared with the thickness of the diffusion layer under stationary conditions. Thus the measured current on an HPLC voltammetric detector reaches a higher value than in a purely diffusion-controlled instrument. In practice, the working electrode is maintained at a preselected potential relative to a reference electrode at or near the limiting current plateau for the solute. The selected potential is determined from the hydrodynamic voltammogram obtained for a flowing sample solution. After a constant background current is established, the current caused by the reduction or oxidation of the solute as it flows past the working electrode is recorded as a function of time. The resulting current is proportional to the concentration of the solute in the column effluent.

The advantages of electrochemical detection over other detection methods are high sensitivity (with minimum detection limits 1000 times lower than those of photometric detectors in some cases), high selectivity (especially for organic compounds in biological matrices), wide linear range of concentration (typically 4–5 orders of magnitude) and relatively low cost, owing to the direct conversion of chemical signal into an electrical signal with no intermediate optical carrier. Characteristic problems are related to the dependence of current flow per unit concentration on mobile phase flow rate, mobile phase pH and ionic strength, condition of the electrode surface and injection volume. It follows that gradient elution is not normally possible, as the response of the detector is critically dependent upon the ionic constancy of the mobile phase (Rucki, 1980). The mobile phase must be electrically conductive and must contain a supporting electrolyte in order to avoid migration effects. For these reasons, voltammetric detectors are mainly applied in combination with reversed-phase and ion exchange liquid chromatography, in which the buffer salts act as the supporting electrolyte.

Either amperometry or coulometry can be applied to electrochemical detection in HPLC. In amperometry, only a small portion (usually <20%) of the electroactive solute is reduced or oxidized, while in coulometry the solute is completely reduced or oxidized. Amperometric detectors used with solid working electrodes (e.g. carbon paste, glassy carbon or platinum) are presently the more popular, as they are less complex in design, and are generally claimed to be more sensitive than coulometric detectors. Amperometric detectors used with mercury electrodes are referred to as polarographic detectors. Numerous designs of HPLC electrochemical detectors have been described and comparisons made between amperometric and coulometric detectors (Brunt, 1981; Bratin and Kissinger, 1981; Krstulovíc, Colin and Guiochon, 1984; Štulik and Pacaková, 1984; White, 1984).

6.4 APPLICATIONS OF HPLC

HPLC has been applied successfully to the determination of thiamin, riboflavin, niacin, vitamin B_6, folate and vitamin C in foodstuffs. The methodology depends to a large extent upon what is being measured. This can be a given vitamin added in fortification, the total (added plus naturally occurring) content of a given vitamin in a fortified food, or the naturally occurring content of a given vitamin in a non-fortified food. In addition, the extraction of vitamins from milk and other dairy products is simpler than that from animal and plant tissues. The parent forms of the vitamins, as used in fortification, exhibit different stabilities towards air, light, temperature and pH, and water solubilities range from the very soluble ascorbic acid to the hydrophobic, sparingly soluble riboflavin. Nevertheless, the above six vitamins in aqueous solution can be separated isocratically by ion interaction HPLC and detected by UV absorbance (Dong, Lepore and Tarumoto, 1988). Owing to the complexities of the food matrix, the simultaneous determination of added vitamins in fortified foods is usually limited to two or three vitamins (Polesello and Rizzolo, 1990). The situation in non-fortified foods is, of course, far more complicated, owing to the difficulties of quantitatively extracting the vitamins from their various bound forms, and to the lower levels present in such foods. There is, therefore, little scope for determining more than one vitamin at a time, apart from thiamin and riboflavin, which can be coextracted in one operation and chromatographed simultaneously or successively.

In the following part of this chapter, applications are arbitrarily divided into single-vitamin analyses and multiple-vitamin analyses.

6.4.1 THIAMIN

HPLC methods for determining thiamin *per se* are summarized in Table 6.3.

Extraction of the free and protein-bound thiamin in milk and milk-based foods is quite straightforward, as illustrated in the analysis of

Table 6.3 HPLC methods used for the determination of thiamin

Food	Sample preparation	Column	Mobile phase	Compounds separated	Detection	Reference
Normal-phase chromatography						
Liver, semisynthetic animal diet	*Extraction*: digest homogenized sample with 0.1 N HCl at 95–100 °C for 1 h. Cool, adjust pH to 4.5 and incubate with Takadiastase/papain at 45–50 °C for 3 h. Cool, dilute to volume with 0.1 N HCl, centrifuge and filter *Derivatization*: oxidize thiamin to thiochrome with alkaline $K_3Fe(CN)_6$, partition into isobutanol and centrifuge	LiChrosorb Li60 5 μm 25 cm × 4 mm i.d.	$CHCl_3$/MeOH (80 : 20)	Thiochrome	Fluorescence: ex. 375 nm em. 430 nm	Bailey and Finglas (1990)
Reversed-phase chromatography						
Rice flour	*Extraction*: digest sample with 0.1 N HCl at 95–100 °C for 30 min. Cool, adjust pH to 4.0–4.5 and incubate with Takadiastase at 45–50 °C for 3 h. Cool, dilute to volume with water and centrifuge	Nucleosil C_{18} 5 μm 15 cm × 4 mm i.d. $T = 55$ °C	Water containing 0.01 M NaH_2PO_4 and 0.15 M $NaClO_4$ adjusted to pH 2.2	Thiamin	Fluorescence: ex. 375 nm em. 435 nm after post-column derivatization of thiamin to thiochrome with alkaline $K_3Fe(CN)_6$	Ohta, Baba and Suzuki (1984)

Table 6.3 *Continued*

Food	Sample preparation	Column	Mobile phase	Compounds separated	Detection	Reference
Ion interaction chromatography						
Infant formula, milk, low-fat yoghurt, eggs, salad dressing	Stir sample with water. Deproteinize by pH adjustment to 1.7-2.0 and then to 4.0–4.2. Dilute to volume with water and filter	μBondapak C_{18} 10 μm 30 cm × 3.9 mm i.d. T = 50 °C	MeOH/water (20 : 80) containing 0.15% sodium hexane sulphonate, 0.75% HOAc and 0.1% EDTA	Thiamin	UV 248 nm	Nicolas and Pfender (1990)
Legumes, pork muscle, full cream milk powder	*Extraction*: autoclave ground sample with dilute HCl at 121 °C for 15 min. Cool, adjust pH to 4.0–4.5 and incubate with Takadiastase at 48 °C for 3 h. Cool, dilute to volume with water and filter *Clean-up/concentration*: readjust pH of extract to 5.0–5.5 and keep at 0 °C. Pass aliquot of extract through an Amberlite CG-50 ion exchange column, wash column with water, and elute thiamin with 0.15 N HCl. Evaporate eluate to	μBondapak C_{18} 10 μm 30 cm × 3.9 mm i.d. T = 30 °C (legumes) or 50 °C (pork and milk products)	MeOH/water (31 : 69) containing 5 mM sodium hexane sulphonate/ 5 mM sodium heptane sulphonate (75:25) and 0.5% HOAc	Thiamin	UV 254 nm	Vidal-Valverde and Reche (1990a)

	dryness, dissolve residue in water and adjust pH to 5.5–6.0. Pass aliquot of solution through a C_{18} Sep-Pak cartridge, wash cartridge with aqueous 5 mM sodium hexane sulphonate and elute thiamin with methanolic 5 mM sodium hexane sulphonate					
Cyanopropyl-bonded phase chromatography						
Infant formula products	Stir reconstituted sample with water. Deproteinize by pH adjustment to 1.7, and then to 4.6. Dilute to volume with water and filter *Clean-up/concentration*: pass filtrate through strong cation exchange SPE cartridge and wash cartridge sequentially with water, MeOH, water. Elute thiamin with 2 M KCl/MeOH (60 : 40) at 65–75 °C. Cool and dilute to volume with cooled elution solvent	Zorbax-CN 6 μm 25 cm × 4.6 mm i.d.	40 mM Triethylammonium phosphate buffer (pH 7.7)/MeOH (90 + 10)	Thiamin	UV 245 nm	Ayi *et al.* (1985)

Notes and abbreviations: see footnote to Table 6.9.

infant formula products (Ayi *et al.*, 1985). This procedure entailed dissolution of the formula with water, pH adjustment to induce protein precipitation, and filtration. Concentration of the thiamin and clean-up was effected using strong cation exchange solid-phase extraction (SPE). The HPLC system comprised a cyanopropyl-bonded stationary phase, a mobile phase of 40 mM triethylammonium phosphate buffer, pH 7.7/methanol (90 +10) and UV detection at 245 nm. The retention time of thiamin in this system, at a flow rate of 1.5 ml/min, was about 10 min. Naturally occurring thiamin monophosphate, which has no thiamin activity, was eluted near the solvent front, as were other phosphorylated thiamin derivatives, if present. For extracting the added thiamin in enriched cereal products and fortified breakfast cereals, the test material was autoclaved with 0.1 N HCl, and then centrifuged and filtered (Kamman, Labuza and Warthesen, 1980).

When determining the total thiamin content of a food commodity, the test material is extracted by autoclaving with dilute mineral acid (usually 0.1 N HCl) followed by enzymatic hydrolysis, in order to convert protein-bound and phosphorylated forms of the vitamin to free thiamin. Although thiamin exhibits a rather low molar absorptivity (ε = 11 305 at λ_{max} 246 nm), absorbance detection has adequate sensitivity for fortified foods (Kamman, Labuza and Warthesen, 1980; Ayi *et al.*, 1985) and also for foods that are relatively rich in the vitamin, such as legumes and pork muscle (Vidal-Valverde and Reche, 1990a). For other food commodities, absorbance detection is inadequate, and it is necessary to employ the more sensitive fluorescence detection after oxidation of the thiamin to thiochrome by pre- or post-column reaction with alkaline hexacyanoferrate (III) (ferricyanide).

Pre-column derivatization allows the relatively nonpolar thiochrome to be determined using conventional reversed-phase chromatography with its attendant ease of operation and long-term stability. Some workers (Fellman *et al.*, 1982; Reyes and Subryan, 1989; Fernando and Murphy, 1990) add orthophosphoric acid 45 s after treatment with alkaline hexacyanoferrate (III) to minimize formation of thiamin disulphide, a pH-dependent side reaction of the thiamin to thiochrome oxidation. Clean-up of the reaction mixture prior to HPLC has been effected using C_{18} SPE cartridges (Fellman *et al.*, 1982; Hasselmann *et al.*, 1989; Reyes and Subryan, 1989). An alternative approach is to selectively extract the thiochrome into isobutanol, and then to inject an aliquot of the organic solution onto a silica HPLC column eluted with chloroform/methanol (80 : 20) (Bailey and Finglas, 1990). An on-column fluorescence detection limit of 0.05 ng thiamin was reported using this approach (Ang and Moseley, 1980).

If the derivatization is carried out post-column, it is actually thiamin that is being chromatographed, and this compound in the ionized state is not retained during conventional reversed-phase chromatography. However, reversed-phase columns can be utilized for thiamin by means of ion interaction chromatography using hexane (or heptane) sulphonic acid as the ion interaction agent, either after post-column derivatization of thiamin and fluorescence detection, or without derivatization using UV detection. Alternatively, ion suppression chromatography has been employed, but this application requires adjustment of the mobile phase pH to 2.2 (Ohta, Baba and Suzuki, 1984), which is approaching the limit of stability (pH 2) of silica-based column packings. Post-column derivatization is not only more reproducible and convenient than pre-column derivatization, but the alkaline pH of the effluent is more conducive to the fluorimetric detection of thiochrome. This is because the fluorescence intensity of thiochrome is pH-dependent and reaches a steady state at pH above 8 (Ishii *et al.*, 1979).

6.4.2 RIBOFLAVIN

HPLC methods for determining riboflavin *per se* are summarized in Table 6.4.

A standard extraction technique suitable for HPLC, and applicable to any kind of foodstuff, is to convert the bound flavins to free riboflavin by autoclaving the sample with dilute mineral acid, followed by enzymatic digestion at the optimum pH. In some applications the hydrolysed extract is heated with 50% (w/v) trichloroacetic acid (TCA) to deactivate and precipitate the previously added enzyme. The total riboflavin content (excluding covalently bound flavins) is then calculated, based on measurement of the riboflavin peak. The chromatography is capable of separating FMN and riboflavin, so a valid estimate of the total riboflavin using this technique depends upon the conversion of FMN to riboflavin being complete. If the hydrolysis is incomplete, as indicated by the presence of an FMN peak in the sample chromatogram, an alternative enzyme preparation and/or a longer incubation period can be tried. If these steps fail to achieve a complete hydrolysis, the FMN peak must be measured in addition to the riboflavin peak. Summation of FMN and riboflavin peak heights provides a total riboflavin content without significant error, provided that the FMN peak height is <25% of the sum of the FMN and riboflavin peak heights (Reyes *et al.*, 1988). An unavoidable source of error is the formation during acid digestion of isomeric riboflavin monophosphates, which are chromatographically separated from FMN.

The above extraction technique has been used for the determination of total riboflavin in a wide range of foods, and the results compared with a standard microbiological assay using *Lactobacillus casei* (Johnsson and Branzell, 1987). The importance of the enzyme treatment in converting

Table 6.4 HPLC methods used for the determination of riboflavin

Food	Sample preparation	Column	Mobile phase	Compounds separated	Detection	Reference
Reversed-phase chromatography						
Italian cheeses	Homogenize sample with water/MeOH (2 : 1), add HOAc, mix and centrifuge. Resuspend the pellet three times in water/MeOH/HOAc (65 : 25 : 10), dilute the pooled supernatants to volume with the same solvent and recentrifuge	LiChrosorb RP-18 5 µm 25 cm × 4 mm i.d.	Water/MeCN (80 : 20)	Riboflavin	VIS 446 nm	Stancher and Zonta (1986)
Eggs, milk, cheese, yoghurt	Milk: acidify to pH 3 with 50% HOAc, stir for 5 min and centrifuge. Resuspend the pellet twice in 2% HOAc and dilute the pooled supernatants to volume with 2% HOAc Eggs: suspend in water/MeOH (1 : 1), acidify, centrifuge Solid samples: homogenize with water/MeOH (2 : 1), acidify, centrifuge	µBondapak C_{18} 10 µm 30 cm × 3.9 mm i.d.	Water containing 0.1% HOAc/MeOH (68 : 32)	Riboflavin	UV 270 nm	Ashoor *et al.* (1983)
Milk, yoghurt, cheese	*Clean-up/concentration* Milk: pass sample through a C_{18} Sep-Pak cartridge, wash cartridge twice with water and elute riboflavin with 20 mM acetate buffer (pH 4.0)/MeOH (1 + 1)	Bio-Sil ODS-5S 25 cm × 4 mm i.d.	Water containing 0.1% HOAc/MeOH (65 : 35)	Riboflavin	UV 270 nm	Ashoor *et al.* (1985)

	Yoghurt and cheese: blend sample with acetate buffer, filter, then solid-phase extraction as for milk					
Milks (various)	As for Ashoor *et al.* (1983) (see above)	Cosmosil-5 C_{18} (Nakarai Chemicals) 15 cm × 4.6 mm i.d.	Water containing 0.1% HOAc/MeOH (65 : 35)	Riboflavin and its decomposition products	UV 254 nm	Toyosaki, Yamamoto and Mineshita (1986)
Wines, ciders, beers	Ultrasonic degassing *Clean-up*: pass sample through C_{18} Sep-Pak cartridge	μBondapak C_{18} 10 μm 30 cm × 3.9 mm i.d.	Water/MeOH (60 : 40)	Riboflavin	Fluorescence: ex. 450 nm em. 525 nm	Moll (1988)
Milk, yoghurt	Deproteinize by mixing sample with 10% TCA and heating at 85–90 °C for 45 min. Cool, dilute with water and filter	Spherisorb ODS 5 μm 25 cm × 4.6 mm i.d.	Water/MeCN (80 : 20)	Riboflavin	Fluorescence: ex. 453 nm em. 580 nm	Ribarova *et al.* (1987)
Skim milk	Deproteinize sample with 10% acidified lead acetate solution and filter	LiChrosorb RP-18 10 μm 25 cm × 4.6 mm i.d.	Water/MeOH/HOAc (50 : 49 : 1)	Riboflavin	Fluorescence (filters)	Palanuk, Warthesen and Smith (1988)
Pasta (enriched)	*Extraction*: autoclave ground sample with 0.1 N HCl at 121 °C for 30 min, cool and centrifuge. Resuspend the pellet twice in 0.1 N HCl and dilute the pooled supernatants to volume	μBondapak C_{18} 10 μm 30 cm × 3.9 mm i.d.	(i) Water/MeOH/HOAc (56 : 43 : 1) (ii) Water/MeOH/HOAc (50 : 49 :1)	(i) Riboflavin (ii) Lumichrome	Fluorescence: (i) ex. 450 nm, em. 510 nm (filters) (ii) ex. 300–350 nm, em, 479 nm (filters)	Woodcock, Warthesan and Labuza (1982)

Table 6.4 *Continued*

Food	Sample preparation	Column	Mobile phase	Compounds separated	Detection	Reference
Flour, bread, milk, meat and cereal products, eggs, desserts	*Extraction*: autoclave with 0.1 N HCl at 121 °C for 30 min, cool and incubate with buffered Takadiastase for 2 h at 40 °C. Dilute if necessary and filter. Trace enrichment on HPLC guard column for low-potency samples	Magnusil C_{22} Supergrade (Magnus Scientific) 15 cm × 4 mm i.d. and guard column (4 cm × 4 mm i.d.) packed with Spherisorb ODS	MeOH/0.1 M citrate buffer pH 5.8 (2 + 3)	Total riboflavin	Fluorescence: ex. 449 nm em. 520 nm	Lumley and Wiggins (1981)
Baby foods, breakfast cereals, enriched flours, dairy products, health foods	*Extraction*: autoclave with 0.1 N HCl for 30 min at 121 °C and cool. Adjust pH to 4.5 and incubate with acid phosphatase at 45 °C overnight. Deproteinize by mixing extract with 50% TCA and heating at 100 °C for 5 min. Adjust pH to 4.5, dilute to volume with water and filter	Hypersil-ODS 5 μm 25 cm × 4.6 mm i.d.	Water/MeOH (3 + 2) adjusted to pH 4.5 with HOAc	Total riboflavin	Fluorescence: ex. 440 nm em. 520 nm	Johnsson and Branzell (1987) (Figure 6.5)
Milk, whole milk powder, cheese	Homogenize sample with 6% formic acid containing 2 M urea, centrifuge. Mix a 2-ml aliquot with sorboflavin as internal standard (IS) *Clean-up/concentration*: pass solution through C_{18} SPE cartridge, wash cartridge with 10% formic acid and elute with flavins with 10% formic acid/MeOH (4 : 1)	LC-18 3 μm (Supelco) 7.5 cm × 4.6 mm i.d.	14% MeCN in 100 mM KH_2PO_4 (final pH 2.9)	FAD, FMN, riboflavin, sorboflavin (IS)	Fluorescence: ex. 450 nm em. 530 nm	Bilic and Sieber (1990)

Dairy products, meat products, fish, fruit, vegetables, flour, baked products, beer, coffee	*Extraction*: autoclave homogenized sample with 0.1 N H_2SO_4 at 121 °C for 20 min. Cool, adjust pH to 4.5 and incubate with Claradiastase at 45 °C overnight. Cool, dilute to volume and filter *Clean-up/concentration*: pass aliquot of filtrate through C_{18} Sep-Pak cartridge, wash cartridge with water and elute the riboflavin with 40–70% MeOH	Spherisorb ODS-2 5 µm 25 cm × 4.6 mm i.d.	H_2O/MeOH (65 : 35)	Total riboflavin	Fluorescence: ex. 445 mn em. 525 nm	Ollilainen *et al.* (1990)
Raw and cooked meats, dairy products, eggs, cereal products	Homogenize sample with MeOH/CH_2Cl_2 (9 + 10) and internal standard (7-ethyl-8-methyl-riboflavin). Add 100 mM citrate-phosphate buffer, pH 5.5, containing 0.1% sodium azide, and rehomogenize and centrifuge	2 PLRP-S 5 µm (Polymer Laboratories) columns in series 25 cm × 4.6 mm i.d. + 15 cm × 4.6 mm i.d. T = 40 °C	MeCN/0.1% sodium azide in 10 mM citrate-phosphate buffer, pH 5.5, in multistep gradient elution programme	FAD, FMN, riboflavin, 7-Et-8-Me-RF	Fluorescence: ex. 450 nm em. 522 nm	Russell and Vanderslice (1992) (Figure 6.6)
Ion interaction chromatography						
Chick peas, green beans, full cream milk powder	*Extraction*: autoclave ground sample with dilute HCl at 121 °C for 15 min. Cool, adjust pH to 4.0–4.5 and incubate with Takadiastase at 48 °C for 3 h. Cool, dilute to volume with water and filter	µBondapak C_{18} 10 µm 30 cm × 3.9 mm i.d.	(a) Water/MeOH/HOAc (67 : 32 :1) containing 5 mM sodium hexane sulphonate (b) Water/	Total riboflavin	UV 254 nm	Vidal-Valverde and Reche (1990b)

Table 6.4 *Continued*

Food	Sample preparation	Column	Mobile phase	Compounds separated	Detection	Reference
	Clean-up/concentration: readjust pH of extract to 4.0–4.5 and pass through Florisil column. Wash column with water and elute riboflavin with triethylamine/ MeOH/water (7 : 30 : 13). Evaporate eluate to dryness and dissolve residue in MeOH/water (same proportion as mobile phase). Pass aliquot of solution through C_{18} Sep-Pak cartridge, wash cartridge with aqueous 5 mM sodium hexane sulphonate and elute riboflavin with methanolic 5 mM sodium hexane sulphonate		MeOH/HOAc (68.5 : 31 : 0.5) containing 5 mM sodium heptane sulphonate/ 5 mM sodium hexane sulphonate (25 : 75)			
Fresh fruit and vegetables	*Extraction*: digest ground dry sample with 0.1 N HCl at 99 °C for 30 min and cool. Incubate with buffered Mylase at 38 °C overnight. Add 50% TCA and heat at 60 °C for 5 min. Cool, adjust pH to 4.0, dilute to volume with water and filter	Ultrasphere-ODS 5 µm 25 cm × 4.6 mm i.d.	MeOH/H_2O (40 : 60) containing 5 mM sodium heptane sulphonate. Adjusted to pH 4.5 with H_3PO_4	Riboflavin	Fluorescence: ex. 450 nm em. 530 nm	Watada and Tran (1985)

Flour, bread, raw beef, corned beef, chicken liver, mushrooms, milk and milk products, cereals	Defat high fat samples with hexane *Extraction*: autoclave homogenized sample with 0.1 N HCl at 121 °C for 30 min. Adjust pH to 6.0 and then to 4.5. Dilute to volume and filter	LiChrosorb RP-8 10 µm 25 cm × 4.0 mm i.d.	$MeOH/H_2O$ (40 : 60) containing 5 mM sodium hexane sulphonate	FMN, riboflavin	Fluorescence: ex. 440 nm (filter) em. 565 nm (filter)	Reyes *et al.* (1988)

Notes and abbreviations: see footnote to Table 6.9.

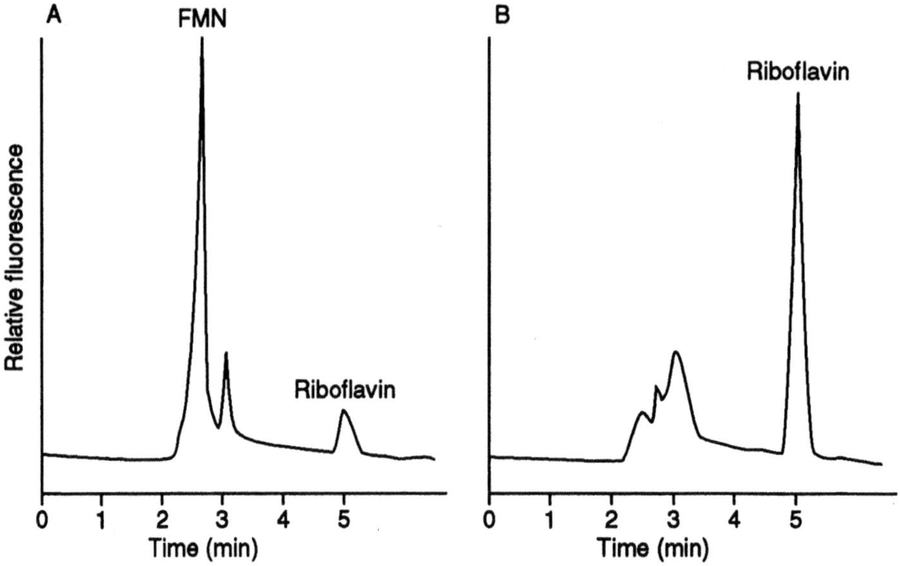

Figure 6.5 Reversed-phase HPLC of the flavins extracted from a typical foodstuff by treatment with (A) 0.1 N hydrochloric acid and (B) acid and enzyme. From Johnsson and Branzell (1987)

FMN to riboflavin is illustrated in Figure 6.5. High correlations were obtained between the two assay techniques for vitamin-enriched samples such as baby foods, gruels, porridges, breakfast cereals and flour ($r = 0.9996$) and for milk and milk products ($r = 0.9999$). This work was reported from Sweden, where FMN, rather than riboflavin, is generally used for enrichment. In contrast, the riboflavin values found with the HPLC method in non-enriched flours and flours with a high rate of extraction were 25–50% lower than those found with the microbiological assay. A possible reason for this disparity was the loss of fluorescence by the inner filter effect. This refers to the absorption of incident or emitted radiation by substances in the complex food matrix which coeluted with riboflavin. Further purification of the filtered extract using C_{18} SPE failed to increase the fluorescence signal, and unchanged results were obtained. Vidal-Valverde and Reche (1990b) reported that C_{18} SPE was inadequate for removing all interfering substances present in hydrolysed food extracts. These authors employed a clean-up procedure involving adsorption chromatography on a Florisil (fuller's earth) column, follwed by C_{18} SPE, which removed the major interfering substances present in legumes, and made absorbance detection at 254 nm sufficiently sensitive for these products (detection limit 0.4 ng/injection).

An alternative technique for determining total riboflavin is to measure the FMN and riboflavin liberated during autoclaving with dilute mineral acid, after precipitation of proteinaceous material by pH adjustment to about 4.5 (as in the AOAC fluorimetric procedure). For acid extracts containing significant amounts of FMN, i.e. where the FMN peak height is >25% of the sum of the FMN and riboflavin peak heights (such as were obtained from raw beef, corned beef, fresh and cooked liver and canned mushrooms), FMN and riboflavin were calculated separately, using their corresponding response factors (ratio of concentration of standard to peak height), and the results were summed to obtain total riboflavin. For smaller amounts of FMN the total riboflavin could be obtained by summation of FMN and riboflavin peak heights without significant error (Reyes *et al.*, 1988). The necessity of applying a correction factor to compensate for the lack of purity of commercial FMN preparations has been stressed by Russell and Vanderslice (1992).

For the analysis of milk, eggs and dairy products, in which free or loosely bound riboflavin is considered to be the predominant naturally occurring flavin present, riboflavin can be determined specifically without the need for acid and enzyme hydrolysis. A common extraction procedure for milk entails precipitation of the protein to below pH 4.5 (the isoelectric point of most proteins) and filtration. This procedure has been employed using acetic acid (Ashoor *et al.*, 1983; Toyosaki, Yamamoto and Mineshita, 1986), TCA (Rhys Williams and Slavin, 1977; Ribarova *et al.*, 1987) and acidified lead acetate solution (Palanuk, Warthesen and Smith, 1988) as the deproteinizing agent.

Most published riboflavin HPLC assays utilize C_{18} stationary phases, either with aqueous/organic mobile phases in the reversed-phase mode or using ion interaction agents (hexane or heptane sulphonic acid). Fluorescence monitoring is the preferred means of detection in most cases. The limits of fluorescence detection at 450/522 nm (ex./em.) for the biologically active flavins at a signal/noise ratio of 3 : 1 were 0.55 pmol or 0.21 ng riboflavin; 1.96 pmol or 0.89 ng FMN; 14.19 pmol or 11.15 ng FAD (Russell and Vanderslice, 1992). The sensitivity can be increased even further to achieve a detection limit of 0.02 ng/injection by irradiating the riboflavin at high pH to form lumiflavin (Ang and Moseley, 1980), but this technique has not been widely adopted. For samples with a low riboflavin content (<10 μg/100 g), Lumley and Wiggins (1981) employed a trace-enrichment technique based on the extremely long retention time of riboflavin on a reversed-phase column when pure water was used as a mobile phase. Concentration was achieved by loading successive 100-μl volumes of sample extract onto the guard column whilst eluting with water. The riboflavin, which concentrated at the column head, could then be eluted as a tight band by changing to the methanol/water mobile phase. The use of a 254-nm fixed-wavelength absorbance detector provided a minimum on-column detection limit of 0.4 ng riboflavin (Vidal-Valverde and Reche, 1990b), which was adequate for the analysis of legumes and full cream milk powder. Absorbance monitoring at 270 nm was also sufficiently sensitive for the analysis of milk and milk products after clean-up and concentration using C_{18} SPE (Ashoor *et al.*, 1985) and has the advantage in simultaneously detecting riboflavin decomposition products (Toyosaki, Yamamoto and Mineshita, 1986). Stancher and Zonta (1986) utilized visible absorbance detection at 446 nm to avoid detection interference in the analysis of Italian cheeses. The on-column detection limit of 2.5 ng (cf. 0.1 ng by fluorescence) was more than adequate for determining the relatively high concentration of riboflavin (at least 100 μg/100 g) present in the cheese commodities analysed.

Russell and Vanderslice (1992) employed a non-degradative two-step extraction procedure for the simultaneous quantification of riboflavin, FMN and FAD in a variety of foods. An internal standard, 7-ethyl-8-methyl-riboflavin, was added at the start of the extraction procedure, and separation of the flavins and internal standard was accomplished with a polymer-based column packing and a multistep gradient elution programme (Figure 6.6). Appropriate correction factors were applied to account for the impurities in the commercial FMN and FAD standards. Bilic and Sieber (1990) extracted riboflavin, FMN and FAD from dairy products by homogenization with 6% formic acid containing 2 M urea in the presence of sorboflavin added as an internal standard. Sorboflavin contains a glucityl side chain instead of a ribityl chain on the isoalloxazine ring. The two riboflavin analogues used as internal standards in the above applications possess the required chemical similarities and elution properties, but neither compound is commercially available at present.

6.4.3 NIACIN

HPLC methods for determining niacin are summarized in Table 6.5.

The free nicotinamide and nicotinic acid naturally present in fresh meat, as well as that possibly added, can be extracted quantitatively with water or methanol and determined by HPLC with reasonable precision. Strong cation exchange chromatography permits the separation of the two vitamers, together with ascorbic acid and sorbic acid, in aqueous extracts of meat (Hamano *et al.*, 1988). Comparison of the HPLC method proposed by Hamano *et al.* with a standard colorimetric method (König reaction; see section 5.4.1) indicated poor agreement, attributed to deficiencies in the latter method. Other investigators have used ion interaction chromatography for determining the niacin compounds. Takatsuki *et al.* (1987) found it necessary to use two

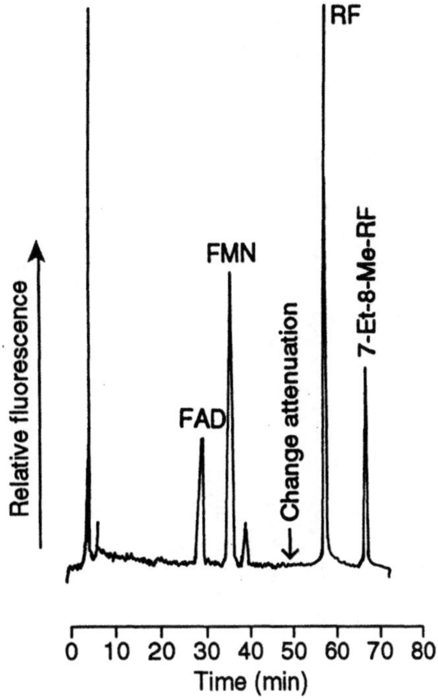

Figure 6.6 Reversed-phase HPLC of the flavins extracted from hamburger. Conditions as given in Table 6.4. (From Russell and Vanderslice (1992). Copyright © 1991 by Department of Agriculture, Government of Canada.)

different mobile phases for determining each compound in deproteinized aqueous extracts of meat; methanol/water (1 + 9) containing buffered tetrabutylammonium ion was used for nicotinic acid, and water containing buffered heptane sulphonic acid for nicotinamide. The detection limit for a 10-g sample was 1 mg/100 g for nicotinic acid and nicotinamide. Results greater than 20 mg/100 g indicated the illegal addition of either vitamer. Tsunoda *et al.* (1988) reported the simultaneous determination of the two vitamers in methanolic extracts of meat and fish using dodecylsulphate as the ion interaction agent. Oishi *et al.* (1988) obtained nicotinic acid and nicotinamide fractions from methanolic extracts of fresh meat by selective elution from an alumina SPE cartridge, and chromatographed each fraction using tetrabutylammonium ion in the mobile phase.

The added nicotinamide was extracted from fortified food products by heating the test material with 2 N H_2SO_4 acid on a boiling water bath for 30 min, and then determined (along with pyridoxine) by ion interaction chromatography (Rees, 1989). The extraction procedure caused a 6% conversion of nicotinamide to nicotinic acid, but this was

Table 6.5 HPLC methods used for the determination of niacin compounds

Food	Sample preparation	Column	Mobile phase	Compounds separated	Detection	Reference
Strong cation exchange chromatography						
Fresh meat (test for added niacin)	Homogenize sample in water, then boil, cool and filter	Partisil SCX 10 µm 25 cm × 4.6 mm i.d.	50 mM phosphate buffer (pH 3.0)	Nicotinic acid, nicotinamide, ascorbic acid, sorbic acid	UV 260 nm	Hamano *et al.* (1988)
Ion interaction chromatography						
Cereal products	*Extraction*: heat sample at 95–100 °C with water and $Ca(OH)_2$ suspension for 30 min, then autoclave at 121 °C for 30 min. Cool and dilute to volume with water. Refrigerate overnight and centrifuge *Clean-up/concentration*: pass aliquot of extract through an AG1-X8 (Bio-Rad) anion exchange column, wash column with water, and elute nicotinic acid with 5% HOAc followed by water. Treat eluate with 1% aqueous $KMnO_4$ at 95–100 °C. Cool, dilute to volume with water and pass through C_{18} Sep-Pak cartridge	µBondapak C_{18} 10 µm 30 cm × 3.9 mm i.d.	$MeOH/H_2O$ (5 : 95) containing tetrabutyl-ammonium phosphate (PIC-A)	Nicotinic acid (representing total niacin)	UV 254 nm	Tyler and Shrago (1980) (Figure 6.7)

Beef, semolina, cottage cheese	*Extraction*: blend sample with water and $Ca(OH)_2$ mixture, then autoclave at 121 °C for 15 min. Cool to 0 °C, filter, adjust to pH 6.5–7.0 with oxalic acid, filter. Pass 10 ml of filtrate through C_{18} Sep-Pak cartridge. Discard first 6 ml of eluate and collect next 3.5 ml. Add 1 drop 85% H_3PO_4 and mix	C_{18} LC-18-DB 5 μm (Supelco) 15 cm × 4.6 mm i.d.	23% MeCN, 0.10% H_3PO_4, 0.10% sodium dodecylsulphate in water (final pH 2.8)	Nicotinic acid (representing total niacin)	UV 254 nm	Tyler and Genzale (1990) (Figure 6.8)
Legumes, lyophilized pork muscle	*Extraction*: autoclave ground sample with dilute HCl at 121 °C for 15 min and cool. Adjust pH to 4.0–4.5 and incubate with Takadiastase at 48 °C for 3 h. Cool, filter and dilute to volume with water *Clean-up/concentration*: re-adjust pH of extract to 4.7 ± 0.02 and pass an aliquot through a Dowex 1-X8 (Bio-Rad) anion exchange column. Wash column with water, and elute nicotinic acid with 0.15 N HCl. Evaporate eluate to dryness and dissolve residue in MeOH/0.1 M acetate buffer of the required pH to obtain a final pH of 4.7–4.9	μBondapak C_{18} 10 μm 30 cm × 3.9 mm i.d.	10 mM sodium acetate buffer (pH 4.66)/ MeOH (9 : 1) containing 5 mM tetra-butylammonium bromide (final pH 4.72)	Nicotinic acid (representing free niacin)	UV 254 nm	Vidal-Valverde and Reche (1991)

Table 6.5 *Continued*

Food	Sample preparation	Column	Mobile phase	Compounds separated	Detection	Reference
Instant coffee	Dissolve sample in hot water, cool, dilute to volume and filter *Clean-up*: pass through Sep-Pak C_{18} cartridge	Spherisorb ODS-2 15 cm × 5 mm i.d.	MeOH/water (8 : 92) containing 5 mM tetrabutylammonium hydroxide (final pH adjusted to 7.0)	Nicotinic acid	UV 254 nm	Trugo, Macrae and Trugo (1985)
Fresh beef and pork, fresh fish, fish products (test for added niacin)	Homogenize sample in water and dilute to volume. Centrifuge and filter. Deproteinize aliquot of the filtrate with saturated zinc sulphate followed by 1 N NaOH. Dilute to volume with water, let stand for 30 min and filter	Radial-PAK μBondapak C_{18} 10 μm 10 cm × 8 mm	(i) 5 mM tetrabutylammonium phosphate (PIC-A) in MeOH/water (1 + 9) (ii) 10 mM heptane sulphonic acid (PIC-B7) in water	(i) Nicotinic acid (ii) Nicotinamide	UV 263 nm	Takatsuki *et al.* (1987)
Beef, pork, tuna (test for added niacin)	Add H_3PO_4 to homogenized sample, then extract with MeOH and filter	Shim-Pack FLC ODS 5 cm × 4.6 mm i.d. $T = 50$ °C	1 mM sodium dodecylsulphate and 20 mM H_3PO_4 /MeOH (7 : 3) pH 2.4	Nicotinic acid, nicotinamide	UV 261 nm	Tsunoda *et al.* (1988)

Fresh meat (test for added niacin)	Extract homogenized sample with MeOH *Clean-up*: Sep-Pak alumina N cartridge eluting nicotinamide with MeOH and nicotinic acid with 0.1 M $NaHCO_3$	LiChrosorb RP-18	MeOH/acetate buffer pH 5 (2 : 10) containing 0.1 M NaOAc and 0.01 M tetrabutylammonium hydroxide	Nicotinic acid, nicotinamide (separate chromatograms)	UV 261 nm	Oishi *et al.* (1988)
Reversed-phase chromatography						
Cereal products, mushrooms	*Acid extraction*: autoclave sample with 0.2 N H_2SO_4 at 1 bar for 1 h and cool. Incubate with buffered Clarase at 45 °C for 3 h. Cool, dilute to volume and filter. *Alkaline extraction*: heat sample with $Ca(OH)_2$ suspension at 95–100 °C for 30 min, then autoclave at 1 bar for 30 min. Cool and dilute to volume. Refrigerate overnight and centrifuge	Nicotinic acid fraction transferred from reversed-phase column (Nucleosil C_{18} 5 µm) to anion exchange column (Nucleosil SB 5 µm) using *automatic* column switching. Both columns 15 cm × 4.6 mm i.d.	(A) 0.57% acetic acid adjusted to pH 3.0 with NaOH to elute the nicotinic acid from the C_{18} column and to place it onto the anion exchange column (B) Mobile phase A/MeOH (5 : 95) to flush the C_{18} column (C) 2.28% acetic acid adjusted to pH 3.0 with NaOH to elute the nicotinic acid from the anion exchange column	Nicotinic acid (representing total niacin)	UV 254 nm	van Niekerk *et al.* (1984)

Notes and abbreviations: see footnote to Table 6.9.

accounted for by subjecting the nicotinamide standard to the same treatment. Nicotinamide was chromatographed using a column packing of Partisil ODS, which is a non-endcapped material containing 50% residual silanol groups. The retention times of nicotinamide and pyridoxine on this column were 8.0 and 5.8 min, respectively. Nicotinamide was less retained on a fully endcapped material (Ultrasphere ODS), so that it eluted before pyridoxine (4.2 and 8.6 min). The limit of detection for a 10-g sample was 0.1 mg/100 g for nicotinamide. HPLC results for milk powder, high-protein meal powder and diet meal powder were in good agreement with results obtained by microbiological assay using *Lactobacillus plantarum*.

In determining the naturally occurring niacin in foodstuffs, it must be decided whether to estimate total niacin or free ('available') niacin (see discussion in section 4.2.3). In addition to the extraction problem, it is necessary to purify sample extracts prior to HPLC because the absorbance detection usually employed is not highly selective. Kral (1983) used pulsed amperometric detection for the analysis of fruit juices subjected to acid hydrolysis but, despite the improved selectivity, it was still necessary to employ cation exchange chromatography as a clean-up step.

Tyler and Shrago (1980) extracted the total niacin from fortified cereal products by autoclaving samples dispersed in calcium hydroxide solution. This procedure releases the naturally occurring bound nicotinic acid, whilst also hydrolysing the added nicotinamide to nicotinic acid. Clean-up of the hydrolysate was effected by anion exchange open-column chromatography, followed by treatment with 1% aqueous potassium permanganate to oxidize pigments and other remaining substances and, finally, passage through a C_{18} SPE cartridge. Figure 6.7 shows chromatograms of purified extracts of semolina and bread samples analysed by ion interaction chromatography and photometric detection at 254 nm. A less laborious, yet more efficient, means of purifying alkaline digests of three major food representatives (beef, semolina and cottage cheese) was reported by Tyler and Genzale (1990). After autoclaving with calcium hydroxide solution, digests were cooled in an ice bath, filtered, and then adjusted to pH 6.5–7.0 with oxalic acid to precipitate the excess calcium. An aliquot (10 ml) of the filtered suspension was loaded onto a C_{18} SPE cartridge, the first 6 ml of effluent was discarded, and the remaining effluent was collected and acidified with phosphoric acid. Analysis of the purified extracts was performed by ion interaction chromatography at acidic pH using sodium dodecylsulphate as the ion interaction agent. A feature of this method is the unusually sharp nicotinic acid peak, which resulted from the injection of the analyte in a large volume (200 μl) of dilute phosphoric acid, and which led to a detection limit of *c.* 0.5 mg/100 g. The high efficiency of

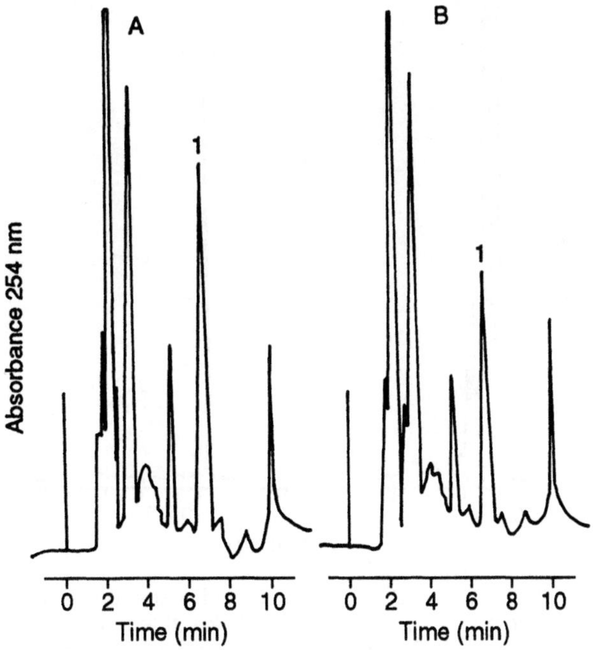

Figure 6.7 Ion interaction HPLC of nicotinic acid (peak 1) extracted from semolina (A) and bread (B) samples after ion exchange and permanganate clean-up. Conditions as given in Table 6.5. (Reprinted from Tyler and Shrago (1980), p. 276, by courtesy of Marcel Dekker, Inc.)

the purification step is evident from the lack of irrelevant peaks in the chromatogram obtained for semolina (Figure 6.8) compared with the many peaks in the chromatogram obtained for semolina after clean-up by anion exchange chromatoraphy, permanganate oxidation and Sep-Pak filtration at acid pH (Figure 6.7). The superior efficiency of the single clean-up step is attributable to the amphoteric nature of nicotinic acid. At pH 7, nicotinic acid is not retained on the C_{18} Sep-Pak cartridge, but a large number of pigmented compounds are retained. Conversely, nicotinic acid is strongly retained on the C_{18} analytical column at acidic pH in the presence of an ion interaction agent, whereas many polar interferences elute in the dead volume. Tyler and Genzale (1990) compared HPLC results with results using a microbiological assay. Agreement between the two methods was obtained for the analysis of beef, semolina and cottage cheese, but certain food samples (e.g. instant coffee) gave higher niacin values using HPLC. On the other hand, Finglas and Faulks (1984a), using gradient elution programmes and strong anion exchange HPLC to determine nicotinic acid in raw and cooked potatoes, reported values that were approximately 50% lower

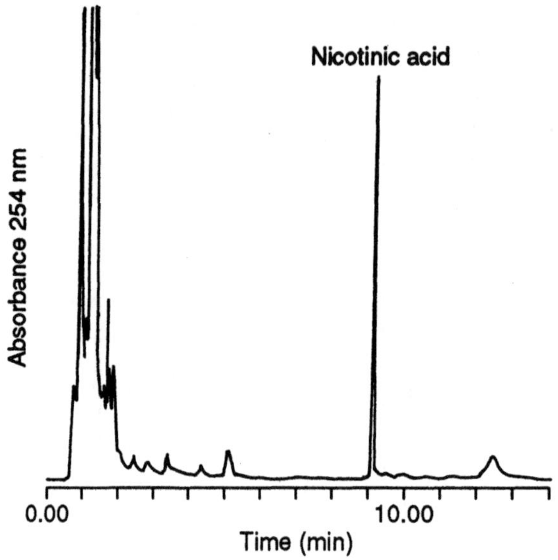

Figure 6.8 Ion interaction HPLC of nicotinic acid extracted from semolina after Sep-Pak C_{18} clean-up and acidification of Sep-Pak effluent. Conditions as given in Table 6.5. (From Tyler and Genzale (1990). Reprinted from the *Journal of the AOAC*, Vol. 73, No. 01, pp. 467–9, 1990. Copyright 1990 by AOAC International.)

than those published in food tables, which were obtained by the AOAC chemical or microbiological methods. The results were, however, in good agreement with the literature value (Burton, 1966) of 0.5 mg/100 g for niacin in old, raw potatoes.

Van Niekerk *et al.* (1984) did not include a clean-up step in their assay procedure for the analysis of cereal products and mushrooms subjected to acid or alkaline hydrolysis. They employed, instead, on-line multidimensional HPLC, whereby the nicotinic acid fraction was transferred from a reversed-phase column to an anion exchange column. The HPLC method gave lower values for the acid extracts than for the alkaline extracts (except for the standard), whereas results obtained microbiologically on both acid and alkaline extracts showed no difference. This suggests that part of the nicotinic acid in the acid extract was present in a bound form that was available to the assay organism (*Lactobacillus plantarum*). The HPLC method had a detection limit of 0.5 mg of nicotinic acid per 100 g of sample when a 5-g sample was extracted and diluted to 100 ml.

For the estimation of free ('available') niacin in legumes and meat (Vidal-Valverde and Reche, 1991), samples (1–10 g, equivalent to 10–100 μg of niacin) were autoclaved with 0.1 N HCl (30 ml) and 6 N

HCl (1 ml) at 121 °C for 15 min. The acid digest was then adjusted to pH 4.0–4.5 and incubated with Takadiastase to hydrolyse the starch present in the legumes. The extracts were purified by strong anion exchange chromatography, and then analysed by ion interaction HPLC. The shape and retention times of the nicotinic acid peak were extremely sensitive to the pH of the mobile phase and, consequently, to column temperature, because of the amphoteric nature of nicotinic acid. Each different food required a trial and error procedure to ascertain the column temperature required for optimum separation.

6.4.4 VITAMIN B_6

Vitamin B_6 is the generic descriptor for a group of 3-hydroxy-2-methylpyridine derivatives, which comprises pyridoxine (PN), pyridoxal (PL), pyridoxamine (PM) and their corresponding 5′-phosphorylated forms, PNP, PLP and PMP. The major end-product of vitamin B_6 metabolism is 4-pyridoxic acid (4-PA). In foods of animal origin, PL, PLP, PM and PMP are found as a result of interconversion of aldehyde and amine forms during processing and storage. Plant-derived foods contain mostly PN, a significant proportion of which may be present as PN-glucoside. PNP does not occur to any significant extent in natural products. Using non-hydrolytic extraction techniques, all six B_6 vitamers, together with 4-PA, can be separated and quantified by HPLC. Accurate quantification of these compounds is an essential prerequisite in biochemistry for studying the metabolism of vitamin B_6, but for routine food analysis it is customary to hydrolyse the phosphorylated forms and to determine PN, PL and PM, each of which represents the sum of the phosphorylated and nonphosphorylated forms. This approach is valid because, in humans, all six vitamers exhibit equal biological activity on a molar basis. The chromatographic separation of three compounds, rather than six, is obviously less demanding of the HPLC system, and the problem of the weakly fluorescent phosphorylated forms is circumvented. Moreover, the data obtained can be compared with data obtained by microbiological (yeast) assay, in which dephosphorylation is obligatory.

HPLC methods for determining vitamin B_6 are summarized in Table 6.6.

Animal and plant tissues differ greatly with respect to the forms of vitamin B_6 contained in them, and this creates the problem of selecting a suitable extraction procedure for food composites. The HPLC method for vitamin B_6 recommended by COST 91 (Brubacher, Müller-Mulot and Southgate, 1985) advocates autoclaving the homogenized test material in a medium of 0.2 N H_2SO_4 for 30 min at 121 °C. Standard solutions of PN, PL and PM are subjected to the same conditions (external

Table 6.6 HPLC methods used for the determination of vitamin B_6 compounds

Food	Sample preparation	Column	Mobile phase	Compounds separated	Detection	Reference
Strong cation exchange chromatography						
Milk (bovine, caprine, human)	Deproteinize with 20% TCA, centrifuge, extract supernatant with diethyl ether and discard the ether. Filter the aqueous portion (0.45-μm membrane). Add 2-amino-5-chlorobenzoic acid as internal standard to an aliquot of filtrate immediately before injection	Vydac 401TP-B 10 μm silica-based cation exchanger 30 cm × 4.6 mm i.d.	Ternary gradient elution Solvent A: 0.02 N HCl Solvent B: 0.1 M NaH_2PO_4 (pH 3.3) Solvent C: 0.5 M NaH_2PO_4 (pH 5.9)	PLP, PNP, 4-PA, PMP, internal standard, PL, PN, PM	Fluorescence: ex. 330 nm em. 400 nm after post-column addition of buffered sodium bisulphite	Coburn and Mahuren (1983)
Reversed-phase chromatography						
Food composites, vegetables, meat and meat products, complete meals	*Extraction*: homogenize sample in a medium of 0.1 N H_2SO_4 and autoclave at 121 °C for 30 min. Cool, dilute to volume with water and filter	Spherisorb RB ODS 5 μm 25 cm × 4 mm i.d.	0.04 M H_2SO_4	PM, PL, PN	Fluorescence: ex. 290 nm em. 395 nm	Brubacher, Müller-Mulot and Southgate (1985)
Fortified breakfast cereals	Sonicate sample with 0.5 M KOAc, pH 4.5, centrifuge. Deproteinize the supernatant by heating at 50 °C with 33.3% w/v TCA and centrifuging	μBondapak C_{18} 10 μm 30 cm × 3.9 mm i.d.	33 mM KH_2PO_4 buffer (pH 2.2)	PM, PL, PN (only PN present at any significant level in breakfast cereals)	Fluorescence: ex. 295 nm em. 405 nm (filters)	Gregory (1980)

Human milk	Dilute sample with 33 mM KH_2PO_4 buffer. Deproteinize by treating with 60% TCA and centrifuging. Dilute supernatant with equal volume of buffer. Remove remaining lipid and TCA by washing with diethyl ether. Remove ether with N_2	Biosphere ODS 5 μm (Bioanalytical Systems)	33 mM KH_2PO_4 buffer (pH 2.9) containing 3% MeOH	PMP, PM, PLP, PL, PN	Fluorescence: ex. 330 nm em. 400 nm after post-column reaction with buffered $NaHSO_3$	Hamaker *et al.* (1985)
Chicken tissues (raw and cooked)	Homogenize with HPO_3 solution, heat to 100 °C, then cool to 0 °C and centrifuge	BioSil ODS-5S 5 μm 25 cm × 4 mm i.d.	66 mM KH_2PO_4 buffer (pH 3.0)	PM, PMP, PL, PLP	Fluorescence: ex. 290 nm em. 395 nm (raw samples) ex. 280 nm em. 395 nm (cooked samples)	Ang, Cenciarelli and Eitenmiller (1988)
Ground beef, lima beans, whole wheat flour, non-fat dry milk	Partially defat sample by cold extraction with $CHCl_3$/petroleum ether (1 : 2), air dry, store overnight at −40 °C. Slurry in water, acidify to pH 2.0, digest with pepsin (37 °C for 3 h), adjust pH to 8.0, digest with pancreatin (37 °C for 12 h). Add TCA and then MeOH, mix and centrifuge. Resuspend pellet in HPLC mobile phase and recentrifuge. Pass combined supernatants through C_{18} Sep-Pak cartridge	μBondapak C_{18} 10 μm 30 cm × 3.9 mm i.d.	75 mM KH_2PO_4 containing monochloroacetic acid at 1.5 g/l and acidified to pH 2.75 with H_3PO_4	PMP, PM, PLP, PL, PN representing biologically available vitamin B_6	Fluorescence: ex. 310 nm em. 390 nm after post-column addition of buffered sodium bisulphite	Ekanayake and Nelson (1988)

Table 6.6 *Continued*

Food	Sample preparation	Column	Mobile phase	Compounds separated	Detection	Reference
Beef, liver, milk	Homogenize beef and liver with 0.1 M KH_2PO_4 buffer (pH 7). Deproteinize the homogenate or the milk sample with 3 N $HClO_4$ and centrifuge. Resuspend the pellet in 1 N $HClO_4$ and recentrifuge. Adjust pH of combined supernatants to 6–7. Heat aliquot with 0.5 M sodium glyoxylate to convert PM and PMP to PL and PLP, respectively *Derivatization*: heat with semicarbazide to form semicarbazones	Ultrasphere IP C_{18} 5 μm 25 cm × 4.6 mm i.d.	33 mM KH_2PO_4 buffer (pH 2.2) containing 2.5% MeCN	Semicarbazones of PL and PLP. Quantification of PL, PLP, PM and PMP is based on assays with and without glyoxylate treatment	Fluorescence: ex. filter 365 nm transmission max.; em. filter > 400 nm transmission	Gregory, Manley and Kirk (1981)
Ion interaction chromatography						
Human milk	Add 4′-deoxypyridoxine (4-dPN) as internal standard to milk sample. Incubate with buffered phosphohydrolase at 37 °C for 1 h. Deproteinize by heating with TCA. Defat with CH_2Cl_2. Centrifuge and adjust pH to 5.2	μBondapak C_{18} 10 μm 30 cm × 3.9 mm i.d.	Gradient elution programme. *Solvent A*. MeOH/water (85 : 15) *Solvent B*. 1% HOAc containing 5 mM sodium heptane sulphonate (PIC-B7)	PL, PN, PM, 4-dPN (internal standard)	Fluorescence: ex. 300 nm em. 375 nm	Morrison and Driskell (1985)

Pork, broccoli, milk	Homogenize pork and broccoli with 5% sulphosalicylic acid (SSA) and 4′-deoxypyridoxine (4-dPN) as internal standard, add CH_2Cl_2, homogenize, centrifuge. Blend milk with 20% SSA and 4-dPN, add CH_2Cl_2, blend, centrifuge *Preparative HPLC*: AG2-X8, Cl^- form (Bio-Rad) anion exchange column (25 cm × 9 mm i.d.) eluted with 0.1 N HCl, fluorescence detection	C_{18} (Perkin-Elmer) 3 μm 3 cm × 4.6 mm i.d.	Linear gradient with 33 mM KH_2PO_4 buffer (pH 2.2) containing 8 mM octane sulphonic acid and increasing percentage of 2-PrOH	PLP, PMP, PL, PN, 4-dPN (internal standard), PM	Fluorescence: ex. 330 nm em. 400 nm after post-column reaction with buffered sodium bisulphite to form fluorescent hydroxy-sulphonate derivatives of PLP and PL; native fluorescence of PMP, PM, PN and 4-dPN	Gregory and Feldstein (1985)
Potatoes	Mix sample with 5% sulphosalicylic acid (SSA) plus 4′-deoxypyridoxine (4-dPN) as internal standard and centrifuge *Clean-up*: SSA removed by passage through a 4 cm × 8 mm i.d. 100–120 mesh AG1-X8 anion exchange column (Bio-Rad)	Radial-PAK C_{18} 4 μm 10 cm × 8 mm	Binary step gradient *Solvent A*. Water containing 0.033 M H_3PO_4, 4 mM octane and heptane sulphonic acid (pH 2.2)/ 2-PrOH (97.5 : 2.5) *Solvent B*. Water containing 0.33 M H_3PO_4	PLP, PMP, PN-glucoside, PL, PN, 4-dPN (internal standard), PM	Fluorescence: ex. 338 nm em. 425 nm after post-column reaction with buffered sodium bisulphite to form fluorescent hydroxy-sulphonate derivatives of PLP and	Addo and Augustin (1988) (Figure 6.9)

Table 6.6 *Continued*

Food	Sample preparation	Column	Mobile phase	Compounds separated	Detection	Reference
			(pH 2.2)/ 2-PrOH (82.5 : 17.5) Equilibrate column with B for 1 h; switch to A 10 min before injection, then to B 3 min after injection		PL; native fluorescence of PMP, PM, PN and 4-dPN	
Pork liver (raw), milk	To minced liver sample or to milk add 4′-deoxypyridoxine (4-dPN) as internal standard and homogenize with ice-cold 0.1–0.5 M $HClO_4$. Centrifuge, adjust pH to 7.5, filter and readjust pH to 4	LiChrosphere RP-18 5 µm 12.5 cm × 4 mm i.d.	Gradient elution programme *Solvent A*. MeOH *Solvent B*. 30 mM KH_2PO_4 buffer (pH 2.7) containing 4 mM octane sulphonic acid Linear gradient: 90% (B) to 60% (B) to 90% (B)	PLP, 4-PA, PMP, PL, PN, 4-dPN (internal standard), PM	Fluorescence: ex. 330 nm em. 400 nm after post-column reaction with buffered sodium bisulphite	Bitsch and Möller (1989)

Notes and abbreviations: see footnote to Table 6.9.

standardization). HPLC is performed under reversed-phase ion suppression conditions using a C_{18} stationary phase, a mobile phase of 0.08 N H_2SO_4, and a fluorescence detector. PM, PL and PN are separated (in that order of elution) within 10 min and quantified, and the amounts of each vitamer are totalled to give the vitamin B_6 content expressed in mg PN/100 g of sample. The small molecular weight differences (1 mg of PN ≡ 1.008 mg of PM ≡ 1.012 mg of PL) are ignored. The detection limits are 10 μg of PM, 30 μg of PL and 30 μg of PN in a 100-g sample.

For the analysis of human milk, Morrison and Driskell (1985)

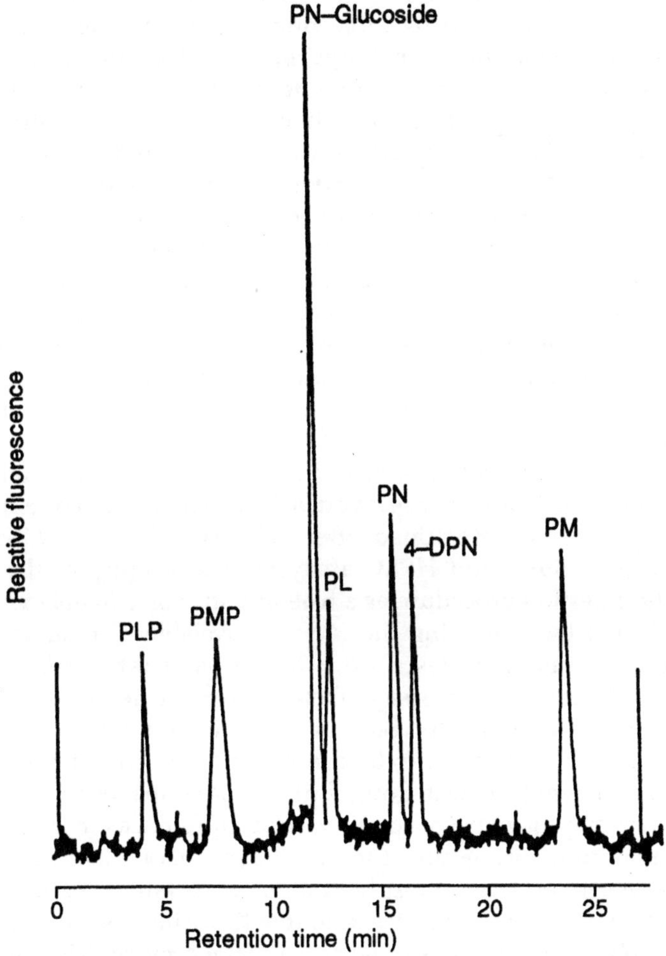

Figure 6.9 Ion interaction HPLC of vitamin B_6 vitamers extracted from potatoes. Conditions as given in Table 6.6. (Reprinted from Addo and Augustin (1988) *J. Fd Sci.*, **53**, 749–52.) Copyright © by Institute of Food Technologists).

hydrolysed the phosphorylated B_6 vitamers with phosphohydrolase, and then determined the PL, PN and PM by means of ion interaction chromatography with a gradient elution programme. The vitamin B_6 antagonist 4′-deoxypyridoxine (4-dPN), which is commercially available as the hydrochloride salt, was used as an internal standard. With the aid of fluorescence detection, the minimum detectable limits for PM and PN were 1 ng/injection, which was equivalent to 6 μg/litre of milk. Excellent correlations between HPLC and microbiologically derived data were observed for PL and total vitamin B_6, but not for PM and PN, where several values were observed to be below minimum detectable limits.

Ekanayake and Nelson (1988) estimated the biologically available vitamin B_6 content of foods by subjecting partially defatted samples to a two-stage enzymatic digestion (pepsin/pancreatin), followed by treatment with TCA and then methanol to terminate the hydrolysis reaction and precipitate the proteins. The hydrolysates were centrifuged at 28 000**g**, and the supernatant fraction was transferred to a hypodermic syringe. The pellet was resuspended in HPLC mobile phase and centrifuged. The supernatant was collected in the same syringe, and the pooled fractions were passed through a Sep-Pak C_{18} cartridge. The purified extracts were analysed by reversed-phase HPLC with ion suppression, using post-column reaction with buffered sodium bisulphite to enhance the fluorescence of PLP. To calculate the available vitamin B_6, nonphosphorylated vitamer equivalents were calculated from the phosphorylated forms by using the molarity conversion factors of 0.6764 for PLP to PL and 0.6777 for PMP to PM. Transamination of PLP to PMP and PL to PM occurred on digestion and was taken into account when calculating the recoveries. Total vitamin B_6 contents of the food samples were determined after acid hydrolysis (AOAC microbiological procedure) and HPLC analysis. The validity of the *in vitro* enzymatic digestion procedure as a true measure of available vitamin B_6 was evaluated by comparing the ratio of available to total vitamin B_6 obtained by the methods described, with the same ratio obtained by rat bioassay and yeast growth assay taken from published data. When the 95% confidence intervals for each of the ratios for a given food were compared, they were found to be comparable for ground beef, non-fat dry milk and whole wheat flour, but not for lima beans. The latter discrepancy may have been due to varietal differences in lima beans.

The extraction procedure for the subsequent determination of phosphorylated and nonphosphorylated B_6 vitamers usually entails precipitation of the protein by treatment with trichloroacetic, perchloric, metaphosphoric or sulphosalicylic acid followed by centrifugation.

The first successful separation of all six B_6 vitamers, plus 4-PA, was accomplishedd by Vanderslice, Stewart and Yarmas (1979) using a 55 °C-thermostatted column packed with Aminex A-25 (Bio-Rad) strong anion exchange resin. All six vitamers, plus 3-hydroxypyridine, were eluted isocratically within 80 min using a pH 10, 0.4 M sodium chloride/0.01 M glycine buffer solution. Two fluorescence monitors were employed, one being dedicated to detecting the weakly fluorescent PLP. In a modified procedure to improve separations and enhance sensitivity (Vanderslice and Maire, 1980; Vanderslice *et al.*, 1981), two A-25 columns maintained at different temperatures (50 °C and 18 °C) were selected singly or in series by programmed operation of a six-way switching valve. Semicarbazide was added to the pH 10 buffer solution to convert the PL and PLP to their respective semicarbazones, which were detected at different wavelengths to the nonderivatized vitamers using a wavelength-programmable spectrofluorimeter. 4-PA could be eluted 20 min after elution of the vitamers by switching to a pH 2.5 buffer. This procedure was utilized to determine PMP, PM, PNP, PN, PLP and PL in pork, fish, hamburger and dried skimmed milk, and PN in fortified breakfast cereals (Vanderslice *et al.*, 1980; Vanderslice, Maire and Yakupkovic, 1981) using 3-hydroxypyridine as an internal standard. Samples were extracted by homogenizing with sulphosalicylic acid, which denatures the protein and releases the B_6 vitamers present. Removal of the sulphosalicylic acid was effected by preparative anion exchange HPLC before the final analysis. If not removed, the sulphosalicylic acid would bind very tightly to the analytical anion exchange column, causing the elution times of the vitamers to change after a series of runs. Sulphosalicylic acid is also highly fluorescent and would create a high fluorescent background on eventual elution. Vanderslice, Maire and Yakupkovic (1981) compared the PN values obtained by HPLC for fortified breakfast cereals with results obtained by the AOAC microbiological assay using *Saccharomyces carlsbergensis* and a radiometric–microbiological assay devised by Guilarte, Shane and McIntyre (1981). Samples analysed by the AOAC assay yielded results that ranged from 62% to 136% of the values obtained by HPLC. Values obtained by the radiometric method agreed to within 5% of HPLC results for four cereal samples, but three other cereal samples were 130% of the values obtained by HPLC. Unfortunately, the separations obtained can no longer be reproduced on Aminex A-25 due to a change in the resin's characteristics brought about by a change in the manufacturing process (Vanderslice, Brownlee and Cortissoz, 1984).

For the determination of PL, PLP, PM and PMP, the major B_6 vitamers in foods of animal origin (Gregory, Manley and Kirk, 1981), beef and liver homogenates or milk samples were deproteinized by treatment with 3 N perchloric acid followed by centrifugation. Duplicate portions of each extract were transferred to test tubes and diluted with phosphate buffer. Water (0.1 ml) or aqueous 0.5 N sodium glyoxylate was added and the tubes were incubated in a boiling water bath for 15 min. The purpose of the glyoxylate treatment was to convert PM and PMP to PL and PLP, respectively. After cooling, semicarbazide (0.5 ml of a 0.2 M aqueous solution) was added to each tube, followed by a 5-min incubation in a boiling water bath. Treatment with semicarbazide converts the aldehydic B_6 vitamers to their semicarbazone derivatives. Semicarbazide treatment is also capable of breaking the Schiff base linkage between PLP and protein lysine residues, allowing the estimation of both free and protein-bound PLP (Dakshinamurti and Chauhan, 1981). The derivatization was employed because PLP-semicarbazone exhibits greater retention and fluorescence than underivatized PLP. The semicarbazone derivatization procedure does not allow the determination of PN and PNP. However, data obtained by microbiological assay show that tissue PN and PNP levels are minimal and insignificant. The derivatized solutions were filtered (0.45 μm) prior to HPLC analysis. The separation of PL- and PLP-semicarbazones was accomplished using reversed-phase HPLC with ion suppression. Quantification of the individual B_6 vitamers (PL, PLP, PM and PMP) was based on the differences in height of the PL- and PLP-semicarbazone peaks in the presence and absence of glyoxylate. Vitamin B_6 values were expressed as micrograms of free base per gram of sample, permitting the addition of values for phosphorylated and nonphosphorylated vitamers. The limit of detection was *c.* 20 μg/100 g for each vitamer in animal tissue samples, and 5 μg/100 ml for milk samples. This sensitivity was sufficient for the analysis of all tissues examined, but the quantification of certain milk samples was difficult because of the low vitamin B_6 content. For comparative microbiological (yeast) assay, the perchloric acid extracts of a limited number of samples were treated with acid phosphatase, and the individual PL, PN and PM fractions were collected manually by HPLC. Reasonable correlation was obtained between the results of the semicarbazone HPLC and microbiological procedures for the individual B_6 vitamers and total vitamin B_6, which supported the accuracy of the HPLC assay.

Coburn and Mahuren (1983) accomplished the separation of all six B_6 vitamers, plus 4-PA, using a single silica-based strong cation exchange column and a ternary gradient elution programme. Post-column addition of pH 7.5 buffer and sodium bisulphite permitted the fluorimetric detection of all B_6 compounds at the same wavelength. The method was capable of measuring nanogram quantities of each B_6 compound in bovine, caprine and human milk. An internal standard (2-amino-5-chlorobenzoic acid) was added to deproteinize milk samples immediately before injection. This compound, which eluted after the fourth peak of interest (PMP), could not be added to the sample at the start of the analysis, and hence served only to compensate for changes in the chromatographic conditions. 4-dPN was not used as an internal standard because it eluted after the last vitamer (PM) and therefore would increase the running time. Bisulphite was chosen over semicarbazide as the derivatizing agent because it gave better detection sensitivity under the acidic conditions of the system. The pH 7.5 buffer was added to the bisulphite to facilitate the detection of PNP, which is not fluorescent under acidic conditions at the wavelengths selected. PNP, which has never been detected in biological samples, sometimes interfered with the quantitation of the first B_6 vitamer peak (PLP), and therefore it was not routinely included in the standards. The absence of a PNP peak might permit the use of 4′-deoxypyridoxine 5′-phosphate (4-dPNP) as an internal standard, as this analogue elutes between the PLP peak and the next peak of interest (4-PA) (Shephard, Louw and Labadarios, 1987). These authors used 4-dPNP as an internal standard to monitor sample preparation and chromatography in the analysis of human plasma using the HPLC technique of Coburn and Mahuren (1983).

Hamaker *et al.* (1985) reported the reversed-phase isocratic separation and quantification of PMP, PM, PLP, PL and PN in human milk using fluorimetric detection after post-column addition of pH 7.5 buffer and sodium bisulphite. Separation of the PL and PLP was shown to be dependent specifically on the presence of TCA, and not on the final pH of the sample extract. PLP, PL and PN were detectable to at least 30 pmol/ml milk, and PM and PMP were detectable to 5 pmol/ml milk. Correlation between the HPLC results and the *S. carlsbergensis* growth assay was significant at $r = 0.87$.

Ang, Cenciarelli and Eitenmiller (1988) proposed a rapid method for the determination of B_6 vitamers in raw and cooked chicken tissues using metaphosphoric acid as the extracting agent. For raw samples the quantification limits per 20 µl injection were 0.10, 0.05, 1.00 and 0.1 ng for PMP, PM, PLP and PL, respectively. The fluorescence detection settings were adjusted to give more sensitivity for measuring the lower amounts of PLP and PL in cooked samples; this reduced the quantification limits of these vitamers to *c.* 0.30 and 0.03 ng, respectively. Recoveries of added vitamers in cooked tissues were between 90% and 107.8%, except in a few cases where the values were only 76.9–79.9% for PL and PLP.

Gregory and Feldstein (1985) determined the major B_6 vitamers in foods using a C_{18} analytical column and linear gradient elution with a phosphate buffer mobile phase containing octane sulphonic acid as an ion interaction agent and an increasing percentage of organic modifier (isopropanol). Food samples were extracted with sulphosalicylic acid in the presence of 4-dPN as internal standard, and subjected to the preparative anion exchange chromatographic technique devised by Vanderslice *et al.* (1980). Post-column addition of a strongly buffered solution of sodium bisulphite converted PL and PLP to their highly fluorescent hydroxysulphonate derivatives, and permitted the detection of the native fluorescence of PMP, PM, PN and 4-dPN at the same excitation and emission wavelengths. Low recoveries were obtained for PLP and PL in pork loin (78.7% and 86.7%, respectively), as also reported by Ang, Cenciarelli and Eitenmiller (1988) for cooked chicken tissues after extraction with metaphosphoric acid. It appears that the aldehydic B_6 vitamers undergo limited entrapment or binding by muscle protein, even in the presence of the deproteinizing agent. PNP was not evaluated in this study because of its minor significance as a naturally occurring form of vitamin B_6. The metabolite 4-PA could be separated and detected by the HPLC system, but could not be quantified, as it is retained by the anion exchange resin used in the preparative system. Bitsch and Möller (1989) used perchloric acid rather than sulphosalicylic acid in their extraction procedure, which permitted the quantification of 4-PA.

The inclusion of PN-glucoside in the chromatographic assay is desirable, as the proportion of glycosylated vitamin B_6 in the sample is a determinant of net bioavailability. Gregory and Ink (1987) used the HPLC analytical system described by Gregory and Feldstein (1985) with a slightly modified gradient elution programme to determine PLP, PMP, PL, PN-glucoside, PN, 4-dPN (internal standard) and PM in plant-derived foods. A similar procedure using a mixture of ion interaction agents (octane and heptane sulphonic acids) was reported by Addo and Augustin (1988) for the analysis of potatoes.

An HPLC method for determining ε-pyridoxyllysine in infant formula products was reported by Grün *et al.* (1991).

6.4.5 FOLATE

Naturally occurring folate in most plant and animal tissues comprises mainly tetrahydrofolic acid (THF), 5-methyl-THF and 10-formyl-THF. Folic acid (pteroylmonoglutamic acid, PGA) and dihydrofolic acid (DHF) do not occur naturally in biological tissues, but they may be detected in trace amounts as oxidation products of THF in food samples stored under conditions that permit exposure to oxygen (Gregory, 1984). PGA is the form added in food fortification, because of its comparative stability.

HPLC methods for determining PGA and the principal naturally occurring folates in foods are summarized in Table 6.7.

To determine the added PGA in fortified breakfast cereals and infant formula products, Day and Gregory (1981) extracted the PGA by homogenization or dilution in a pH 7.0 phosphate buffer containing ascorbate as an antioxidant. Cereal extracts were centrifuged directly,

Table 6.7 HPLC methods used for the determination of folate compounds

Food	Sample preparation	Column	Mobile phase	Compounds separated	Detection	Reference
Fortified milk and soy-based infant formula	Disperse powders in water plus 0.05 M phosphate/citrate buffer (pH 8.0) containing ascorbate. Incubate with papain at 40 °C overnight, then centrifuge and filter. Resuspend pellet in 0.005 M phosphate-citrate buffer (pH 8.0) and rinse filter with the diluted buffer *Clean-up/concentration*: pass extract through a DEAE cellulose column, wash column with 0.05 M phosphate buffer (pH 7.0) and elute folate with 0.1 M phosphate buffer (pH 7.0) containing 0.5 M NaCl	Spherisorb ODS 10 μm 25 cm × 4.6 mm i.d.	30-min linear gradient from 2% to 30% MeCN in 0.1 M acetate buffer, pH 4.0	PGA	UV 280 nm	Hoppner and Lampi (1982)
Fortified break-fast cereal, fortified liquid infant formula	Cereal: homogenize in pH 7.0 phosphate/ascorbate buffer, centrifuge, filter Formula: dilute with pH 7.0 phosphate/ascorbate buffer, adjust to pH 4.5, centrifuge, filter	Ultrasphere ODS 5 μm 25 cm × 4.6 mm i.d. coupled with μBondapak Phenyl 10 μm 30 cm × 3.9 mm i.d.	0.033 M potassium phosphate (pH 2.3) containing 9.5% MeCN	PGA	Fluorescence (ex. filter 365 nm max, em. filter > 415 nm) after post-column oxidation of PGA to pterin fragment with calcium hypochlorite reagent	Day and Gregory (1981) (Figure 6.10)

Table 6.7 *Continued*

Food	Sample preparation	Column	Mobile phase	Compounds separated	Detection	Reference
Cabbage, cows' milk, calf liver, orange juice, whole-wheat flour	*Extraction and deconjugation*: blend samples with 0.05 M acetate buffer (pH 4.9) containing 1% ascorbic acid. Heat at 100 °C for 1 h in sealed N_2-flushed tubes, then cool on ice and centrifuge at 2 °C. Incubate supernatant with hog kidney conjugase at 37 °C for 1 h in sealed N_2-flushed tubes *Clean-up*: adjust pH of deconjugated extract to 7.0 and apply to DEAE-Sephadex A-25 (Pharmacia) anion exchange column. Wash column with 0.01 M phosphate buffer (pH 7.0) containing ascorbate, then with 0.2 M phosphate buffer (pH 7.0) containing ascorbate and 1 M sodium sulphate. Elute monoglutamyl folate with additional phosphate/ascorbate/sulphate solution	μBondapak Phenyl 10 μm 30 cm × 3.9 mm i.d.	15-min linear gradient from 7.2 to 11.3% MeCN in 0.033 M sodium phosphate, pH 2.3	THF, 5-CH_3-THF, DHF, 5-CHO-THF, PGA	Fluorescence (ex. 295 nm, em. 365 nm) for THF, 5-CH_3-THF and 5-CHO-THF Fluorescence (2nd detector) (ex. filter 365 nm max, em. filter > 415 nm) after post-column oxidation of DHF, THF and PGA to pterin fragments with calcium hypochlorite reagent	Gregory, Sartain and Day (1984) (Figure 6.11)

Milk, dairy products	Homogenize solid products, adjust to pH 4.5 with acetic acid and centrifuge. Add phosphate buffer (pH 4.5) containing 10% ascorbate and 1 M 2-mercaptoethanol. Incubate with hog kidney conjugase at 37 °C for 2 h and centrifuge	C_{18} Microsorb 3 μm (Rainin) 10 cm × 4.6 mm i.d.	MeOH/phosphate buffer (pH 6.8) containing tetrabutylammonium phosphate at 50 ml/l delivered by high-pressure mixing of MeOH/buffer (50 : 50) and 100% aqueous buffer	THF, 5-CHO-THF, DHF, PGA, 5-CH_3-THF	Fluorescence: (ex. 238 nm, em. filter > 340 nm) after post-column pH adjustment of the eluent with 4.25% (v/v) phosphoric acid for the reduced forms of the vitamin. PGA requires oxidation with buffered hypochlorite (pH 3.0)	Holt, Wehling and Zeece (1988)
Orange juice, grapefruit juice	*Deconjugation*: centrifuge and adjust pH to 5.0. Incubate with hog kidney conjugase at 37 °C for 1 h. Cool on ice and centrifuge at 2 °C *Clean-up*: pass supernatant through phenyl SPE cartridge, wash cartridge with 0.05 M phosphate/acetate buffer (pH 5) containing 5 mM tetrabutylammonium phosphate, followed by the buffer/TBAP containing 10% MeOH. Elute folate with the buffer containing 30% MeOH without TBAP	Zorbax ODS 25 cm × 4.6 mm i.d.	25% MeOH in phosphate/acetate buffer (pH 5.5)	5-CH_3-THF	Amperometric: glassy carbon electrode, +0.2 V vs Ag/AgCl	White (1990)

Table 6.7 *Continued*

Food	Sample preparation	Column	Mobile phase	Compounds separated	Detection	Reference
Orange juice, grapefruit juice	*Deconjugation*: as for White (1990) (see above) except longer (90 min) incubation with conjugase *Clean-up*: Direct injection of deconjugated sample onto a Nova-PAK C_{18} 4μm pre-column (7.5 cm × 3.9 mm i.d.) followed by automatic backflush of the analyte to the analytical column	Zorbax ODS 25 cm × 4.6 mm i.d.	(A) 10% MeOH in phosphate/acetate buffer (pH 5.0) containing 5 mM tetrabutylammonium phosphate for pre-column elution. (B) Similar to A but containing 30% MeOH for back-flushing and analysis	5-CH_3-THF	As above	White, Lee and Krüger (1991)

Notes and abbreviations: see footnote to Table 6.9.

while formula extracts were adjusted to pH 4.5 to precipitate the proteins, and then centrifuged. The extracts were analysed by isocratic reversed-phase HPLC using a C_{18} column and a phenyl column connected in series. Fluorimetric detection was achieved using in-line post-column chemistry to convert PGA to a highly fluorescent pterin compound. The chromatogram of an infant formula (Figure 6.10) shows that PGA is the only detectable folate present.

The general approach for extracting naturally occurring folates from food samples is to apply a heat treatment to denature folate-binding proteins and enzymes that may catalyse folate degradation or interconversion, followed by deconjugation of the folate polyglutamates to

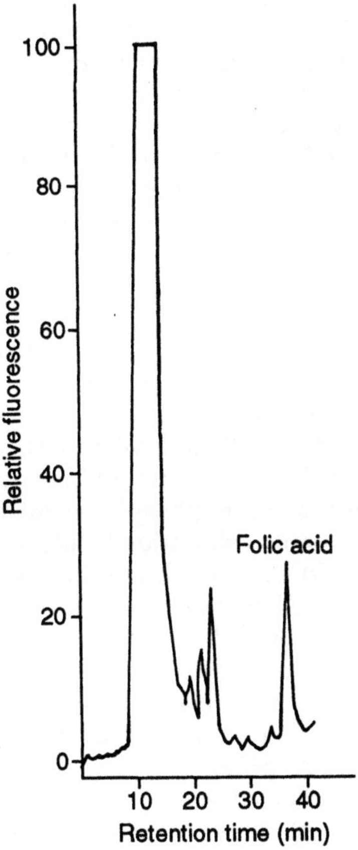

Figure 6.10 Reversed-phase HPLC of folic acid in liquid infant formula. Conditions as given in table 6.7. (Reprinted with permission from Day, B.P. and Gregory, J.F. (1981) Determination of folacin derivatives in selected foods by high-performance liquid chromatography. *J. Agric. Fd Chem.*, **29**, 374–7. Copyright (1981) American Chemical Society.)

their monoglutamyl forms by incubation with a partially purified hog kidney conjugase preparation. Gregory, Sartain and Day (1984) employed such a procedure in which the mildly acidic (pH 4.9) extraction conditions were favourable to the stability of ascorbate and also to the subsequent enzymatic deconjugation step. A prolonged (1 h) heating time was employed to intentionally convert 10-formyl-THF to 5-formyl-THF, as a means of simplifying the quantification of formyl tetrahydrofolates by HPLC. No degradation of 5-methyl-THF occurred during the heat treatment, while less than 10% loss of THF was observed. The resulting extracts were purified by anion exchange chromatography on DEAE-Sephadex A-25 columns, and then analysed by single-column reversed-phase HPLC using a linear gradient elution programme. Determination of THF and its substituted derivatives was accomplished by monitoring the fluorescence produced by excitement at 290–295 nm in the acidic environment of the mobile phase. A fluorimetric detector which is capable of extremely high sensitivity is required for this purpose. Because of the much greater fluorescence of THF and 5-methyl-THF compared with 5-formyl-THF, a change in excitation and emission slit widths was necessary before elution of 5-formyl-THF to maintain adequate detector response. With the aid of a second fluorescence detector, PGA, DHF and also THF could be measured after post-column derivatization to pterin compounds. Chromatograms showing the naturally occurring folates in rat liver, cabbage, milk and orange juice are depicted in Figure 6.11. The suitability of the method was supported by recovery data and fluorescence spectral studies, and by its application to a wide range of biological materials.

Holt, Wehling and Zeece (1988) achieved the separation of THF, 5-formyl-THF, DHF, PGA and 5-methyl-THF using ion interaction HPLC with tetrabutylammonium phosphate and a mobile phase pH of 6.8. The use of post-column acidification to allow fluorimetric detection of reduced folates would extend column life, as acidic mobile phases gradually erode silica-based column packings.

A method developed by White (1990) for the determination of 5-methyl-THF in citrus juice involved centrifugation, adjustment to pH 5.0 and treatment with conjugase, followed by SPE using a phenyl-bonded phase with the aid of an ion interaction agent (tetrabutyl-ammonium phosphate). At pH 5.0, 5-methyl-THF is essentially anionic, and the use of the ion interaction agent improved its retention on the phenyl-bonded phase. HPLC was performed using a C_{18} column, a methanol/buffer mobile phase of pH 5.5, and amperometric detection; the detection limit was in the low nanogram range. Ascorbic acid, which is present in natural orange juice at a concentration roughly 1000 times that of 5-methyl-THF, is easily oxidized at the operating potential of +0.2 V, and the detector response was found to be about equal for the two compounds. SPE was capable of lowering the ascorbate to a residual concentration of only about 10 times that of 5-methyl-THF. Without SPE, the ascorbate, although not retained on the HPLC column, caused severe tailing, which swamped the detector signal and obscured the 5-methyl-THF peak. The standard was prepared to contain ascorbate at 10 times the concentration of 5-methyl-THF. In an automated HPLC method for the determination of 5-methyl-THF in citrus juice (White, Lee and Krüger, 1991), sample clean-up took place on a C_{18} pre-column, followed by backflush of the analyte to the C_{18} analytical column.

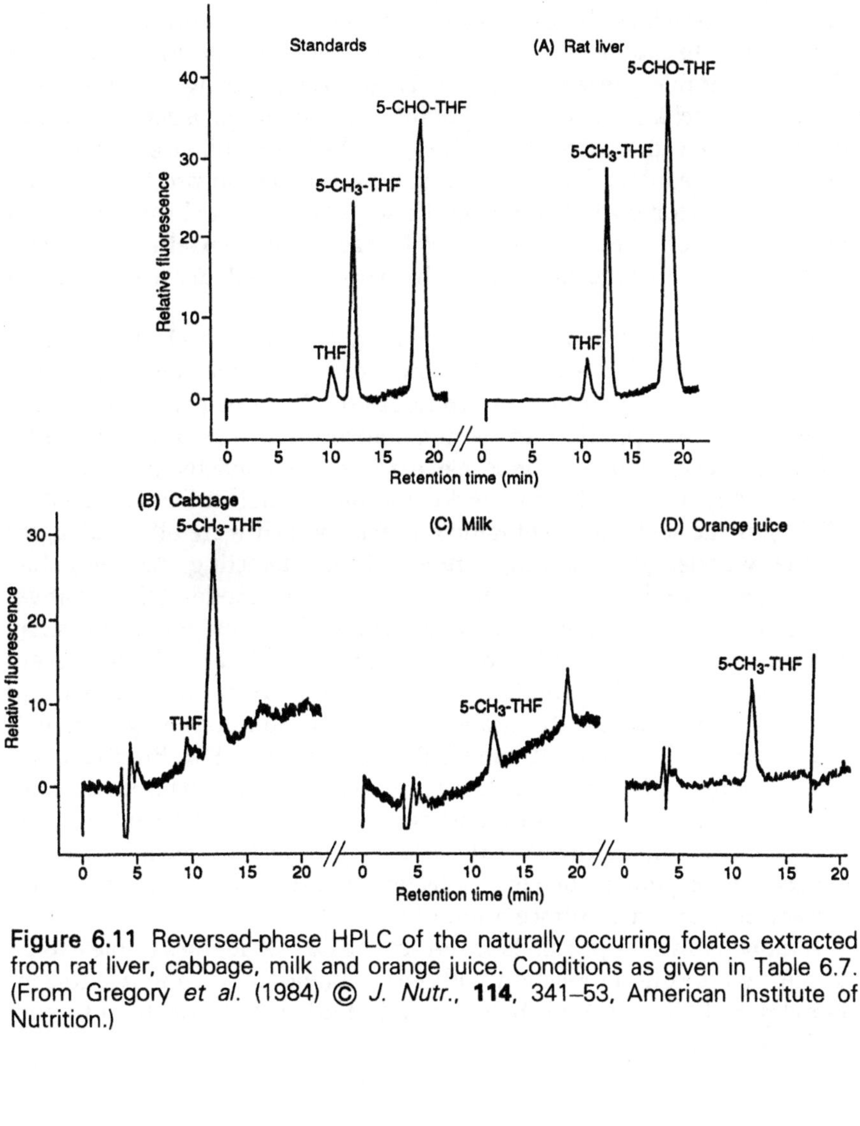

Figure 6.11 Reversed-phase HPLC of the naturally occurring folates extracted from rat liver, cabbage, milk and orange juice. Conditions as given in Table 6.7. (From Gregory *et al.* (1984) © *J. Nutr.*, **114**, 341–53, American Institute of Nutrition.)

6.4.6 VITAMIN C

General considerations

In food analysis, a method for determining total vitamin C must, by definition, account for L-ascorbic acid (AA) and its reversible oxidation product of equal biopotency, L-dehydroascorbic acid (DHAA). In addition, the ability to distinguish AA from its epimer D-isoascorbic acid (erythorbic acid, EA) is important in the analysis of processed foods. EA is a permitted food antioxidant in some countries as a cheaper alternative to AA, but it possesses only 5% of the vitamin C activity of AA in guinea pigs. The ability to separate and detect these epimers by HPLC also provides the opportunity to use EA as an internal standard for the quantification of AA, provided it is shown that EA is absent in the food sample presented for analysis. HPLC, using a weak anion exchange mechanism, has the potential to separate, isocratically, not only AA from its oxidation products, DHAA and diketogulonic acid, but, simultaneously, EA from its analogous oxidation products, DHEA and diketogluconic acid (Doner and Hicks, 1981). Other chromatographic modes, in addition to weak anion exchange, facilitate useful separations and are utilized in accordance with the particular analytical requirements (Table 6.8).

AA can be detected directly either by absorbance or electrochemical monitoring, and fluorescence detection can be utilized after chemical derivatization to a fluorescent compound. The detection of DHAA, however, poses a problem as the molar absorptivity of this compound is relatively very weak and it is electrochemically inactive. Doner and Hicks (1981) used a refractive index monitor to detect DHAA, DHEA, diketogulonic acid and diketogluconic acid, which were all transparent at the wavelength (268 nm) employed for detecting AA and EA. Refractive index detection is nonselective and only moderately sensitive, and hence it has no utility in the accurate measurement of the small amounts of DHAA and other oxidation products that might be present in foods. Some HPLC methods for analysing fruits, fruit juices and vegetables have employed dual absorbance detection, AA being measured at 254 nm and DHAA at 210 nm (Finley and Duang, 1981; Bradbury and Singh, 1986) or 214 nm (Wimalasiri and Wills, 1983). This dual detector technique is simple to perform and does not involve the analytes in any chemical reactions. However, the accuracy of DHAA measurement is expected to be poor at such low detection wavelengths, unless DHAA is present in more than a trace amount.

A more popular approach is to reduce the DHAA in the sample extract to AA by pre-column reaction with either DL-homocysteine (Dennison, Brawley and Hunter, 1981; Behrens and Madère, 1987) or dithiothreitol

Table 6.8 HPLC methods used for the determination of vitamin C compounds

Food	Sample preparation	Column	Mobile phase	Compounds separated	Detection	Reference
Strong anion exchange chromatography						
Orange juice	Centrifuge, add cyclopentanone as internal standard	Yanaco SAX-801 10 µm 25 cm × 2.2 mm i.d.	0.1 M $NaNO_3$	AA, three reductones, cyclopentanone (internal standard)	UV 260 nm	Obata, Tsuchihashi and Tokuyama (1980)
Fresh and processed fruit and vegetables	Homogenize with 6% HPO_3, centrifuge and filter. Repeat extraction, add benzoic acid solution as internal standard and dilute to volume with 6% HPO_3. Pass through C_{18} SPE cartridge	Partisil 10 SAX 25 cm × 4.6 mm i.d.	0.1 M sodium acetate buffer (pH 4.25)	AA, benzoic acid (internal standard)	UV 250 nm	Rizzolo, Forni and Polesello (1984)
Whole fruit, fruit juice, cereals, milk products	Fruits, cereals: extract with 3% HPO_3/8% HOAc, centrifuge. Milk products: deproteinize with cold 0.05 M $HClO_4$, centrifuge	Zipax SAX 50 cm × 2.1 mm i.d. $T = 25\,°C$	70 mM acetate buffer (pH 4.75)	AA	Amperometric: carbon paste electrode +0.8 V vs Ag/AgCl	Pachla and Kissinger (1976)
Fruit juices, fruits, vegetables	Homogenize, add pyrogallol and 0.1 M citric acid, vortex under N_2. Add CH_2Cl_2 to remove fat, centrifuge and pass through C_{18} Sep-Pak cartridge	DA-X8-11 (Dionex) SAX column 15 cm × 5 mm i.d.	0.1 M citrate buffer (pH 3.8) containing 10 mM NaCl and 5 mM EDTA	AA and DHAA	Fluorescence (filters) through post-column derivatization (oxidation of AA to DHAA plus reaction with OPDA to form the DFQ fluorophore)	Vanderslice and Higgs (1984)

Table 6.8 *Continued*

Food	Sample preparation	Column	Mobile phase	Compounds separated	Detection	Reference
Weak anion exchange chromatography						
Wheat flours, bread dough conditioners	Homogenize with 0.7 mM dithiothreitol, centrifuge, filter	μBondapak-NH_2 10 μm Two 30 cm × 3.9 mm i.d. columns connected in series	10 mM NaH_2PO_4 buffer (pH 4.46)/ MeOH/MeCN (30 : 35 : 35)	AA (representing total vitamin C)	UV 254 nm	Lookhart Hall and Finney (1982)
Non-fat dry milk	Dissolve in water containing 1 mg/ml dithiothreitol (DTT), stir, add 12% HPO_3, stir, add 2 ml MeCN, stir, centrifuge	μBondapak-NH_2 30 cm × 7.8 mm i.d. T = 21 °C	MeCN/5 mM KH_2PO_4 (70 + 30) + 0.125 ml/l of mercapto-ethanol	AA (representing total vitamin C)	UV 268 nm	Margolis and Black (1987)
Fruits, vegetables	Homogenize with 3% citric acid, dilute to volume and filter. Pass through C_{18} Sep-Pak cartridge	μBondapak-NH_2 10μm 30 cm × 3.9 mm i.d.	MeCN/10 mM $NH_4H_2PO_4$ buffer (pH 4.3) (70 : 30)	AA, DHAA	Dual UV 254 nm (AA) 214 nm (DHAA)	Wimalasiri and Wills (1983)
Tropical root crops	Homogenize with 5% HPO_3 and filter	μBondapak-NH_2 in Z-module cartridge	MeCN/5 mM KH_2PO_4 buffer (pH 4.6) (70 : 30)	AA, DHAA	Dual UV 210 nm (DHAA) 254 nm (AA)	Bradbury and Singh (1986)

Orange juice, soft drinks, protein-fortified drinks	*For AA* deproteinize (if necessary) with 12.5% TCA, centrifuge, filter *For total vitamin C* adjust filtrate to pH 7.0 with 45% KH_2PO_4, add 0.8% homocysteine solution (allow 15 min reaction time), filter	μBondapak-NH_2 30 cm × 3.9 mm i.d.	MeOH/0.25% KH_2PO_4 buffer (pH 3.5) (50 : 50)	AA (representing total vitamin C if DHAA is reduced with homocysteine)	UV 244 nm	Dennison, Brawley and Hunter (1981)
Fresh apple and potato	*For AA* blend with 2.5% HPO_3, and mobile phase, filter through Celite, refilter, pass through C_{18} Sep-Pak cartridge *For total vitamin C* treat second filtrate with dithiothreitol (DTT) after adjusting to pH 6 (allow 30 min reaction time at ambient temperature), pass through C_{18} Sep-Pak cartridge	Dynamax-60A-NH_2 8 μm (Rainin) 25 cm × 4.6 mm i.d.	MeCN/50 mM KH_2PO_4 (70 : 25)	AA (representing total vitamin C if DHAA is reduced with DTT), ascorbic acid-2-phosphate	UV 254 nm	Sapers *et al.* (1990)
Frozen apples, potato products, concentrated fruit and vegetable juices, frozen juices, natural and artificially flavoured drink mixes, Hi-C drinks, cured meat products	Suspend blended sample in water or EtOH (potato products), filter, pass through C_{18} Sep-Pak cartridge. Add dithiothreitol (DTT) to one portion of each sample to obtain total vitamin C and total isovitamin C	LiChrosorb-NH_2 25 cm × 4 mm i.d.	MeCN/50 mM KH_2PO_4 buffer (pH 5.95) (75 : 25)	AA and EA (representing total vitamin C and isovitamin C, respectively, if DHAA and DHEA are reduced with DTT)	UC 268 nm	Tuan, Wyatt and Anglemier (1987)

Table 6.8 *Continued*

Food	Sample preparation	Column	Mobile phase	Compounds separated	Detection	Reference
Fresh fruit and vegetables, fruit drinks	Homogenize with 3% HPO_3, filter, pass through C_{18} Sep-Pak cartridge	NH_2-phase (Alltech)	MeCN/50 mM KH_2PO_4 buffer (pH 5.9) (75 : 25)	AA, DHAA	UV 254 nm (AA) Fluorescence (DHAA) through post-column derivatization (reaction with OPDA to form the fluorophore)	Kacem *et al.* (1986)
Ion-exclusion partition chromatography						
Citrus fruit juices, fruits, vegetables	Dilute or extract with 0.05% EDTA in 0.1 M H_2SO_4, filter or centrifuge	Aminex HPX-87 SCX sulphonated PS-DVB resin 30 cm × 7.8 mm i.d.	4.5 mM H_2SO_4	AA	UV 245 nm	Ashoor, Monte and Welty (1984)
Potatoes	Homogenize with 95% EtOH/water containing 0.2% conc. H_2SO_4 (60 : 40), filter	Aminex HPX-87 SCX sulphonated PS-DVB resin 9 μm 30 cm × 7.8 mm i.d.	9 mM H_2SO_4	AA, oxalic acid, citric acid, malic acid, fumaric acid	UV 260 nm (AA) UV 210 nm (other acids)	Bushway, Bureau and McGann (1984)
Milk (fluid and powdered)	Powdered milk: dilute with 1% HPO_3, centrifuge Fluid milk: centrifuge	SCX sulphonated PS-DVB resin, H^+-form (Bio-Rad) 9 μm 10 cm × 7.8 mm i.d.	1 mM H_2SO_4	AA	Amperometric: glassy carbon electrode, +0.70 V vs Ag/AgCl	Mannino and Pagliarini (1988)

Fresh fruits, fruit juices, dry mixed fruits, potatoes	Homogenize solid samples or dilute liquid samples with 5 mM H_2SO_4 (pH 2) + 10 mM mannitol, centrifuge, filter (0.45 μm) or (for some fresh fruits) pass through C_{18} Sep-Pak cartridge	Polypore H 10 μm (Bioanalytical Systems) 10 cm × 4.6 mm i.d.	10 mM H_2SO_4 + 10 mM mannitol	AA, free sulphite	Amperometric dual electrode Free sulphite: Pt, +0.70 V AA: glassy carbon, +0.80 V vs Ag/AgCl	Huang, Duda and Kissinger (1987)
Fruits, fruit drinks, vegetables	Dilute or homogenize with 20 mM H_2SO_4, centrifuge, filter (0.45 μm). Mix with 50 mM phosphate buffer (pH 7) and 10 mM dithiothreitol (2 min reaction time at ambient temp.)	SCX sulphonated PS-DVB resin (Wescan) 10 cm × 4.6 mm i.d.	20 mM H_2SO_4	AA (representing total vitamin C)	Amperometric: Pt electrode, +0.60 V or +0.80 V vs Ag/AgCl	Kim (1989)
Reversed-phase chromatography						
Fresh citrus fruit juices	Dilute with mobile phase, filter	PLRP-S 100 Å 5 μm (Polymer Laboratories) 25 cm × 4.6 mm i.d.	0.2 M NaH_2PO_4 buffer (pH 2.14)	AA, EA	UV 244 nm (AA) UV 220 nm (AA, EA)	Lloyd *et al.* (1988a, b) (Figure 6.13)
Fruits, vegetables, juices	Homogenize with 0.2 M phosphate buffer (pH 2.0) and extract with 3% HPO_3, centrifuge	PLRP-S 100 Å 5 μm 25 cm × 4.6 mm i.d.	1.8% THF and 0.3% HPO_3 in water	AA	UV 244 nm	Bushway *et al.* (1988)
Fruits, vegetables	Extract with 6% HPO_3 containing 1 μM EDTA and 0.1 μM diethylthiocarbamate	μBondapak C_{18} 10 μm in a 10 cm × 8 mm radial compression module (Waters)	1.5% $NH_4H_2PO_4$ buffer (pH 3)	AA	UV 254 nm	Watada (1982)

Table 6.8 *Continued*

Food	Sample preparation	Column	Mobile phase	Compounds separated	Detection	Reference
Citrus juices	Mix with 5% HPO_3, centrifuge, pass through C_{18} SPE cartridge, add quinic acid as internal standard	Zorbax ODS 25 cm × 4.6 mm i.d.	2% KH_2PO_4 buffer (pH 2.4)	AA, quinic acid (internal standard)	UV 245 nm	Lee and Coates (1987)
Candies and soft drinks fortified with vitamin C	Dissolve in 2% HPO_3, centrifuge (candies), pass through C_{18} SPE cartridge	Inertsil ODS (Gasukurokogyo Co.) 15 cm × 4.6 mm i.d. $T = 35$ °C	0.1% v/v phosphoric acid (pH 2.2)	AA	UV 254 nm	Maeda *et al.* (1988)
Rose hips	Extract with 1% HPO_3, pass through C_{18} SPE cartridge	LiChrosorb RP-18 5 µm 25 cm × 4 mm i.d.	0.25% HPO_3	AA, DHAA	UV 267 nm for both peaks after post-column reduction of DHAA to AA with dithiothreitol at 50 °C	Ziegler, Meier and Sticher (1987)
Orange juice	Centrifuge, mix 1 : 1 with 6% HPO_3, filter	Brownlee RP-18 5µm 22 cm × 4.6 mm i.d. (or 10 cm × 4.6 mm i.d.)	2% $NH_4H_2PO_4$ (pH 2.8)	AA	Amperometric: glassy carbon electrode, +0.6 V vs Ag/AgCl	Wilson and Shaw (1987)

Citrus juices, vegetables	*For total vitamin C and total isovitamin C*: blend with 0.3 M TCA, dilute to volume and filter. Add 4.5 M acetate buffer (pH 6.2), incubate at 37 °C for 5 min with ascorbate oxidase. Add 0.1% OPDA, react at 37 °C for 30 min *For DHAA and DHEA*: as above, but omit enzymatic oxidation	Hypersil – ODS 3μm 12.5 cm × 4.6 mm i.d.	80 mM KH_2PO_4/MeOH (80 : 20) final pH 7.8	Quinoxaline derivatives of DHAA and DHEA representing total vitamin C (AA + DHAA) and total isovitamin C (EA + DHEA) respectively	Fluorescence: ex. 365 nm (filter) em. 418 nm (filter)	Speek, Schrijver and Schreurs (1984)
Ion interaction chromatography						
Fruit, fruit juices, vegetables, infant formula	Homogenize and dilute to volume with 6% HPO_3, filter	μBondapak C_{18} 30 cm × 3.9 mm i.d.	MeOH/H_2O containing 1 mM tridecylammonium formate, adjusted to pH 5 (1 + 1)	AA	UV 254 nm	Sood *et al.* (1976)
Raw potatoes, potato products	Homogenize with 6% HPO_3, filter, add EtOH, centrifuge	μBondapak C_{18} 30 cm × 3.9 mm i.d.	MeOH/H_2O (60 : 40) containing 0.5 mM tridecylammonium formate, adjusted to pH 4.5	AA	UV 254 nm	Augustin, Beck and Marousek (1981)

Table 6.8 *Continued*

Food	Sample preparation	Column	Mobile phase	Compounds separated	Detection	Reference
Fresh tomatoes	Homogenize with 6% HPO_3, mix aliquot of slurry with MeOH, add 0.5% pentanophenone as internal standard, centrifuge, dilute with MeOH containing 1.5 mM pyrogallol	Vydac 201-HS C_{18} 10μm 25 cm × 4.6 mm i.d.	MeOH/H_2O/MeCN (60 + 40 + 1) containing 0.5 mM tridecylammonium formate, adjusted to pH 4.25	AA	UV 247 nm	Russell (1986)
Meat products	Extract with 6% HPO_3	μBondapack C_{18} 30 cm × 3.9 m i.d.	3 mM trioctylmethylammonium chloride in MeOH/H_2O, (1 : 1), final pH 5.05	AA	UV 255 nm	Parolari (1982)
Fruits, fruit juice products, vegetables	Dilute or extract with 6% HPO_3/EtOH (10 : 90), filter (paper), centrifuge, filter (0.45 μm membrane), pass through Sep-Pak C_{18} cartridge	Spherisorb ODS 10 μm 25 cm × 4 mm i.d.	(i) 0.1 M phosphate buffer (pH 4.2) containing 5 mM tetrabutylammonium hydroxide (ii) 0.2 M phosphate buffer (pH 4.2) containing 10 mM hexadecyltrimethylammonium bromide/MeOH (1 + 1)	AA	UV 254 nm	Moledina and Flink (1982)

Cured meats	Homogenize with 6% HPO_3, filter through glass wool and pass through Sep-Pak C_{18} cartridge	μBondapak C_{18} 30 cm × 3.9 mm i.d.	5 mM tetrabutylammonium formate (pH 4.77)	EA	UV 254 nm	Lee and Marder (1983)
Fruit juices, ham	Dilute or homogenize with HPO_3, filter	LiChrosorb RP-8 or RP-18 15 or 20 cm × 4.6 mm i.d.	0.1 M phosphate buffer containing 5 mM cetyltrimethylammonium bromide/MeOH (9 : 1)	AA, EA	UV 264 nm	Coustard and Sudraud (1981)
Fruits, fruit juices, vegetables	Extract with HPO_3/HOAc solution, filter, pass through C_{18} SPE cartridge	Two 30 cm × 3.9 mm i.d. μBondapak C_{18} columns connected in series	8 mM phosphate buffer, pH 5.3 containing 0.7 ml/l tri-n-butylamine	AA, DHAA, DKGulA	UV 210 nm and 254 nm	Finley and Duang (1981)
Fruits, infant foods, milk	Fruits, infant foods: extract with 3% HPO_3/8% HOAc, centrifuge, dilute to volume with cold 50 mM $HClO_4$. Milk: dilute to volume with cold 50 mM $HClO_4$, centrifuge	LiChrosorb RP-18 15 cm × 4.6 mm i.d.	80 mM acetate buffer containing 1 mM tridecylamine and 15% MeOH (final pH 4.5)	AA	Amperometric: carbon paste electrode, +0.7 V vs Ag/AgCl	Pachla and Kissinger (1979)
Bread	Grind freeze-dried bread, extract with 3% HPO_3, centrifuge, dilute to volume with cold 0.05 M $HClO_4$	Alltech C-18 5 μm 25 cm × 4.6 mm i.d. $T = 25$ °C	80 mM acetate buffer, pH 4.2 containing 0.1 mM disodium EDTA and 1 mM octyltriethylammonium phosphate	AA	Amperometric: glassy carbon electrode, +0.72 V, vs Ag/AgCl	Hung, Seib and Kramer (1987)

Table 6.8 *Continued*

Food	Sample preparation	Column	Mobile phase	Compounds separated	Detection	Reference
Beers	Ultrasonic degassing	μBondapak C_{18} 30 cm × 3.9 mm i.d.	Citrate buffer pH 4.4 containing 0.5 mM EDTA and 1 mM *N*-methyl-dodecylamine	AA	Amperometric: glassy carbon electrode, +0.60 V vs Ag/AgCl	Moll and Joly (1987)
Orange juice, milk	Dilute with cold 50 mM $HClO_4$ and centrifuge	Ultrasphere ODS 5 μm 25 cm × 4.6 mm i.d.	40 mM acetate buffer containing 1 mM decylamine and 15% MeOH	AA, EA	Amperometric: carbon paste electrode, +0.7 V vs Ag/AgCl	Tsao and Salimi (1982)
Beer	Ultrasonic degassing	Zorbax ODS 25 cm × 4.6 mm i.d.	0.1 M acetate buffer pH 5.5 containing 200 mg/l disodium EDTA and 1 mM octylamine	AA or EA	Amperometric: glassy carbon electrode, +0.60 V vs Ag/AgCl	Knudson and Siebert (1987)

Vegetables, milk, infant formula, apple juice, orange juice	Homogenize in cold 17% HPO_3, centrifuge *For AA*: dilute with phosphate buffer (pH 9.8) to give a final pH of 7.1. After 30 min at 25 °C further dilute with cold 0.85% HPO_3. Dilute an aliquot with acetate buffer (pH 4.8) containing 15% MeOH *For total vitamin C (AA + DHAA)*: dilute with 1% homocysteine in phosphate buffer (pH 9.8) to give a final pH of 7.1. Then as for AA.	RP C_{18} 5 μm (unspecified) 25 cm × 4.6 mm i.d.	80 mM acetate buffer containing 1 mM n-octylamine, 15% MeOH and 0.015% HPO_3 (final pH 4.6)	AA (determine DHAA by subtracting AA value from total vitamin C value)	Amperometric: glassy carbon electrode, +0.7 V vs Ag/AgCl	Behrens and Madère (1987)
Infant formula	As above	As above	As above	As above	As above	Behrens and Madère (1989)
Canned food, frozen concentrated orange juice	As above	As above	As above	As above	As above	Behrens and Madère (1990)
Cured meats	Grind with 5% HPO_3 containing 0.1 mg/ml disodium EDTA, centrifuge and dilute with mobile phase	Ultrasphere ODS 5 μm 25 cm × 4.6 mm i.d. $T = 30$ °C	40 mM acetate buffer containing 5 mM tetrabutylammonium phosphate and 0.2 mg/ml disodium EDTA (final pH 5.25)	AA, EA	Amperometric: glassy carbon electrode, +0.6 V vs Ag/AgCl	Kutnink and Omaye (1987)

Table 6.8 *Continued*

Food	Sample preparation	Column	Mobile phase	Compounds separated	Detection	Reference
Milk, whey, whey beverages	*For AA*: dilute with 3% HPO_3, centrifuge *For DHAA*: dilute with 3% HPO_3, centrifuge, react with 0.2% OPDA in water/MeOH (1 + 1)	Polygosil 60 C_{18} 7 µm 25 cm × 4.6 mm i.d. T = 30 °C	2 mM hexadecyltrimethylammonium bromide in 0.1% $NaH_2PO_4.H_2O$ (pH 3.8)/MeOH (1 + 1)	AA, DHAA (as DFQ derivative)	*AA*: UV 248 nm *DFQ*: Fluorescence ex. 350 nm, em, 430 nm	Kneifel and Sommer (1985)
Processed meat	Homogenize with 0.5% HPO_3 and centrifuge. Dilute with 0.5% HPO_3, add MeOH to give a 4% final concentration	Hypersil ODS 5 µm 25 cm × 4 mm i.d.	H_2O/MeOH/acetate buffer/1, 5-dimethylhexylamine (945 + 40 + 15 + 1.5)	AA, EA	UV 254 nm	Schüep and Keck (1990)
Fresh fruits	Homogenize with 0.4% HPO_3 and dilute to volume. Filter (0.2 µm), pass through C_{18} Sep-Pak cartridge (if coloured)	µBondapak C_{18} 10 µm 30 cm × 3.9 mm i.d.	0.1 M KH_2PO_4 MeOH (9 : 1) containing 5 mM cetyltrimethylammonium bromide	AA	UV 265 nm	Diop *et al.* (1988)

Cyanopropyl-bonded phase chromatography						
Citrus juices	Dilute with H_2O, filter	μBondapak-CN 30 cm × 3.9 mm i.d.	2% HOAc/ MeOH (95 : 5)	AA, sorbic acid, benzoic acid	UV 254 nm (AA) 230 nm (sorbic and benzoic acids)	Carnevale (1980)
Hydrophilic gel chromatography						
Orange juice	Pass through mixed Amberlite CG50 and XAD-2 ion exchange column	Asahipak GS-320 (hydrophilic gel) (Asahi Chemical) 50 cm × 7.6 mm i.d. $T = 30$ °C	15 mM tartrate buffer, pH 3.0 containing 2 mM EDTA and 0.05% β-thiodiglycol	AA, DHAA, DKG, glucose	Fluorescence (ex. 325 nm; em. 400 nm) through post-column derivatization at 90 °C with benzamidine at alkaline pH in the presence of K_2SO_3	Seki *et al.* (1985)

Notes and abbreviations: see footnote to Table 6.9.

(Lookhart, Hall and Finney, 1982; Margolis and Black, 1987; Tuan, Wyatt and Anglemier, 1987; Kim, 1989; Sapers *et al.*, 1990) and then to determine the AA (representing total vitamin C) by HPLC analysis using absorbance or electrochemical detection. The DHAA value can be calculated by subtracting the AA value (obtained without reduction) from the total vitamin C value, but the error will be appreciable if the concentration of DHAA is very low relative to that of AA. Diop *et al.* (1988) referred to previous work that reported an incomplete reduction of DHAA by DL-homocysteine (55% instead of 97.8% claimed by Dennison, Brawley and Hunter, 1981), and which led to a low (50%) recovery of DHAA as measured by spiking. Ziegler, Meier and Sticher (1987) determined DHAA directly, in addition to AA, by separating the two compounds using reversed-phase HPLC with ion suppression, and reducing DHAA to AA with dithiothreitol in a post-column in-line reaction system. This technique enabled the DHAA to be measured photometrically (267 nm) at the same sensitivity as AA with a detection limit of 1.4 ng per 10 μl injection volume (signal/noise ratio of 2 : 1). Attempts to use electrochemical detection were unsuccessful, owing to a high background signal and electrode poisoning that resulted from the excess dithiothreitol. Karp, Ciambra and Miklean (1990) extended the system of Ziegler, Meier and Sticher (1987) by reacting the excess dithiothreitol with *N*-ethylmaleimide, thereby permitting the electrochemical detection of both AA and DHAA with a detection limit of 0.3 ng per 20 μl injection volume.

An alternative approach is to oxidize the AA in the sample extract to DHAA and then to react the DHAA with *o*-phenylenediamine (OPDA) to form the fluorescent quinoxaline derivative 3-(1,2-dihydroxyethyl) furo[3,4-*b*]quinoxaline-1-one (DFQ) (Figure 6.12). HPLC analysis of the resulting solution, with fluorescence detection of the DFQ, gives the total vitamin C value, while DHAA can be determined directly in a separate analysis by omitting the oxidation step. Speek, Schrijver and Schreurs (1984) determined total vitamin C and total isovitamin C (EA + DHEA) in citrus juices and vegetables, after enzymatic oxidation of AA to DHAA and EA to DHEA, through fluorimetric detection of the corresponding DFQ fluorophores separated by reversed-phase HPLC.

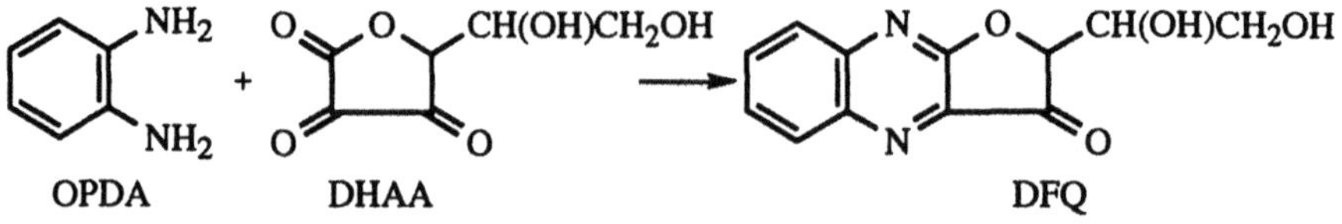

Figure 6.12 Reaction between dehydroascorbic acid and *o*-phenylenediamine to form the quinoxaline derivative (DFQ).

Stability studies showed that the quinoxaline derivatives of DHAA and DHEA deteriorated rapidly under daylight exposure and in the dark at 22 °C, whereas they were fairly stable in the dark at 4 °C or −20 °C for at least 12 h. Reductones react slowly with OPDA and do not interfere (Jaffe, 1984). Vanderslice and Higgs (1984) separated AA and DHAA by strong anion exchange HPLC, and achieved fluorimetric detection of each compound through post-column in-line chemistry, involving oxidation of AA to DHAA with mercury (II) chloride or copper (II) sulphate, followed by reaction with OPDA to form DFQ. This procedure resulted in a long run time of 30 min and broad peaks. Ion interaction HPLC effected the separation of AA, EA, DHAA and DHEA using three C_{18} columns connected in series, and these compounds were detected after post-column oxidation and derivatization to the DFQ fluorophores. A 50-min run time was required for peak separation under the conditions employed (Vanderslice and Higgs, 1988). Kneifel and Sommer (1985) determined AA and DHAA in milk, whey and whey beverages by separate analysis. For AA, samples were deproteinized and analysed by ion interaction HPLC with UV detection at 248 nm. For DHAA, samples were incubated for 40 min at room temperature with OPDA reagent and analysed on the same HPLC system, but with fluorescence detection of the DFQ. A disadvantage of this technique was that the DFQ peak eluted very close to the void volume, thus making it difficult to guarantee peak purity. AA and DHAA could be detected simultaneously if UV and fluorescence detection were performed in series, but then all samples would have to be incubated for 40 min with possible loss of AA. Kacem *et al.* (1986) separated AA and DHAA by weak anion exchange HPLC, and used absorbance monitoring at 254 nm for detecting AA, and fluorimetric detection of DHAA after post-column derivatization to DFQ. Seki *et al.* (1985) reported the simultaneous determination of AA, DHAA, diketogulonic acid and glucose using fluorimetric detection, after post-column derivatization with benzamidine at alkaline pH in the presence of potassium sulphite.

Electrochemical detection

Hydrodynamic voltammograms for AA show that the peak current reaches a plateau at +0.8 V using either a platinum or glassy carbon electrode (Huang, Duda and Kissinger, 1987). An oxidative potential of +0.8 V is relatively high, and the many compounds with lower or very close potentials that are present in biological materials will also be detected. Thus the specificity of the assay relies largely upon the chromatographic separation. In practice, a potential of +0.6 V is frequently chosen which, though not as sensitive as +0.8 V, results in improved selectivity.

DHAA, being electrochemically inactive, must be reduced chemically to AA if it is to be taken into account. These circumstances also apply to EA and its oxidation product, DHEA.

The minimum detection limit of an amperometric detector towards AA, using an oxidation potential of +0.6 V, was reported to be 0.3 ng on-column (based on a signal/noise ratio of 3 : 1), and was an order of magnitude lower than the limit obtained with a photometric detector used for comparison (Karp, Ciambra and Miklean, 1990). The higher sensitivity gives ECD the advantage over absorbance detection for the analysis of foods that contain relatively small amounts of vitamin C.

The response of an electrochemical detector decreases slowly with time as a result of deposition of sample material on the electrode surface. In the absence of an internal standard, this electrode 'poisoning' necessitates frequent injections of standards. Periodic polishing of the electrode surface in accordance with the manufacturer's instructions will restore the detector response to a level approximating to the level it was at the previous time it was polished. Kim (1989) cleaned the platinum electrode at the beginning of a day's experiments by applying −1.0 V for several minutes, followed by +1.8 V for another several minutes before re-equilibrating at the operating potential of +0.8 V. The problem of electrode poisoning can be minimized by avoiding the injection of concentrated solutions. Kim (1989) diluted the sample solution before injection so that the AA concentration lay within the range 0.1–0.5 ppm.

Chromatography

Strong anion exchange (SAX) chromatography

The first published application of HPLC for isolating AA in a food commodity (orange juice) utilized a Zipax SAX column and absorbance detection, but no quantitative data were reported (Williams, Baker and Schmit, 1973). Benzoic acid has been used as an internal standard for the quantification of AA in fresh and processed fruit and vegetables using a Partisil SAX column and absorbance detection (Rizzolo, Forni and Polesello, 1984). Pachla and Kissinger (1976) used a Zipax SAX column and an amperometric detector for the quantitative determination of AA extracted from whole fruit and fortified cereals with 3% metaphosphoric acid/8% acetic acid. This extracting solution, owing to its high ionic strength, would decrease the retention time if injected directly onto an anion exchange column, so sample extracts were diluted with cold 0.05 M perchloric acid for the chromatographic assay. SAX stationary phases cause on-column decomposition of unstabilized AA solutions to DHAA, but a medium of 0.05 M perchloric acid prevents this occurrence during a normal analysis time frame (Veazey and Nieman, 1980).

Obata, Tsuchihashi and Tokuyama (1980) demonstrated the separation of AA, cyclopentanone (internal standard) and three reductones (L-β-3,4-dihydroxyphenylalanine, reductic acid and triose reductone) using a Yanaco SAX-801 column and absorbance detection, and revealed the presence of triose reductone in heat-processed skimmed milk. The separation of AA and EA by SAX chromatography has not been reported and presumably cannot be achieved.

Weak anion exchange (WAX) chromatography

Aminopropyl-bonded stationary phases operated in the weak anion exchange mode have the potential to separate AA, EA, DHAA, DHEA, diketogulonic acid and diketogluconic acid (Doner and Hicks, 1981). Since there is no significant difference in pK_a values of the ionizable protons between AA and EA, one must assume that factors other than degree of ionization affect interactions with the stationary phase. One possible mechanism is hydrogen bonding between hydroxyl protons in the compounds with the neutral amino group in the stationary phase (Donor and Hicks, 1981). For the simultaneous determination of AA and DHAA in fruit and vegetables (Wimalasiri and Wills, 1983), citric acid, rather than metaphosphoric acid, was used as the extracting medium, as metaphosphoric acid had a similar retention time to DHAA and absorbed strongly at its detection wavelength of 214 nm. For the determination of total vitamin C (AA + DHAA) and/or total isovitamin C (EA + DHEA) after pre-column reduction of the oxidized forms, the reducing agent dithiothreitol elutes near the solvent front, and hence does not interfere in the determination (Margolis and Black, 1987). An alternative reducing agent, DL-homocysteine, produced a strongly absorbing doublet peak in front of the AA peak, and so would mask the EA peak. Tuan, Wyatt and Anglemier (1987) determined total vitamin C or total isovitamin C in a variety of foods, using dithiothreitol as a reducing agent. Phenylalanine could be used as an internal standard for determining total vitamin C in fruit and vegetable samples, but could not be used for determining total isovitamin C in meat products, owing to the presence of interfering peaks. Sapers *et al.* (1990) stressed that neutralization of metaphosphoric acid to pH 6 in sample extracts was essential in order to obtain a quantitative recovery of DHAA; recovery was only 14% in non-neutralized extracts (pH 2.9) and 45% at pH 4. The column life of aminopropyl-bonded phases is somewhat limited compared to that of reversed phases, owing to the loss of the amine function when it reacts irreversibly with the carbonyl groups of reducing sugars or other compounds to form Schiff bases. Bui-Nguyên (1985) reported that the resolution of AA and EA decreased after 50–100 AA assays using an aminopropyl-bonded column. The resolution was not significantly improved by increasing the percentage of methanol in the mobile phase (decreasing the polarity), but increasing the column temperature from 35 to 60 °C restored the separation.

Ion exclusion partition chromatography

Kim and Kim (1988) employed ion exclusion chromatography with amperometric detection to determine AA in foods and beverages. The method was rapid (total analysis time, 5 min), sensitive (<0.1 mg/100 g food sample detectable) and selective. The coefficient of variation for the analysis was approximately 5%. A useful feature of this technique is its ability to simultaneously determine the sulphite present in fruit juices and instant mashed potato. The results obtained for these commodities using the AOAC titrimetric method with 2,6-dichlorophenolindophenol (DCPIP) were higher than those obtained chromatographically, due to the interference by free sulphite. A disadvantage of ion exclusion chromatography is that AA and EA cannot be separated. The method was extended to include the determination of DHAA after reduction to AA with dithiothreitol (Kim, 1989). Dithiothreitol is electrochemically active, but its peak appears well after the AA peak in the chromatogram, so it does not hinder the quantitative determination. Huang, Duda and Kissinger (1987) determined free sulphite and AA in lemon juice simultaneously, using amperometry with a dual electrode configuration, platinum for sulphite and glassy carbon for AA. Bushway, Bureau and McGann (1984) determined the major organic acids, including AA, in potatoes. Malic acid was not completely resolved from AA, but this problem was obviated by allowing the AA to oxidize to DHAA overnight at room temperature.

Reversed-phase chromatography

Lloyd *et al.* (1988a, b) examined the effects of changing ionic strength and pH upon the separation of AA and EA on a PLRP-S 100 Å 5-μm PS–DVB column operated in the reversed-phase mode. The optimum mobile phase composition was found to be 0.2 M NaH_2PO_4, with the pH adjusted to 2.14 using 0.5 N HCl. This pH value is 2 pH units below the pK_a of 4.17 for AA, in accordance with the principle of ion suppression chromatography. Under these conditions small changes in mobile phase buffer salt composition and pH would have a negligible effect on the solute capacity factor (k) and selectivity (α). This optimized system was applied to the routine determination of AA in fresh citrus fruit juices using absorbance detection at 220 nm (Figure 6.13).

Reversed-phase chromatography at around neutral pH (i.e. without ion suppression) can be utilized if the quinoxaline fluorophore is chromatographed after pre-column oxidation of AA and derivatization (Speek, Schrijver and Schreurs, 1984).

Ion interaction chromatography

The tetrabutylammonium salts that are generally popular as ion interaction agents cause a relatively poor retention of AA, but they have been used without an organic modifier to determine AA and EA in meat products (Lee and Marder, 1983; Kutnink and Omaye, 1987; Vanderslice and Higgs, 1988). These reagents have been reported (Carnevale, 1980) to be unsuitable for the analysis of citrus juices, because the relatively high concentration of ionizable material (mostly citric acid) exceeds their ion interaction capacity, resulting in loss of resolution, distortion of peak shapes and changes in elution volume. Most published ion interaction chromatographic methods for determining vitamin C and related compounds use a more hydrophobic reagent with longer aliphatic chains, and methanol as organic modifier to achieve the desired separation and to impart the required solubility. The reagents represent a variety of primary, secondary or tertiary amines. Some ion interaction agents, namely n-octylamine, n-decylamine, hexadecyltrimethylammonium bromide (Kutnink and Omaye, 1987) and tridecylammonium formate (Watada, 1982; Lee and Marder, 1983), reportedly form precipitates (presumably phosphate complexes) when mixed with dilute (5% or 6%) metaphosphoric acid used in the extraction procedure. This precipitation causes the problem of pressure build-up within the HPLC

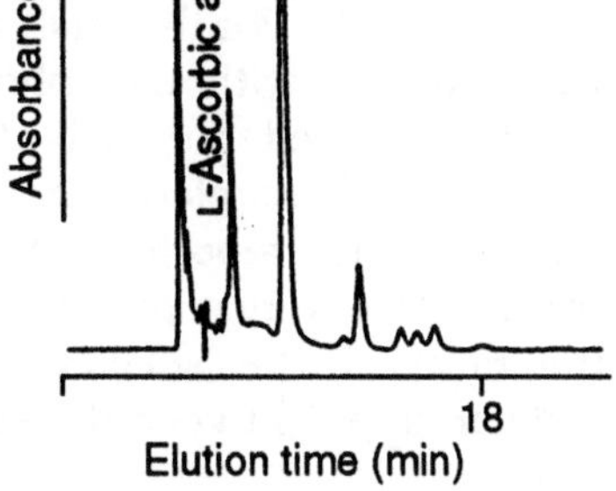

Figure 6.13 Reversed-phase HPLC of ascorbic acid in fresh orange juice. Conditions as given in Table 6.8 (From Lloyd *et al.* (1988b).)

system, which is not prevented by the addition of methanol to the mobile phase.

Moledina and Flink (1982) showed that buffering of the mobile phase to pH 4.2 (the pK_{a1} value of AA) was essential for obtaining a sharp, well-defined AA peak. Maintaining the pH between 4.2 and 4.5 with a buffer salt would ensure that the AA and the ion interaction agent are in the ionic form, whilst also ensuring a sufficiently acidic medium in the interest of AA stability. Potatoes and green bell peppers were the only samples among the fruits, juices and vegetables tested where the AA values obtained by HPLC and titrometry (DCPIP method) were essentially equal. These results could be due to a lack of reducing compounds in these products or to coeluting substances, which absorb at the detection wavelength (254 nm).

The separation of AA and EA has been achieved in meat products using tetrabutylammonium phosphate in acetate buffer (with no problem of precipitation) (Kutnink and Omaye, 1987), cetyltrimethylammonium bromide in phosphate buffer/methanol (Coustard and Sudraud, 1981) and 1,5-dimethylhexylamine in acetate buffer/methanol (Schüep and Keck, 1990). The separation of AA, EA and their respective oxidation products, DHAA and DHEA, has been achieved using tetrabutylammonium phosphate as the ion interaction agent (Vanderslice and Higgs, 1988), but it was necessary to employ three 25-cm ODS columns connected in series.

Finley and Duang (1981) reported the simultaneous assay of AA, DHAA and diketogulonic acid in fruit, juices and vegetables using two 30-cm C_{18} columns connected in series. Tri-n-butylamine, rather than tetrabutylammonium phosphate, was used as the ion interaction agent, as the latter displayed a high UV absorbance at the low wavelength (210 nm) necessary to detect DHAA and diketogulonic acid.

Augustin, Beck and Marousek (1981) reported that data obtained by HPLC and titrometry (DCPIP method) compared favourably for the analysis of raw potatoes and potato products (flakes, granules and French fries), but titrimetric values for potato chips (crisps) were more than twice those obtained by HPLC. For the analysis of fresh tomatoes, Russell (1986) included methanol with metaphosphoric acid in the extraction procedure, which allowed the early addition of pentanophenone as an internal standard. Precipitation problems using tridecylammonium formate, although not reported by Augustin, Beck and Marousek (1981) or Russell (1986), were experienced by Lee and Marder (1983). The latter authors used the smaller molecule, tetrabutylammonium formate, to determine EA in cured meats without incurring precipitation.

Pachla and Kissinger (1979) used the classical extracting solution, 3% metaphosphoric acid/8% acetic acid, in the analysis of fruits, infant foods and milk. Because of the high acidity and ionic strength of this solution, the extracts were diluted with cold 50 mM perchloric acid prior to HPLC. Archer (1981) avoided the use of such acids by stabilizing sample solutions with EDTA and citric acid as a means of chelating divalent metal ions and protecting AA from metal-catalysed oxidation. Morawski (1984) precipitated the proteins in milk by extraction with acetonitrile containing thiourea as antioxidant to provide a protein-free extract, which was compatible with the HPLC mobile phase.

Cyanopropyl-bonded phase chromatography

The separation of AA, sorbic acid and benzoic acid in citrus juices was effected using a μBondapak-CN column and a 2% acetic acid/methanol (95 : 5) mobile phase (Carnevale, 1980); a C_{18}-bonded phase did not effect the separation using the same mobile phase.

Hydrophilic gel chromatography

The separation of glucose, diketogulonic acid, DHAA and AA (in that order of elution) was obtained within 30 min on a 50 cm × 7.6 mm i.d. Asahipak GS-320 column maintained at 30 °C and eluted with an aqueous buffer of pH 3.0 (Seki *et al.*, 1985). The GS-320 column packing material is a cross-linked vinyl copolymer, which separates polar compounds by means of hydrophilic interactions. Fluorescence detection through post-column derivatization with benzamidine allowed the determination of nanogram amounts of AA, DHAA and diketogulonic acid. The method was applied to the determination of AA in orange juice after ion exchange chromatographic clean-up.

6.4.7 MULTIPLE VITAMIN ANALYSES

Ion interaction HPLC eliminates the differences in ionization between the various vitamins, and permits their isocratic elution in the sequence of ascorbic acid, nicotinic acid, nicotinamide, pyridoxine, folic acid, thiamin and riboflavin. The technique is routinely applied to the analysis of pharmaceutical multivitamin preparations (Jenkins, 1982) and has also been applied to the determination of thiamin, riboflavin, pyridoxine and nicotinic acid in infant formula premixes and vitamin supplements using *m*-hydroxybenzoic acid as an internal standard (Chase and Soliman, 1990). Dong, Lepore and Tarumoto (1988) systematically evaluated the factors controlling the above separation, and found that a mobile phase of water containing 15% methanol, 5 mM hexane sulphonic acid, 1% acetic acid and 0.13% triethylamine yielded an excellent separation with several C_8 and C_{18} columns. Triethylamine was used as a mobile phase additive to reduce the peak tailing of the strongly basic thiamin.

HPLC methods for the simultaneous or successive determination of two or more vitamins are summarized in Table 6.9.

Thiamin and riboflavin

Autoclaving food samples with dilute mineral acid, followed by enzymatic hydrolysis, will convert protein-bound thiamin pyrophosphate (TPP) and other bound forms of thiamin to free thiamin. This treatment will also convert protein-bound FAD and FMN to free riboflavin. Thus the total extractable thiamin and the total extractable riboflavin can be determined from one sample hydrolysate with a considerable saving of time and effort.

For the analysis of fortified foods, such as breakfast cereals, thiamin and riboflavin can be determined simultaneously (i.e. in one chromatographic run), and without the need for derivatization, by ion interaction chromatography and photometric detection at 254 nm (Kamman, Labuza and Warthesen, 1980). Most applications, however, use fluorescence detection as a means of obtaining adequate sensitivity for thiamin after conversion to thiochrome. The chromatographic mode employed depends upon whether the derivatization is carried out pre-column or post-column. Pre-column derivatization provides the opportunity for detecting thiochrome and riboflavin simultaneously using simple reversed-phase chromatography. This technique has been carried out using a single fluorescence detector equipped with suitable excitation and emission filters to obtain adequate responses for each compound (Fellman *et al.*, 1982; Reyes and Subryan, 1989). In order to obtain the optimum wavelength settings to achieve maximum sensitivity for each compound, it would be necessary to install a wavelength-programmable spectrofluorimeter or two fluorescence monitors connected in series. It is usually preferred to determine thiochrome and riboflavin successively (i.e. in two successive chromatographic runs) so that the optimum detection parameters can be selected (Finglas and Faulks, 1984b; Hasselmann *et al.*, 1989; Fernando and Murphy, 1990). Although the separation of thiochrome from riboflavin might seem to be unnecessary if they are to be determined successively, it is in fact essential. If these compounds coeluted, the radiation emitted by thiochrome could be reabsorbed by riboflavin by the inner filter effect, causing a diminished fluorescent signal.

With post-column derivatization, thiamin and riboflavin can be chromatographed simultaneously using ion interaction chromatography. This technique, used with two fluorescence detectors, has been applied to the analysis of a wide range of foods (Mauro and Wetzel, 1984; Wills,

Table 6.9 HPLC methods used for multiple vitamin analyses

Food	Sample preparation	Column	Mobile phase	Compounds separated	Detection	Reference
Reversed-phase chromatography						
Raw and cooked potatoes	*Extraction*: reflux sample with 0.1 N HCl for 30 min and cool to below 50 °C. Incubate with buffered (pH 4.5) Takadiastase at 45–50 °C for 2 h. Cool, dilute to volume with water and filter Derivatization: oxidize thiamin to thiochrome with alkaline $K_3Fe(CN)_6$	μBondapak C_{18} 10 μm 30 cm × 3.9 mm i.d.	Water/MeOH (70 : 30)	Thiochrome Riboflavin (separate chromatograms)	*Thiochrome* Fluorescence: ex. 365 nm em. 435 nm *Riboflavin* Fluorescence: ex. 450 nm em. 510 nm	Finglas and Faulks (1984b)
Dietetic foods	*Extraction*: digest sample with 0.1 N HCl at 95–100 °C for 30 min and cool. Adjust pH to 4.5 and incubate with *β*-amalase and Takadiastase at 37 °C overnight. Dilute to volume with water and filter (0.2 μm) *For riboflavin*: use filtrate directly *For thiamin*: convert to thiochrome by treating aliquot of filtrate with alkaline $K_3Fe(CN)_6$. Pass solution through C_{18} Sep-Pak cartridge, wash cartridge with 50 mM sodium acetate, then elute thiochrome with $MeOH/H_2O$ (60 : 40)	μBondapak C_{18} 10 μm 30 cm × 3.9 mm i.d.	50 mM acetate buffer (pH 4.5)/MeOH (40 : 60)	Thiochrome Riboflavin (separate chromatograms)	*Thiochrome* Fluorescence: ex. 366 nm em. 435 nm *Riboflavin* Fluorescence: ex. 422 nm em. 522 nm	Hasselmann *et al.* (1989)

Table 6.9 *Continued*

Food	Sample preparation	Column	Mobile phase	Compounds separated	Detection	Reference
Soy products	*Extraction*: hydrate dry samples and heat at 90 °C for 30 min. Adjust pH of medium to 2 with 5 N HCl and autoclave at 20 lb/in^2 for 15 min. Adjust pH of cooled extract to 4.5, centrifuge and filter *For riboflavin*: use filtrate directly *For thiamin*: oxidize to thiochrome by treating aliquot of filtrate with alkaline $K_3Fe(CN)_6$ and neutralizing with conc. H_3PO_4 after 45 s	Ultrasphere C_{18} 5 μm 15 cm × 4.6 mm i.d.	10 mM acetate buffer/(pH 5.5)/MeCN (87 : 13)	Thiochrome Riboflavin (separate chromatograms)	*Thiochrome* Fluorescence (filters) *Riboflavin* Fluorescence: ex. 436 nm em. 535 nm (filters)	Fernando and Murphy (1990)
Peas, beans, liver, skim milk, whole and enriched wheat flour	*Extraction*: autoclave samples with dilute HCl at 121 °C for 15 min and cool. Adjust pH to 4.0–4.5 and incubate with Takadiastase at 48 °C for 3 h. Deproteinize by adding 50% TCA and heating at 95–100 °C for 15 min. Cool, adjust pH to 3.5, dilute to volume with water and filter *Derivatization*: oxidize thiamin to thiochrome by treatment with alkaline $K_3Fe(CN)_6$ followed by conc H_3PO_4	Radial-PAK C_8 10 μm 10 cm × 8 mm	10 mM phosphate buffer (pH 7.0)/MeOH (63 : 37)	Thiochrome and riboflavin (in same chromatogram)	Fluorescence: *Thiochrome and riboflavin* ex. 360 nm em. 415 nm (filters) *Riboflavin alone* ex. 450 nm em. 530 nm (filters)	Fellman *et al.* (1982)

	Clean-up/concentration: pass the oxidized extract through an activated C_{18} Sep-Pak cartridge and wash the cartridge sequentially with 10 mM phosphate buffer (pH 7.0) and 10 mM phosphate buffer/MeOH (95 : 5). Elute the vitamins with 50% aqueous MeOH and dilute to volume					
Cereal products	*Extraction*: autoclave ground sample with 0.1 N HCl at 121 °C for 30 min and cool. Adjust pH to 4.0–4.5 and incubate with Takadiastase at 50 °C for 3 h (minimum). Cool and dilute to volume with water *Derivatization and clean-up/concentration*: as for Fellman *et al*. (1982) (see above)	Radial PAK C_{18} 10 μm 10 cm × 8 mm	5 mM phosphate buffer (pH 7.0)/MeOH (65 : 35)	Thiochrome and riboflavin (in same chromatogram)	Fluorescence (filters)	Reyes and Subryan (1989)
Ion interaction chromatography						
Cereal products, fortified breakfast cereals	*Extraction*: autoclave sample with 0.1 N HCl at 121 °C for 30 min, cool and centrifuge	μBondapak C_{18} 10 μm 30 cm × 3.9 mm i.d.	10 mM phosphate buffer (pH 7.0)/MeCN (12.5 : 87.5) containing 5 mM sodium heptane sulphonate	Thiamin and riboflavin (in same chromatogram)	UV 254 nm	Kamman, Labuza and Warthesen (1980)

Table 6.9 *Continued*

Food	Sample preparation	Column	Mobile phase	Compounds separated	Detection	Reference
Cereal products, fresh meat and meat products, fresh fruit and vegetables, eggs, milk, yoghurt	*Extraction*: digest sample with 0.1 N HCl at 95–100 °C for 30 min, cool and dilute to volume. Adjust pH of aliquot to 4.0–4.5 and incubate with Clarase at 45–50 °C for 3 h. Cool and filter *Clean-up/concentration*: pass filtrate through Sep-Pak C_{18} cartridge, wash cartridge with aqueous 5 mM sodium hexane sulphonate and elute the vitamins with methanolic 5 mM sodium hexane sulphonate	Radial-PAK C_{18} 10 μm 10 cm × 8 mm	MeOH/water (40 : 60) containing 5 mM hexane sulphonic acid	Thiamin and riboflavin (in same chromatogram)	*Thiochrome* Fluorescence: ex. 360 nm em. 425 nm (filters) after post-column derivatization with alkaline $K_3Fe(CN)_6$ *Riboflavin* Fluorescence: ex. 360 nm em. 500 nm (filters)	Wimalasiri and Wills (1985) Wills, Wimalasiri and Greenfield (1985)
Enriched cereal-based products	*Extraction*: digest sample with 0.1 N H_2SO_4 at 95–100 °C for 10 min and cool. Incubate with buffered Mylase at 56 °C for 1 h. Cool, dilute to volume and filter	μBondapak C_{18} 10 μm 30 cm × 3.9 mm i.d.	MeOH/water (36 : 64) containing 5 mM hexane sulphonic acid and 1% HOAc	Thiamin and riboflavin (in same chromatogram)	*Thiochrome* Fluorescence: (filters) after post-column derivatization with alkaline $K_3Fe(CN)_6$ *Riboflavin* Fluorescence (2nd detector)	Mauro and Wetzel (1984) (Figure 6.14)

Infant formula (fortified)	Extract sample with water. Deproteinize by pH adjustment to 1.7 and then to 4.6, dilute to volume with water and filter	Spherisorb ODS-1 5 μm 15 cm × 4.6 mm i.d.	40 mM triethylammonium phosphate buffer (pH 3.0) containing 7.5 mM sodium octane sulphonate, 10% MeOH and 5% MeCN	Pyridoxal, pyridoxine, riboflavin	Fluorescence: ex. 285 nm em. 546 nm (filter)	Ayi, Yuhas and Deangelis (1986) (Figure 6.15)
Fortified foods (e.g. milk products, powdered meals)	*Extraction*; digest sample with 2 N H_2SO_4 at 95–100 °C for 30 min. Cool, dilute to volume with water and filter	Partisil ODS 10 μm or Ultrasphere ODS 5 μm	2.5 M sodium acetate (80 ml), HOAc (50 ml) and water (25 ml) containing 1.1 g sodium heptane sulphonate. Mixture diluted to 1 litre with water	Nicotinamide and pyridoxine	*Nicotinamide* UV 260 nm *Pyridoxine* Fluorescence: ex. 296 nm em. 396 nm Detectors connected in series	Rees (1989)

Table 6.9 *Continued*

Food	Sample preparation	Column	Mobile phase	Compounds separated	Detection	Reference
Fortified cereal products	*Extraction*: digest ground sample with 0.1 N H_2SO_4 at 95–100 °C or 30 min and cool. Incubate with buffered Clarase at 55 °C for 1 h, centrifuge and dilute to volume	μBondapak C_{18} 10 μm 25 cm × 4.6 mm i.d. and 5 cm × 4.6 mm i.d. short column. Sample clean-up achieved by column switching	MeOH/water HOAc (30 : 69 : 1) containing 5 mM sodium hexane sulphonate	Pyridoxine, riboflavin and thiamin	Dual fluorescence *Pyridoxine and riboflavin* 1st detector: ex. 288 nm em. 418 nm (cut-off filter) *Thiochrome* 2nd detector: ex. 360 nm em. 460 nm (cut-off filter) after post-column oxidation of thiamin with alkaline $K_3Fe(CN)_6$ to form thiochrome	Wehling and Wetzel (1984)

μ-Bondapak, Porasil, Radial-PAK, Nova-PAK (Waters Associates); LiChrosorb (Merck); Spherisorb (Phase Separations); Nucleosil, Polygosil (Macherey-Nagel); Bio-Sil, Aminex (Bio-Rad); Hypersil (Shandon); Ultrasphere (Altex); Supelcosil (Supelco); Vydac (Separations Group); Partisil (Whatman); Zipax, Zorbax (Du Pont).
MeOH (methanol); EtOH (ethanol); MeCN (acetonitrile); HOAc (acetic acid); HPO_3 (metaphosphoric acid); $HClO_4$ (perchloric acid).

Wimalasiri and Greenfield, 1985; Wimalasiri and Wills, 1985). A chromatogram of the two vitamins extracted from a sample of enriched corn (maize) flour is depicted in Figure 6.14.

Riboflavin and pyridoxine

Ayi, Yuhas and Deangelis (1986) developed a comparatively simple method for the simultaneous determination of supplemental riboflavin and PN in fortified milk-based and soy-based infant formula products. The method took advantage of the natural fluorescence of these vitamins and was performed using a single fluorescence detector equipped with carefully selected filters. The ion interaction mode of chromatography was capable of isolating PN from the other B_6 vitamers and from 4-PA. Similarly, riboflavin was well separated from its potential degradation products, lumiflavin and lumichrome. A chromatogram of a milk-based infant formula product is depicted in Figure 6.15.

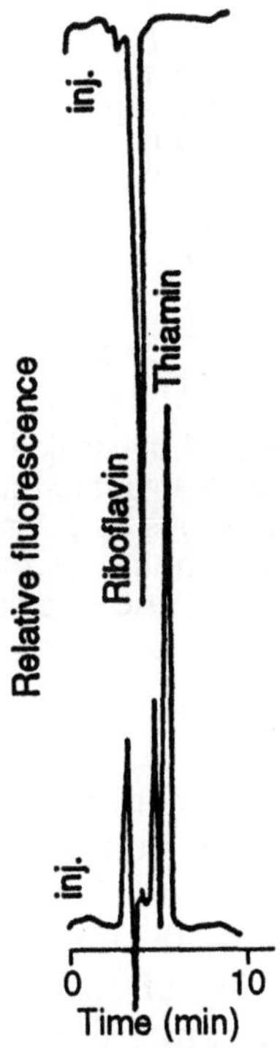

Figure 6.14 Ion interaction HPLC of riboflavin and thiamin (after post-column oxidation to thiochrome) extracted from enriched corn (maize) flour. Conditions as given in Table 6.9. (From Mauro and Wetzel, 1984.)

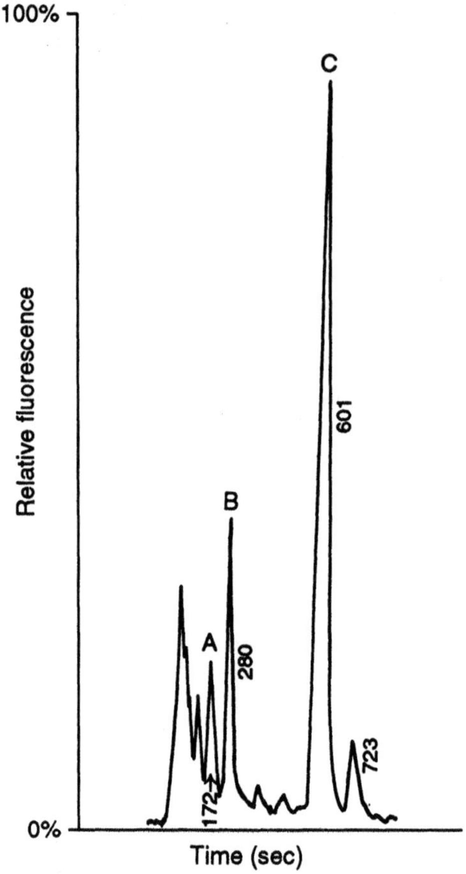

Figure 6.15 Ion interaction HPLC of pyridoxine and riboflavin extracted from a fortified milk-based liquid concentrate infant formula product. Peaks: (A) pyridoxal; (B) pyridoxine; (C) riboflavin. Conditions as given in Table 6.9. (From Ayi, Yuhas and Deangelis (1986). Reprinted from the *Journal of the AOAC*, Vol. 69, No. 01, pp. 56–9, 1986. Copyright 1986 by AOAC International.)

Nicotinamide and pyridoxine

Rees (1989) used ion interaction chromatography, and absorbance and fluorescence detectors connected in series, for the simultaneous determination of nicotinamide and PN, respectively, in fortified food products. The extraction process (heating with 2 N H_2SO_4 for 30 min at 100 °C) caused a 6% conversion of nicotinamide to nicotinic acid, but this was catered for by subjecting both the standard and the sample extract to the same treatment. An ODS column containing residual free silanol groups was used for routine analyses and gave retention times of 8.0 and 5.8 min for nicotinamide and PN, respectively. If a new product was being analysed, or it was known that the PN peak was subject to interference from other peaks, the analysis was repeated using a fully endcapped ODS column. On this column, the order of elution was reversed, nicotinamide and PN having retention times of 4.2 and 8.6 min respectively. The detection limit for nicotinamide was 0.1 mg/100 g, and that for PN was 0.01 mg/100 g. PN is usually present in fortified food products at levels 10 times lower than those of nicotinamide, and hence the higher sensitivity of detection for PN was fortuitous.

Thiamin, riboflavin and pyridoxine

Wehling and Wetzel (1984) accomplished the simultaneous determination of thiamin, riboflavin and PN in fortified cereal products after extraction of the samples by heating with 0.1 N H_2SO_4, followed by Clarase treatment to break down the starch. Ion interaction chromatography with isocratic elution separated the three vitamins within 20 min, but more strongly retained components took up to 50 min to elute. The 50-min chromatographic analysis time was halved by the use of on-line sample clean-up, utilizing a short (5 cm) C_{18} column in addition to the C_{18} analytical (25 cm) column, and a column switching arrangement. Aliquots of the test extract were injected onto the short column, with the effluent being routed directly to waste. Solvent flow through the analytical column and detector was maintained independently by a second pump. At 0.60 min after injection, the fraction of effluent containing the vitamins was diverted onto the analytical column, and at 3.50 min the valve was switched back to its original position. During the remaining time, as the vitamins were undergoing analysis, the more strongly retained components were eluted from the short column directly to waste. Fluorescence detection was used to measure the native fluorescence of PN and riboflavin. Thiamin, in the form of thiochrome, was detected by a second fluorescence monitor after post-column derivatization, the strong alkaline conditions suppressing the fluorescence of PN and riboflavin. The concentration of potassium hexacyanoferrate (III) added for post-column thiochrome formation was decreased significantly from levels used in previous procedures in order to minimize the quenching effect of excess reagent during detection. Detection limits were 2 μg/g for PN and 1 μg/g for both riboflavin and thiamin.

REFERENCES

Adams, R.F. (1985) Ion-pair chromatography of pharmaceuticals. In *Ion-pair Chromatography. Theory and Biological and Pharmaceutical Applications* (ed. M.T.W. Hearn), Marcel Dekker, Inc., New York, pp. 141–207.

Addo, C. and Augustin, J. (1988) Changes in the vitamin B-6 content in potatoes during storage. *J. Fd Sci.*, **53**, 749–52.

Ang, C.Y.W., Cenciarelli, M. and Eitenmiller, R.R. (1988) A simple liquid chromatographic method for determination of B_6 vitamers in raw and cooked chicken. *J. Fd Sci.*, **53**, 371–5.

Ang, C.Y.W. and Moseley, F.A. (1980) Determination of thiamin and riboflavin in meat and meat products by high-pressure liquid chromatography. *J. Agric. Fd Chem.*, **28**, 483–6.

Arai, Y. and Hanai, T. (1988) Capability of a photodiode array detector for vitamin analysis. *J. Liquid Chromat.*, **11**, 2409–18.

Archer, A.W. (1981) Stability of aqueous solutions of ascorbic acid prepared for analysis by high performance liquid chromatography. *J. Ass. Publ. Analysts*, **19**, 91–3.

Ashoor, S.H., Monte, W.C. and Welty, J. (1984) Liquid chromatographic determination of ascorbic acid in foods. *J. Ass. Off. Analyt. Chem.*, **67**, 78–80.

Ashoor, S.H., Seperich, G.J., Monte, W.C. and Welty, J. (1983) HPLC determination of riboflavin in eggs and dairy products. *J. Fd Sci.*, **48**, 92–4, 110.

Ashoor, S.H., Knox, M.J., Olsen, J.R. and Deger, D.A. (1985) Improved liquid chromatographic determination of riboflavin in milk and dairy products. *J. Ass. Off. Analyt. Chem.*, **68**, 693–6.

Augustin, J., Beck, C. and Marousek, G.I. (1981) Quantitative determination of ascorbic acid in potatoes and potato products by high performance liquid chromatography. *J. Fd Sci.*, **46**, 312, 313, 316.

Ayi, B.K., Yuhas, D.A. and Deangelis, N.J. (1986) Simultaneous determination of vitamins B_2 (riboflavin) and B_6 (pyridoxine) in infant formula products by reverse phase liquid chromatography. *J. Ass. Off. Analyt. Chem.*, **69**, 56–9.

Ayi, B.K., Yuhas, D.A., Moffett, K.S., Joyce, D.M. and Deangelis, N.J. (1985) Liquid chromatographic determination of thiamine in infant formula products by using ultraviolet detection. *J. Ass. Off. Analyt. Chem.*, **68**, 1087–92.

Bailey, A.L. and Finglas, P.M. (1990) A normal phase high performance liquid chromatographic method for the determinaiton of thiamin in blood and tissue samples. *J. Micronutr. Anal.*, **7**, 147–57.

Bakalyar, S.R. and Henry, R.A. (1976) Variables affecting precision and accuracy in high-performance liquid chromatography. *J. Chromat.*, **126**, 327–45.

Bartha, A., Vigh, G. and Varga-Puchony, Z. (1990) Basis of the rational selection of the hydrophobicity and concentration of the ion-pairing reagent in reversed-phase ion-pair high-performance liquid chromatography. *J. Chromat.*, **499**, 423–34.

Behrens, W.A. and Madère, R. (1987) A highly sensitive high-performance liquid chromatography method for the estimation of ascorbic and dehydroascorbic acid in tissues, biological fluids, and foods. *Analyt. Biochem.*, **165**, 102–7.

Behrens, W.A. and Madère, R. (1989) Ascorbic and dehydroascorbic acid content of infant formula. *J. Fd Comp. Anal.*, **2**, 48–52.

Behrens, W.A. and Madère, R. (1990) Ascorbic and dehydroascorbic acid contents of canned food and frozen concentrated orange juice. *J. Fd Comp. Anal.*, **3**, 3–8.

Bidlingmeyer, B.A. (1980) Separation of ionic compounds by reversed-phase liquid chromatography: an update of ion-pairing techniques. *J. Chromatogr. Sci.*, **18**, 525–39.

Bidlingmeyer, B.A., Deming, S.N., Price, W.P. Jr, Sachok, B. and Petrusek, M. (1979) Retention mechanism for reversed-phase ion-pair liquid chromatography. *J. Chromat.*, **186**, 419–34.

Bilic, N. and Sieber, R. (1990) Determination of flavins in dairy products by high-performance liquid chromatography using sorboflavin as internal standard. *J. Chromat.*, **511**, 359–66.

Bitsch, R. and Möller, J. (1989) Analysis of B_6 vitamers in foods using a modified high-performance liquid chromatographic method. *J. Chromat.*, **463**, 207–11.

Bradbury, J.H. and Singh, U. (1986) Ascorbic acid and dehydroascorbic acid content of tropical root crops from the South Pacific. *J. Fd Sci.*, **51**, 975–8, 987.

Bratin, K. and Kissinger, P.T. (1981) Reductive LCEC of organic compounds. *J. Liquid Chromat.*, **4**(Suppl. 2), 321–57.

Brubacher, G., Müller-Mulot, W. and Southgate, D.A.T. (1985) *Methods for the Determination of Vitamins in Food. Recommended by COST 91*. Elsevier Applied Science Publishers, London and New York.

Brunt, K. (1981) Electrochemical detectors for high-performance liquid chromatography and flow analysis systems. In *Trace Analysis*, Vol. 1 (ed. J.F. Lawrence), Academic Press, New York, pp. 47–120.

Bui-Nguyên, M.H. (1985) Ascorbic acid and related compounds. In *Modern Chromatographic Analysis of the Vitamins* (eds A.P. De Leenheer, W.E. Lambert and M.G.M. De Ruyter), Marcel Dekker, Inc., New York, pp. 267–301.

Burton, W.G. (1966) *The Potato*, 2nd edn, Veenman, Wageningen.

Bushway, R.J., Bureau, J.L. and McGann, D.F. (1984) Determinations of organic acids in potatoes by high performance liquid chromatography. *J. Fd Sci.*, **49**, 75–7, 81.

Bushway, R.J., King, J.M., Perkins, B. and Krishnan, M. (1988) High performance liquid chromatographic determination of ascorbic acid in fruits, vegetables and juices *J. Liquid Chromat.*, **11**, 3415–23.

Carnevale, J. (1980) Determination of ascorbic, sorbic and benzoic acids in citrus juices by high-performance liquid chromatography. *Fd Technol. Aust.*, **32**, 302, 304–5.

Chase, G.W. Jr and Soliman, A.M. (1990) Analysis of thiamin, riboflavin, pyridoxine and niacin in multivitamin premixes and supplements by high performance liquid chromatography, *J. Micronutr. Anal.*, **7**, 15–25.

Coburn, S.P. and Mahuren, J.D. (1983) A versatile cation-exchange procedure for measuring the seven major forms of vitamin B_6 in biological samples. *Analyt. Biochem.*, **129**, 310–17.

Cooke, N.H.C. and Olsen, K. (1979) Chemically bonded alkyl reversed-phase columns. *Am. Lab.*, **11**, 45, 46, 48, 50, 52–5, 58–60.

Coustard, J.M. and Sudraud, G. (1981) Separation of ascorbic and isoascorbic acids by ion-pair reverse-phase chromatography. *J. Chromat.*, **219**, 338–42 (in French).

Dakshinamurti, K. and Chauhan, M.S. (1981) Chemical analysis of pyridoxine vitamers. In *Methods in Vitamin B-6 Nutrition. Analysis and Status Assessment* (eds J.E. Leklem and R.D. Reynolds), Plenum Press, New York, pp. 99–122.

Dawkins, J.V., Lloyd, L.L. and Warner, F.P. (1986) Chromatographic characteristics of polymer-based high-performance liquid chromatography packings. *J. Chromat.*, **352**, 157–67.

Day, B.P. and Gregory, J.F. (1981) Determination of folacin derivatives in selected foods by high-performance liquid chromatography. *J. Agric. Fd Chem.*, **29**, 374–7.

Dennison, D.B., Brawley, T.G. and Hunter, G.L.K. (1981) Rapid high-performance liquid chromatographic determination of ascorbic acid and combined ascorbic acid-dehydroascorbic acid in beverages. *J. Agric. Fd Chem.*, **29**, 927–9.

Diop, P.A., Franck, D., Grimm, P. and Hasselmann, C. (1988) High-performance liquid chromatographic determination of vitamin C in fresh fruits from West Africa. *J. Fd Composition Anal.*, **1**, 265–9.

Doner, L.W. and Hicks, K.B. (1981) High-performance liquid chromatographic separation of ascorbic acid, erythorbic acid, dehydroascorbic acid, dehydroerythorbic acid, diketogulonic acid, and diketogluconic acid. *Analyt. Biochem.*, **115**, 225–30.

Dong, M.W., Lepore, J. and Tarumoto, T. (1988) Factors affecting the ion-pair chromatography of water-soluble vitamins. *J. Chromat.*, **442**, 81–95.

Drouen, A.C.J.H., Billiet, H.A.H. and De Galan, L. (1984) Dual-wavelength absorbance ratio for solute recognition in liquid chromatography. *Analyt. Chem.*, **56**, 971–8.

Ekanayake, A. and Nelson, P.E. (1988) Applicability of an *in vitro* method for the estimation of vitamin B_6 biological availability. *J. Micronutr. Anal.*, **4**, 1–15.

Fellman, J.K., Artz, W.E., Tassinari, P.D., Cole, C.L. and Augustin, J. (1982) Simultaneous determination of thiamin and riboflavin in selected foods by high-performance liquid chromatography. *J. Fd Sci.*, **47**, 2048–50, 2067.

Fernando, S.M. and Murphy, P.A. (1990) HPLC determination of thiamin and riboflavin in soybeans and tofu. *J. Agric. Fd. Chem.*, **38**, 163–7.

Finglas, P.M. and Faulks, R.M. (1984a) Nutritional composition of UK retail potatoes, both raw and cooked. *J. Sci. Fd Agric.*, **35**, 1347–56.

Finglas, P.M. and Faulks, R.M. (1984b) The HPLC analysis of thiamin and riboflavin in potatoes. *Fd Chem.*, **15**, 37–44.

Finley, J.W. and Duang, E. (1981) Resolution of ascorbic, dehydroascorbic and diketogulonic acids by paired-ion reversed-phase chromatography. *J. Chromat.*, **207**, 449–53.

Froehlich, P. and Wehry, E.L. (1981) Fluorescence detection in liquid and gas chromatography. Techniques, examples, and prospects. In *Modern Fluorescence Spectroscopy*, Vol. 3 (ed. E.L. Wehry) Plenum Press, New York, pp. 35–94.

Gloor, R. and Johnson, E.L. (1977) Practical aspects of reverse phase ion pair chromatography. *J. Chromatogr. Sci.*, **15**, 413–23.

Gregory, J.F. (1980) Comparison of high-performance liquid chromatographic and *Saccharomyces uvarum* methods for the determination of vitamin B_6 in fortified breakfast cereals. *J. Agric. Fd Chem.*, **28**, 486–9.

Gregory, J.F. (1984) Determination of folacin in foods and other biological materials. *J. Ass. Off. Analyt. Chem.*, **67**, 1015–19.

Gregory, J.F. and Feldstein, D. (1985) Determination of vitamin B-6 in foods and other biological materials by paired-ion high-performance liquid chromatography. *J. Agric. Fd Chem.*, **33**, 359–63.

Gregory, J.F. and Ink, S.L. (1987) Identification and quantification of pyridoxine-β-glucoside as a major form of vitamin B_6 in plant-derived foods. *J. Agric. Fd Chem.*, **35**, 76–82.

Gregory, J.F., Manley, D.B. and Kirk, J.R. (1981) Determination of vitamin B-6 in animal tissues by reverse-phase high-performance liquid chromatography. *J. Agric. Fd Chem.*, **29**, 921–7.

Gregory, J.F., Sartain, D.B. and Day, B.P.F. (1984) Fluorometric determination of folacin in biological materials using high performance liquid chromatography. *J. Nutr.*, **114**, 341–53.

Grün, I.U., Barbeau, W.E., Chrisley, B. and Driskell, J.A. (1991) Determination of vitamin B_6, available lysine, and ε-pyridoxyllysine in a new instant baby food product. *J. Agric. Fd Chem.*, **39**, 102–8.

Guilarte, T.R., Shane, B. and McIntyre, P.A. (1981) Radiometric-microbiologic assay of vitamin B-6: application to food analysis. *J. Nutr.*, **111**, 1869–75.

Hamaker, B., Kirksey, A., Ekanayake, A. and Borschel, M. (1985) Analysis of B-6 vitamers in human milk by reverse-phase liquid chromatography. *Am. J. Clin. Nutr.*, **42**, 650–5.

Hamano, T., Mitsuhashi, Y., Aoki, N. and Yamamoto, S. (1988) Simultaneous determination of niacin and niacinamide in meats by high-performance liquid chromatography. *J. Chromat.*, **457**, 403–8.

Hasselmann, C., Franck, D., Grimm, P., Diop, P.A. and Soules, C. (1989) High-performance liquid chromatographic analysis of thiamin and riboflavin in dietetic foods. *J. Micronutr. Anal.*, **5**, 269–79.

Henry, R.A., Schmit, J.A. and Williams, R.C. (1973) Application of a new chemically bonded, superficially porous anion-exchange packing to nucleotide analysis. *J. Chromatogr. Sci.*, **11**, 358–65.

Holt, D.L., Wehling, R.L. and Zeece, M.G. (1988) Determination of native folates in milk and other dairy products by high-performance liquid chromatography. *J. Chromat.*, **449**, 271–9.

Hoppner, K. and Lampi, B. (1982) The determination of folic acid (pteroylmonoglutamic acid) in fortified products by reversed phase high pressure liquid chromatography. *J. Liquid Chromat.*, **5**, 953–66.

Horvath, C. and Melander, W. (1977) Liquid chromatography with hydrocarbonaceous bonded phases; theory and practice of reversed phase chromatography. *J. Chromatogr. Sci.*, **15**, 393–404.

Horvath, C.G., Preiss, B.A. and Lipsky, S.R. (1967) Fast liquid chromatography: an investigation of operating parameters and the separation of nucleotides on pellicular ion exchangers. *Analyt. Chem.*, **39**, 1422–8.

Huang, T., Duda, C. and Kissinger, P.T. (1987) LCEC determination of sulphite in food. *Current Separations* (Bioanalytical Systems, Inc., West Lafayette, IN), **8**, 49–52.

Hung, T.-H.T., Seib, P.A. and Kramer, K.J. (1987) Determination of L-ascorbyl 6-palmitate in bread using reverse-phase high-performance liquid chromatography (HPLC) with electrochemical (EC) detection. *J. Fd Sci.*, **52**, 948–53, 974.

Ishii, K., Sarai, K., Sanemori, H. and Kawasaki, T. (1979) Analysis of thiamine and its phosphate esters by high-performance liquid chromatography. *Analyt. Biochem.*, **97**, 191–5.

Iskandarani, Z. and Pietrzyk, D.J. (1982) Ion interaction chromatography of organic anions on a poly(styrene-divinylbenzene) adsorbent in the presence of tetraalkylammonium salts. *Analyt. Chem.*, **54**, 1065–71.

Jaffe, G.M. (1984) Vitamin C. In *Handbook of Vitamins. Nutritional, Biochemical, and Clinical Aspects* (ed. L.J. Machlin), Marcel Dekker, Inc., New York, pp. 199–244.

Jenkins, C. (1982) An HPLC method for the separation and quantitation of water-soluble vitamins in vitamin-mineral formulations. *Pharm. Technol.*, **6**(3), 53–6, 59, 61–5.

Johnson, E.L. and Stevenson, R. (1978) *Basic Liquid Chromatography*, Varian Associates, Inc., Ca.

Johnsson, H. and Branzell, C. (1987) High performance liquid chromatographic determination of riboflavin in food – a comparison with a microbiological method. *Int. J. Vitam. Nutr. Res.*, **57**, 53–8.

Jones, D.G. (1985) Photodiode array detectors in UV-VIS spectroscopy: Part I. *Analyt. Chem.*, **57**, 1057A, 1058A, 1060A, 1062A, 1064A, 1066A, 1068A, 1070A, 1073A.

Kacem, B., Marshall, M.R., Matthews, R.F. and Gregory, J.F. (1986) Simultaneous analysis of ascorbic acid and dehydroascorbic acid by high-performance liquid chromatography with postcolumn derivatization and UV absorbance. *J. Agric. Fd Chem.*, **34**, 271–4.

Kamman, J.F., Labuza, T.P. and Warthesen, J.J. (1980) Thiamin and riboflavin analysis by high performance liquid chromatography. *J. Fd Sci.*, **45**, 1497–9, 1504.

Karp, S., Ciambra, C.M. and Miklean, S. (1990) High-performance liquid chromatographic post-column reaction system for the electrochemical detection of ascorbic acid and dehydroascorbic acid. *J. Chromat.*, **504**, 434–40.

Khym, J.X. (1974) *Analytical Ion-exchange Procedures in Chemistry and Biology. Theory, Equipment, Techniques*, Prentice-Hall, Inc., Englewood Cliffs, NJ.

Kim, H.-J. (1989) Determination of total vitamin C by ion exclusion chromatography with electrochemical detection. *J. Ass. Off. Analyt. Chem.*, **72**, 681–6.

Kim, H.-J. and Kim, Y.-K. (1988) Analysis of ascorbic acid by ion exclusion chromatography with electrochemical detection. *J. Fd Sci.*, **53**, 1525–7.

Kneifel, W., and Sommer, R. (1985) An HPLC method for the determination of vitamin C in milk, whey and whey beverages. *Z. Lebensmittelunters u.-Forsch.*, **181**, 107–10.

Knudson, E.J. and Siebert, K.J. (1987) The determination of ascorbates in beer by liquid chromatography with electrochemical detection. *J. Am. Soc. Brewing Chem.*, **45**, 33–7.

Kral, K. (1983) Determination of nicotinic acid in fruit juices by HPLC with amperometric detection at a SMDE. *Z. Analyt. Chem.*, **314**, 479–82 (in German).

Krstulović, A.M., Colin, H. and Guiochon, G.A. (1984) Electrochemical detectors for liquid chromatography. *Adv. Chromat.*, **24**, 83–124.

Kutnink, M.A. and Omaye, S.T. (1987) Determination of ascorbic acid, erythorbic acid, and uric acid in cured meats by high performance liquid chromatography. *J. Fd Sci.*, **52**, 53–6.

Lee, D.P. (1982) Reversed-phase HPLC from pH 1 to 13. *J. Chromatogr. Sci.*, **20**, 203–8.

Lee, H.S. and Coates, G.A. (1987) Liquid chromatographic determination of vitamin C in commercial Florida citrus juices. *J. Micronutr. Anal.*, **3**, 199–209.

Lee, K. and Marder, S. (1983) HPLC determination of erythorbate in cured meats. *J. Fd Sci.*, **48**, 306, 308.

Lloyd, L.L., Warner, F.P., Kennedy, J.F. and White, C.A. (1988a) Quantitative analysis of vitamin C (L-ascorbic acid) by ion suppression reversed phase chromatography. *Fd Chem.*, **28**, 257–68.

Lloyd, L.L., Warner, F.P., Kennedy, J.F. and White, C.A. (1988b) Ion suppression reversed-phase high-performance liquid chromatography method for the separation of L-ascorbic acid in fresh fruit juice. *J. Chromat.*, **437**, 447–52.

Locke, D.C. (1973) Chemically bonded stationary phases for liquid chromatography. *J. Chromatogr. Sci.*, **11**, 120–8.

Lookhart, G.L., Hall, S.B. and Finney, K.F. (1982) Determination of ascorbic acid in wheat flours, bread dough conditioners, and commercial vitamin C tablets by high-performance liquid chromatography. *Cereal Chem.*, **59**, 69–71.

Lumley, I.D. and Wiggins, R.A. (1981) Determination of riboflavin and flavin mononucleotide in foodstuffs using high-performance liquid chromatography and a column-enrichment technique. *Analyst, Lond.*, **106**, 1103–8.

Maeda, Y., Ochi, S., Masui, T. and Matubara, S. (1988) Liquid chromatographic determination of L-ascorbic acid in candies and soft drinks. *J. Ass. Off. Analyt. Chem.*, **71**, 502–4.

Majors, R.E. (1972) High performance liquid chromatography on small particle silica gel. *Analyt. Chem.*, 44, 1722–6.

Majors, R.E. (1975) Recent advances in high performance liquid chromatography packings and columns. *Am. Lab.*, **7**, 13, 14, 16, 18, 20–2, 24, 26, 28, 30–4, 36–9.

Majors, R.E. (1980a) Multidimensional high performance liquid chromatography. *J. Chromatogr. Sci.*, **18**, 571–9.

Majors, R.E. (1980b) Practical operation of bonded-phase columns in high-performance liquid chromatography. In *High-performance Liquid Chromatography, Advances and Perspectives*, Vol. 1 (ed. C. Horvath), Academic Press, New York, pp. 75–111.

Mannino, S. and Pagliarini, E. (1988) A rapid HPLC method for the determination of vitamin C in milk. *Lebensm.-Wiss. u.-Technol.*, **21**, 313–4.

Margolis, S.A. and Black, I. (1987) Stabilization of ascorbic acid and its measurement by liquid chromatography in nonfat dry milk. *J. Ass. Off. Analyt. Chem.*, **70**, 806–9.

Mauro, D.J. and Wetzel, D.L. (1984) Simultaneous determination of thiamine and riboflavin in enriched cereal based products by high-performance liquid chromatography using selective detection. *J. Chromat.*, **299**, 281–7.

Meyer, V.R. (1988) *Practical High-performance Liquid Chromatography*, John Wiley & Sons, Chichester.

Moledina, K.H. and Flink, J.M. (1982) Determination of ascorbic acid in plant food products by high performance liquid chromatography. *Lebensm.-Wiss. u.-Technol.*, **15**, 351–8.

Moll, N. (1988) Reversed-phase high performance liquid chromatographic determination of riboflavin (vitamin B2) in alcoholic beverages. *Dev. Fd Sci.*, **17**, 753–69.

Moll, N. and Joly, J.P. (1987) Determination of ascorbic acid in beers by high-performance liquid chromatography with electrochemical detection. *J. Chromat.*, **405**, 347–56.

Morawski, J. (1984) Analysis of dairy products. *Fd Technol.*, **38**(4), 70, 72, 74–8.

Morrison, L.A. and Driskell, J.A. (1985) Quantities of B_6 vitamers in human milk by high-performance liquid chromatography. *J. Chromat. Biomed. Appl.*, **337**, 249–58.

Nicolas, E.C. and Pfender, K.A. (1990) Fast and simple liquid chromatographic determination of nonphosphorylated thiamine in infant formula, milk, and other foods. *J. Ass. Off. Analyt. Chem.*, **73**, 792–8.

Obata, H., Tsuchihashi, W. and Tokuyama, T. (1980) Determination of reductones by high-pressure liquid chromatographic method. *Agric. Biol. Chem.*, **44**, 1435–6.

Ohta, H., Baba, T. and Suzuki, Y. (1984) High-performance liquid chromatographic analysis of thiamine in rice flour with fluorimetric post-column derivatization. *J. Chromat.*, **284**, 281–4.

Oishi, M., Amakawa, E., Ogiwara, T. *et al.* (1988) Determination of nicotinic acid and nicotinamide in meats by high performance liquid chromatography and conversion of nicotinamide in meats during storage. *J. Fd Hyg. Soc. Japan*, **29**, 32–7 (in Japanese).

Ollilainen, V., Mattila, P., Varo, P., Koivistoinen, P. and Huttunen, J. (1990) The HPLC determination of total riboflavin in foods. *J. Micronutr. Anal.*, **8**, 199–207.

Pachla, L.A. and Kissinger, P.T. (1976) Determination of ascorbic acid in foodstuffs, pharmaceuticals, and body fluids by liquid chromatography with electrochemical detection. *Analyt. Chem.*, **48**, 364–7.

Pachla, L.A. and Kissinger, P.T. (1979) Analysis of ascorbic acid by liquid chromatography with amperometric detection. *Methods Enzymol.*, **62D**, 15–24.

Palanuk, S.L., Warthesen, J.J. and Smith, D.E. (1988) Effect of agitation, sampling location and protective films on light-induced riboflavin loss in skim milk. *J. Fd Sci.*, **53**, 436–8.

Parolari, G. (1982) Ascorbic acid in meat products. Analysis by reversed phase ion pair high-pressure liquid chromatography. *Industria Conserve*, **57**, 19–22 (in Italian).

Polesello, A. and Rizzolo, A. (1990) Application of HPLC to the determination of water-soluble vitamins in foods: 2 (a review 1985–9). *J. Micronutr. Anal.*, **8**, 105–88.

Rees, D.I. (1989) Determination of nicotinamide and pyridoxine in fortified food products by HPLC. *J. Micronutr. Anal.*, **5**, 53–61.

Reyes, E.S.P. and Subryan, L. (1989) An improved method of simultaneous HPLC assay of riboflavin and thiamin in selected cereal products. *J. Fd Comp. Anal.*, **2**, 41–7.

Reyes, E.S.P., Norris, K.M., Taylor, C. and Potts, D. (1988) Comparison of paired-ion liquid chromatographic method with AOAC fluorometric and microbiological methods for riboflavin determination in selected foods. *J. Ass. Off. Analyt. Chem.*, **71**, 16–19.

Rhys Williams, A.T. and Slavin, W. (1977) Determination of riboflavin in milk and riboflavin clearance into urine using HPLC with fluorescence detection. *Chromatogr. Newslett.*, **5**, 9–11.

Ribarova, F., Shishkov, S., Obretenova, N. and Metchkueva, L. (1987) Comparative determination of riboflavin in milk by HPLC and lumiflavin methods. *Nahrung*, **31**, 77–9.

Rizzolo, A., Forni, E. and Polesello, A. (1984) HPLC assay of ascorbic acid in fresh and processed fruit and vegetables. *Fd Chem.*, **14**, 189–99.

Rucki, R.J. (1980) Electrochemical detectors for flowing liquid systems. *Talanta*, **27**, 147–56.

Russell, L.F. (1986) High performance liquid chromatographic determination of vitamin C in fresh tomatoes. *J. Fd Sci.*, **51**, 1567–8.

Russell, L.F. and Vanderslice, J.T. (1992) Non-degradative extraction and simultaneous quantitation of riboflavin, flavin mononucleotide, and flavin adenine dinucleotide in foods by HPLC. *Fd Chem.*, **43**, 151–62.

Sapers, G.M., Douglas, F.W. Jr, Ziolkowski, M.A., Miller, R.L. and Hicks, K.B. (1990) Determination of ascorbic acid, dehydroascorbic acid and ascorbic acid-2-phosphate in infiltrated apple and potato tissue by high-performance liquid chromatography. *J. Chromat.*, **503**, 431–6.

Schieffer, G.W. (1985) Limitation of assessing high-performance liquid chromatographic peak purity with photodiode array detectors. *J. Chromat.*, **319**, 387–91.

Schüep, W. and Keck, E. (1990) Measurement of ascorbic acid and erythorbic acid in processed meat by HPLC. *Z. Lebensmittelunters u.-Forsch.*, **191**, 290–2.

Seki, T., Yamaguchi, Y., Noguchi, K. and Yanagihara, Y. (1985) Separation of ascorbic acid, dehydroascorbic acid, diketogulonic acid and glucose by isocratic elution from a column of a hydrophilic gel. *J. Chromat.*, **332**, 283–6.

Sepaniak, M.J. and Kettler, C.N. (1986) Fluorometric detection. In *Detectors for Liquid Chromatography* (ed. E.S. Yeung), John Wiley & Sons, New York, pp. 148–203.

Shephard, G.S., Louw, M.E.J. and Labadarios, D. (1987) Analysis of vitamin B_6 vitamers in plasma by cation-exchange high-performance liquid chromatography. *J. Chromat., Biomed. Appl.*, **416**, 138–43.

Snyder, L.R. and Kirkland, J.J. (1979) *Introduction to Modern Liquid Chromatography*, 2nd edn, John Wiley & Sons, Inc., New York.

Sood, S.P., Sartori, L.E., Wittmer, D.P. and Haney, W.G. (1976) High-pressure liquid chromatographic determination of ascorbic acid in selected foods and multivitamin products. *Analyt. Chem.*, **48**, 796–8.

Speek, A.J., Schrijver, J. and Schreurs, W.H.P. (1984) Fluorometric determination of total vitamin C and total isovitamin C in foodstuffs and beverages by high-performance liquid chromatography with precolumn derivatization. *J. Agric. Fd Chem.*, **32**, 352–5.

Stancher, B. and Zonta, F. (1986) High performance liquid chromatographic analysis of riboflavin (vitamin B_2) with visible absorbance detection in Italian cheeses. *J. Fd Sci.*, **51**, 857–8.

Stranahan, J.J. and Deming, S.N. (1982) Thermodynamic model for reversed-phase ion-pair liquid chromatography. *Analyt. Chem.*, **54**, 2251–6.

Štulík, K. and Pacaková, V. (1984) Electrochemical detection in high-performance liquid chromatography. *CRC Crit. Rev. Analyt. Chem.*, **14**, 297–351.

Takatsuki, K., Suzuki, S., Sato, M., Sakai, K. and Ushizawa, I. (1987) Liquid chromatographic determination of free and added niacin and niacinamide in beef and pork, *J. Ass. Off. Analyt. Chem.*, **70**, 698–702.

Toyosaki, T., Yamamoto, A. and Mineshita, T. (1986) Simultaneous analysis of riboflavin and its decomposition products in various milks by high-performance liquid chromatography. *J. Micronutr. Anal.*, **2**, 117–23.

Trugo, L.C., Macrae, R. and Trugo, N.M.F. (1985) Determination of nicotinic acid in instant coffee using high-performance liquid chromatography. *J. Micronutr. Anal.*, **1**, 55–63.

Tsao, C.S. and Salimi, S.L. (1982) Differential determination of L-ascorbic acid and D-isoascorbic acid by reversed-phase high-performance liquid chromatography with electrochemical detection. *J. Chromat.*, **245**, 355–8.

Tsunoda, K., Inoue, N., Iwasaki, H., Akiya, M. and Hasebe, A. (1988) Rapid simultaneous analysis of nicotinic acid and nicotinamide in foods, and their behaviour during storage. *J. Fd Hyg. Soc. Japan*, **29**, 262–6 (in Japanese).

Tuan, S., Wyatt, J. and Anglemier, A.F. (1987) The effect of erythorbic acid on the determination of ascorbic acid levels in selected foods by HPLC and spectrophotometry. *J. Micronutr. Anal.*, **3**, 211–28.

Tyler, T.A. and Genzale, J.A. (1990) Liquid chromatographic determination of total niacin in beef, semolina, and cottage cheese. *J. Ass. Off. Analyt. Chem.*, **73**, 467–9.

Tyler, T.A. and Shrago, R.R. (1980) Determination of niacin in cereal samples by HPLC. *J. Liquid Chromat.*, **3**, 269–77.

Vanderslice, J.T., Brownlee, S.R. and Cortissoz, M.E. (1984) Liquid chromatographic determination of vitamin B-6 in foods. *J. Ass. Off. Analyt. Chem.*, **67**, 999–1007.

Vanderslice, J.T. and Higgs, D.J. (1984) HPLC analysis with fluorometric detection of vitamin C in food samples. *J. Chromatogr. Sci.*, **22**, 485–9.

Vanderslice, J.T. and Higgs, D.J. (1988) Chromatographic separation of ascorbic acid, isoascorbic acid, dehydroascorbic acid and dehydroisoascorbic acid and their quantitation in food products. *J. Micronutr. Anal.*, **4**, 109–18.

Vanderslice, J.T. and Maire, C.E. (1980) Liquid chromatographic separation and quantification of B_6 vitamers at plasma concentration levels. *J. Chromat.*, **196**, 176–9.

Vanderslice, J.T., Maire, C.E. and Yakupkovic, J.E. (1981) Vitamin B_6 in ready-to-eat cereals: analysis by high performance liquid chromatography. *J. Fd Sci.*, **46**, 943–6.

Vanderslice, J.T., Stewart, K.K. and Yarmas, M.M. (1979) Liquid chromatographic separation and quantification of B_6 vitamers and their metabolite, pyridoxic acid. *J. Chromat.*, **176**, 280–5.

Vanderslice, J.T., Maire, C.E., Doherty, R.F. and Beecher, G.R. (1980) Sulfosalicylic acid as an extraction agent for vitamin B_6 in food. *J. Agric. Fd Chem.*, **28**, 1145–9.

Vanderslice, J.T., Brown, J.F., Beecher, G.R., Maire, C.E. and Brownlee, S.G. (1981) Automation of a complex high-performance liquid chromatography system. Procedures and hardware for a vitamin B_6 model system. *J. Chromat.*, **216**, 338–45.

van Niekerk, P.J., Smit, S.C.C., Strydom, E.S.P. and Armbruster, G. (1984) Comparison of a high-performance liquid chromatographic and microbiological method for the determination of niacin in foods. *J. Agric Fd Chem.*, **32**, 304–7.

Veazey, R.L. and Nieman, T.A. (1980) Chemiluminescence high-performance liquid chromatographic detector applied to ascorbic acid determinations. *J. Chromat.*, **200**, 153–62.

Vidal-Valverde, C. and Reche, A. (1990a) An improved high performance liquid chromatographic method for thiamin analysis in foods. *Z. Lebensmittelunters u.-Forsch.*, **191**, 313–18.

Vidal-Valverde, C. and Reche, A. (1990b) Reliable system for the analysis of riboflavin in foods by high performance liquid chromatography and UV detection. *J. Liquid Chromat.*, **13**, 2089–101.

Videl-Valverde, C. and Reche, A. (1991) Determination of available niacin in legumes and meat by high-performance liquid chromatography. *J. Agric. Fd Chem.*, **39**, 116–21.

Watada, A.E. (1982) A high-performance liquid chromatography method for determining ascorbic acid content of fresh fruits and vegetables. *Hort. Sci.*, **17**, 334–5.

Watada, A.E. and Tran, T.T (1985) A sensitive high-performance liquid chromatography method for analyzing riboflavin in fresh fruits and vegetables. *J. Liquid Chromat.*, **8**, 1651–62.

Wehling, R.L. and Wetzel, D.L. (1984) Simultaneous determination of pyridoxine, riboflavin, and thiamin in fortified cereal products by high-performance liquid chromatography. *J. Agric. Fd Chem.*, **32**, 1326–31.

White, D.R. Jr (1990) Determination of 5-methyltetrahydrofolate in citrus juice by reversed-phase high-performance liquid chromatography with electrochemical detection. *J. Agric. Fd Chem.*, **38**, 1515–18.

White, D.R. Jr, Lee, H.S. and Krüger, R.E. (1991) Reversed-phase HPLC/EC determination of folate in citrus juice by direct injection with column switching. *J. Agric. Fd Chem.*, **39**, 714–17.

White, P.C. (1984) Recent developments in detection techniques for high-performance liquid chromatography. Part 1. Spectroscopic and electrochemical detectors. A review. *Analyst, Lond.*, **109**, 677–97.

Williams, R.C., Baker, D.R. and Schmit, J.A. (1973) Analysis of water-soluble vitamins by high-speed ion-exchange chromatography. *J. Chromatogr. Sci.*, **11**, 618–24.

Wills, R.B.H., Wimalasiri, P. and Greenfield, H. (1985) Comparative determination of thiamin and riboflavin in foods by high-performance liquid chromatography and fluorometric methods. *J. Micronutr. Anal.*, **1**, 23–9.

Wilson, C.W. and Shaw, P.E. (1987) High-performance liquid chromatographic determination of ascorbic acid in aseptically packaged orange juice using ultraviolet and electrochemical detectors. *J. Agric. Fd Chem.*, **35**, 329–31.

Wimalasiri, P. and Wills, R.B.H (1983) Simultaneous analysis of ascorbic acid and dehydroascorbic acid in fruit and vegetables by high-performance liquid chromatography. *J. Chromat.*, **256**, 368–71.

Wimalasiri, P. and Wills, R.B.H. (1985) Simultaneous analysis of thiamin and riboflavin in foods by high-performance liquid chromatography. *J. Chromat.*, **318**, 412–16.

Woodcock, E.A., Warthesen, J.J. and Labuza, T.P. (1982) Riboflavin photochemical degradation in pasta measured by high performance liquid chromatography. *J. Fd Sci.*, **47**, 545–9, 555.

Yeung, E.S. and Sepaniak, M.J. (1980) Laser fluorometric detection in liquid chromatography. *Analyt. Chem.*, **52**, 1465A, 1466A, 1471A, 1472A, 1476A, 1478A, 1481A.

Yost, R., Stoveken, J. and Maclean, W. (1977) Positive peak identification in liquid chromatography using absorbance ratioing with a variable-wavelength spectrophotometric detector. *J. Chromat.*, **134**, 73–82.

Ziegler, S.J., Meier, B. and Sticher, O. (1987) Rapid and sensitive determination of dehydroascorbic acid in addition to ascorbic acid by reversed-phase high performance liquid chromatography using a post-column reduction system. *J. Chromat.*, **391**, 419–26.

Microbiological methods for the determination of the B-group vitamins

7

7.1 HISTORY

Microbiological assays for determining the B-group vitamins stem from an important publication by Snell and Strong (1939), which described a method for determining riboflavin in natural materials. The method utilized *Lactobacillus casei* as the test organism and was developed from existing procedures used by dairy bacteriologists to identify the essential growth factors for lactic acid bacteria. Similar procedures for assaying other B-group vitamins using lactic acid bacteria quickly followed, and many of these procedures are in routine use today in the same basic format.

7.2 GENERAL PRINCIPLES

7.2.1 PRINCIPLE OF THE MICROBIOLOGICAL ASSAY

Microbiological methods of vitamin determination are based on the absolute requirement of certain micro-organisms for specific vitamins of the B-group; that is, the organisms can multiply only when the specific vitamin is present in the surrounding medium. Aliquots of a standard solution of the vitamin to be determined, or aliquots of the sample extract containing the vitamin, are added to an initially translucent basal nutrient medium, complete in all respects except for the vitamin in question. Following inoculation with the assay organism, the organism multiplies in proportion to the vitamin content of the standard or sample, and the extent of the growth is ascertained by measuring the turbidity produced. Over a defined concentration range, the measured response will be directly proportional to the amount of vitamin present and, within this range, the sample solution and standard vitamin solution can be compared accurately. The response depends very much upon whether bound forms of the vitamin are released during the extraction stage of the assay.

7.2.2 FACILITIES AND EQUIPMENT

A self-contained work area capable of being darkened or fitted with gold fluorescent tubes is the first essential for carrying out vitamin assays. Microbiological manipulations should be performed well away from the sample preparation area, preferably in a separate room of structural simplicity to facilitate cleaning. Another essential requirement is a readily available supply of fresh glass-distilled water; deionized water is not suitable for folate and vitamin B_{12} assays (Pearson, 1967a). All glassware should be kept exclusively for microbiological assays, and a meticulous washing-up regime is essential to ensure that the glassware is scrupulously clean before use. Glass pipettes, if not disposable, should be soaked in a sterilizing fluid before thorough rinsing with water in a pipette washer, and final rinsing with distilled water. It is usually sufficient to wash test tubes and other glassware in detergent, followed by several rinsings in tap water, with a final rinsing in distilled water. Detergent-washed glassware has been reported to be inadequate for vitamin B_{12} assays; Skeggs (1963a) found it necessary to acid-wash all glassware, followed by rinsing 13 times with tap water and 2 times with distilled water. A similar cleaning regime has also been found necessary for biotin assays (Scheiner and De Ritter, 1975).

Essential equipment is itemized below.

- **Autoclave** – large enough to admit all racks of tubes for a given assay and capable of accurate adjustment to a constant pressure of 15 lb/in^2. A steam-injected rather than electrically heated autoclave is preferable, because it allows steaming at 100 °C and has a more rapid overall operation sequence from heating up to cooling down.
- **Incubators** – forced-draught or circulating water bath capable of maintaining a constant accurate temperature (±0.5 °C) in the range of 27–37 °C. A shaking incubator or water bath is required for assays with yeasts; assays with protozoa require incubation with both shaking and illumination.
- **Nephelometer** – equipped to accept the assay tubes for direct measurement of turbidity. Alternatively, the turbidities may be read in a conventional colorimeter or spectrophotometer by transferring the assay solution to the appropriate tubes or cells.
- **Tubes and tube racks** – uniform, lipless Pyrex test tubes (17 × 150 mm). If it is intended to measure the turbidity directly in the assay tubes, they should be approximately optically matched, and discarded when they become etched. Stainless steel wire racks to hold 6 × 12 tubes.

Other essential items of equipment include a refrigerator, drying oven, centrifuge, balance, vortex mixer, pH meter, automatic dispenser, screw-cap culture tubes, inoculating needle and loop, and assorted pipettes. For assays using yeasts and protozoa, a large quantity of small Erlenmeyer flasks (25–50 ml) is useful.

7.2.3 ASSAY ORGANISMS

Lactic acid bacteria are the most widely used assay organisms, but yeasts and protozoa are also used.

As a group, the lactic acid bacteria approach the ideal for microbiological assay work. Their nutritional requirements are specific and complex, they grow readily in synthetic and semisynthetic media, and they are nonpathogenic. They are not prone to mutation and have maintained their characteristics unimpaired after many years of subculture in the laboratory. Their growth can be easily followed either by turbidity measurement or by titration of the lactic acid produced by their metabolism. The rod forms (genus, *Lactobacillus*) are microaerophilic and the coccus forms (genus, *Enterococcus, Leuconostoc*) are facultative aerobes (Snell, 1950). This ability to grow well in limited amounts of air means that test tubes of medium can conveniently be used for assay purposes.

Lactic acid bacteria do not respond to PN (Snell, 1981), and certain species of yeasts, which respond vigorously to all three vitamin B_6 free bases, are used instead for the determination of total vitamin B_6. Assays using yeasts have also been reported for several other B-group vitamins. Because yeasts grow aerobically, such assays have the inconvenience of requiring constant and uniform shaking during incubation.

Protozoa have more highly developed ingestive and digestive systems than do bacteria and yeasts, which allow them to respond to conjugated forms of vitamins (e.g. folate polyglutamates). Also, fewer problems are encountered with nonspecific stimulation when using protozoa. Because of the more mammalian-like response of protozoa to the various naturally occurring forms of the vitamins, protozoan techniques have routinely been used to evaluate clinical vitamin status since 1968 (Voigt and Eitenmiller, 1978). However, the test growth period for protozoa is longer than that for lactic acid bacteria (3–5 days versus 24–48 h), conditions of growth are more demanding, and growth response is more difficult to measure.

The assay organisms are particular strains obtained from various culture collections. Cultures are despatched in freeze-dried form sealed under vacuum in glass ampoules, which must be opened under strictly aseptic conditions. Growth may be slower than usual immediately after resuscitation, and the culture must be activated by making at least three successive daily transfers in liquid culture medium before preparing agar stab or slope cultures. A list of the commonly used assay organisms with their American Type Culture Collection (ATCC) numbers is given in Table 7.1.

7.2.4 ASSAY MEDIA

Media for the microbiological assay of vitamins are commercially available in a dehydrated form from Difco Laboratories, Michigan, USA. They are reconstituted simply by suspending the required weighed amount in distilled water, heating to effect solution, and autoclaving. The use of dehydrated media allows a fresh batch of medium to be made up in the amount required with the minimum of time and effort.

Table 7.1 Assay parameters for the microbiological assay of the B-group vitamins

Vitamin	Organism (ATCC No.)	Basal medium (Difco Code No.)	[a]Conc. working standard solution (ng/ml)	[a]Assay range (ng/tube)
Thiamin	*L. viridescens* (12706)	Bacto-Thiamin Assay Medium LV (0808)	0.2	0–1
Riboflavin	*L. casei* subsp. *rhamnosus* (7469)	Bacto-Riboflavin Assay Medium (0325)	0.4	0–2
Riboflavin	*E. faecalis* (10100)	According to Barton-Wright (1967)	2	0–10
Niacin (as nicotinic acid)	*L. plantarum* (8014)	Bacto-Niacin Assay Medium (0322)	40	0–200
B_6	*S. carlsbergensis* (9080)	Bacto-Pyridoxine Y Medium (0951)	3	0–12
B_6	*K. apiculata* (9774)	According to Barton-Wright (1971)	4	0–16
Pantothenic acid	*L. plantarum* (8014)	Bacto-Pantothenate Assay Medium (0604)	40	0–200
Biotin	*L. plantarum* (8014)	Bacto-Biotin Assay Medium (0419)	0.2	0–1
Total folate	*L. casei* subsp. *rhamnosus* (7469)	Bacto-Folic Acid Casei Medium (0822)	0.4	0–2
B_{12}	*L. delbrueckii* subsp. *lactis* (4797)	Bacto-Vitamin B_{12} Assay Medium (0360)	0.04	0–0.2
B_{12}	*O. malhamensis* (11532)	According to Ford (1953)	0.2	0–0.8

[a] K.J. Scott (personal communication).

Alternatively, the medium can be prepared in the laboratory from individual ingredients (Association of Vitamin Chemists, Inc., 1966; Pearson, 1967a). The general procedure in this case is to keep most of the constituents as stock solutions in the refrigerator, but solutions of vitamins must always be freshly prepared. The prescribed volumes of these solutions are dispensed into a beaker and the readily soluble major components (e.g. glucose and sodium acetate) are added slowly with stirring. The pH is then adjusted to the desired value (say 6.8) with dilute sodium hydroxide and the solution is made up to the required volume. Media prepared in this manner can be stored for several days in the refrigerator under a layer of toluene or in the frozen state indefinitely.

7.3 GENERAL ASSAY PROCEDURE

7.3.1 INTRODUCTION

All of the assay methods which employ lactic acid bacteria are similar, regardless of the organism being used or the vitamin being determined. In the standard procedure, the appropriate basal medium free of the vitamin to be determined, is prepared at twice its final concentration (double strength). Multiple aliquots of a standard solution of the pure vitamin and of suitably prepared extracts of the test food are added to a series of uniform test tubes in amounts suitable to produce gradations in growth between no growth and maximum growth. The contents of all tubes are diluted with water to the same volume, and an equal volume of the translucent basal medium is added. The tubes are sterilized, cooled to a uniform temperature, and then inoculated with an actively growing culture of the test organism. The assay tubes are incubated for 22–24 h at a constant temperature near the optimum for the test organism until growth has reached the maximum permitted by the limiting vitamin present. The growth response to standard and test extract is then determined by measuring the turbidity produced. The data obtained from the standards are used to construct a standard curve from which the vitamin concentrations of the various sample aliquots are derived. The use of multiple aliquots allows a validity check to be carried out: the vitamin concentration found should be directly proportional to the volume of aliquot taken. The amount of vitamin present in the original sample is then calculated at the different test levels, and the results are averaged to obtain the final result.

In earlier procedures the bacterial response to the vitamins was usually determined by titration of the lactic acid produced after 72 h of incubation. The measurement of turbidity (nephelometry) is nowadays generally preferred to the measurement of metabolic products, as it is simpler and requires shorter incubation times. More recently, alternative means of measuring the bacterial response have been reported. The radiometric microbiological assay (RMA) is based upon the measurement of radioactive $^{14}CO_2$ generated from the metabolism of a ^{14}C-labelled nutrient by the test organism, and has been applied to the determination of niacin (Guilarte and Pravlik, 1983), vitamin B_6 (Guilarte, 1983), biotin (Guilarte, 1985), folate (Chen, Hill and McIntyre, 1983) and vitamin B_{12} (Chen and McIntyre, 1979) in foods, and also to pantothenic acid in human blood and milk (Guilarte, 1989). In these applications, the radioactivity is measured automatically by means of a commercially available gas flow system incorporating an ionization chamber (Guilarte, 1991a). The RMA combines the biological specificity of measuring a vitamin-dependent microbiological metabolic reaction with the sensitivity and accuracy of radioactive decay measurement. Extraction methods suitable for the analysis of thiamin, niacin, pantothenic acid and biotin with the RMA have been discussed by Guilarte (1991b). Sample preparation is simplified due to the fact that coloured, turbid or precipitated debris do not interfere with the $^{14}CO_2$ output or detection; furthermore, the scrupulous cleaning of glassware is unnecessary. A nonradiometric technique for measuring metabolic CO_2 employs an infrared CO_2 analyser, which measures automatically the infrared radiation absorbed by the CO_2 band at 4.2 μm (Goli and Vanderslice, 1989).

The standard assay procedure using lactic acid bacteria can be broken down into a number of steps:

1. maintenance of stock cultures;
2. preparation of the inoculum culture;
3. preparation of the basal medium;
4. extraction of the vitamin from the test material;
5. preparation of vitamin standard solutions;
6. setting up the assay;
7. quantification.

A scheme of steps (1) and (2) is depicted in Figure 7.1. Assay parameters are presented in Table 7.1

7.3.2 MAINTENANCE OF STOCK CULTURES

It is obviously essential to maintain a pure culture of each assay organism and to preserve its viability and sensitivity. It is possible to sustain these requirements over a period of several years by employing a regular schedule of subculturing into a nutrient medium of suitable composition. The frequency of subculturing depends upon the composition of the medium and upon the particular assay organism or group of

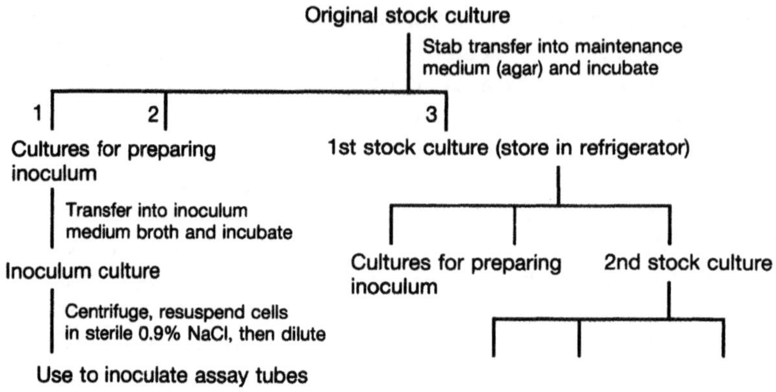

Figure 7.1 Preparation of stock cultures and inocula (standard assay procedure).

organisms used. Stock cultures of lactic acid bacteria are maintained as stab cultures in a semisynthetic agar-based maintenance medium, which contains all of the nutritional factors essential for the organism's normal growth and metabolism. Such media invariably contain yeast extract and glucose plus other nutrients. A buffer salt is included to prevent the pH from rapidly dropping to levels which would inhibit growth, although growth will proceed until a pH of at least 4 is reached (Barton-Wright, 1952). The medium is formulated to give an initial pH (typically 6.8) that is somewhat higher than the optimum pH of 5.5–6.5 for most lactic acid bacteria (Snell, 1948). This is to allow for the production of acid that occurs when the medium is sterilized by autoclaving.

At regular intervals, three fresh stab cultures are prepared in maintenance medium from a stock culture. The usual procedure is to distribute 10-ml quantities of medium into lipless 16–20-mm diameter test tubes and autoclave the plugged tubes for 20 min at 15 lb pressure (121 °C). After cooling, stab inoculations are made into the solidified agar. The tubes are incubated under the appropriate conditions for each vitamin (typically overnight at 37 °C) that produce distinctly visible growth along the line of the stab. Since the growth rate of an organism is a function of temperature, the incubation must be precisely controlled to within ±0.5 °C of the selected temperature. The stab cultures thus prepared are stored in the refrigerator under aseptic conditions. One of these cultures is reserved as the stock culture until the next time for transfer, when it will be used to prepare three more agar stabs. The other two are held available during the interval between transfer for the preparation of inoculum cultures required for assay.

The maintenance of *Lactobacillus delbrueckii* subsp. *lactis* used for the determination of vitamin B_{12} apparently presents occasional problems of lack of growth in subcultures or loss of sensitivity to B_{12} (Bell, 1971). A satisfactory procedure is to maintain *L. delbrueckii* (ATCC No. 7830) as a stock culture in Bacto-Skim Milk Medium (Difco) supplemented with 1% Bacto-Tryptose (Difco) according to the procedure described by Skeggs (1963a). In this procedure, stock cultures are transferred every 6 weeks into freshly prepared skim milk medium, incubated for 24 h at 37 °C, and subcultured in duplicate into tryptose milk medium. After a second incubation, one culture is returned to the refrigerator as the new stock. The second culture is kept available as a working stock for inoculum preparation and subcultured every week or as needed. This rather involved procedure is carried out to rid the stock culture of any toxic materials carried from the old culture.

For the determination of vitamin B_6, Bell (1974) maintained the yeast *Saccharomyces carlsbergensis* (ATCC No. 9080) under aerobic conditions on an agar slope using 10 ml of sterilized Bacto-Lactobacilli Agar AOAC (Difco Code 0900) in a 1-oz McCartney bottle. The yeast was subcultured weekly by taking a loopful of yeast from the current culture onto a fresh agar slope, incubating at 32 °C overnight, and storing in a refrigerator.

7.3.3 PREPARATION OF THE INOCULUM CULTURE

Stab cultures of lactic acid bacteria that have been stored in the refrigerator must be activated by making at least three successive daily stab transfers before preparing the inoculum. The inoculum is prepared the day before the day of the assay by subculturing the activated agar stab into a tube containing sterile inoculum medium. A new inoculum should not be made from a previously prepared inoculum, because of the possible danger of contamination; this practice may also promote changes in the nutritional requirements of the assay organism.

Several different methods of preparing the inoculum have been proposed. The most satisfactory methods take into account the capacity of the assay organism for storing sufficient amounts of vitamins (particularly pantothenic acid, biotin, folate and vitamin B_{12}) to produce considerable growth in the assay blank tubes. Such methods are designed to reduce cellular vitamin accumulation to a minimum, and also to eliminate the risk of carry-over of vitamin and other components of the nutrient medium that might interfere in the subsequent assay. It is important that the inoculum be suitably diluted. If insufficient dilution is made, the blanks may be too high, and slight differences in the drop size of the inoculum may introduce variations in the amount of growth in the assay tubes which are unrelated to the amount of vitamin present in the material being assayed. On the other hand, if the inoculum is too dilute, growth may not be complete by the end of the assay period. It is also desirable to inoculate the assay tubes from inoculum cultures which are in the logarithmic (acceleration) phase of growth.

In methods described by Snell (1950), Barton-Wright (1952) and Strohecker and Henning (1966), the inoculum culture is grown in a liquid basal medium to which has been added the vitamin to be assayed in an amount that barely supports the growth of the assay organism. This depletion technique limits the accumulation of the vitamin in the cells and thus maintains the sensitivity of the organism towards the vitamin. A 10-ml quantity of such a medium can be prepared by taking 5 ml of double-strength basal medium and adding 2.5 ml of standard vitamin solution plus 2.5 ml of distilled water, and then autoclaving. The inoculum broth thus prepared is inoculated with agar stab culture and incubated overnight at 37 °C. The incubation time must not exceed 22–24 h for the lactic acid bacteria or yeasts, or the organism will become attenuated (weakened) and poor growth responses will be encountered. The cells of the resultant culture are washed with isotonic saline (0.9% NaCl solution) to reduce carry-over of vitamin into the assay tubes during the subsequent inoculation. This operation is performed aseptically by centrifuging the tube contents and resuspending the cells in a suitable volume of saline for direct use as an inoculum, or after an appropriate dilution has been made. In some methods, two or even three centrifugal washings are employed for certain vitamins.

Difco supply special dehydrated inoculum media, whose formulations are the same as those of the corresponding maintenance media, except that the agar component is omitted (Difco Laboratories, 1985). The cells grown in such media are harvested by centrifugation and washed with sterile isotonic saline or, in accordance with the United States Pharmacopeia (USP) procedure for determining vitamin B_{12}, with single-strength basal assay medium.

Bell (1974) found that procedures using centrifugal washing gave an inoculum in the lag phase of growth, thus necessitating unduly long assay incubation periods. Problems of airborne bacterial contamination were also encountered. Bell prepared inocula for the determination of riboflavin, niacin, pantothenic acid, biotin, folate and vitamin B_{12} using Bacto-Micro Inoculum Broth (Difco Code 0320) as the inoculum medium. The common procedure for all these determinations was to subculture the assay organism from the most recent agar stab into 5 ml of sterile inoculum broth (Difco) and incubate overnight at 37 °C. The following morning, one drop of this subculture was added to 5 ml of single strength basal medium (basal medium diluted with an equal volume of water) containing a controlled amount of the vitamin being assayed. These amounts were 25 ng nicotinic acid/ml, 20 ng pantothenic acid/ml, 0.05 ng biotin/ml, 2 ng riboflavin/ml, 1.0 ng folic acid/ml, and 0.04 ng cyanocobalamin/ml. Both the inoculum broth and the basal medium were at 37 °C during transfer of the organism. After a further 6 h incubation at 37 °C, two drops of the resultant culture were transferred to 10 ml of single-strength basal medium (without added vitamin). This final suspension was used as the inoculum and contained cells in the logarithmic growth phase.

The inoculum for the determination of thiamin using *L. viridescens* was prepared in a similar manner to that described above, except that the inoculum medium was Bacto-APT Broth (Difco Code 0655) and the incubation temperature was 30 °C.

To prepare the inoculum for the determination of vitamin B_6, a loop of *S. carlsbergensis* from the agar slope was added to 5 ml of single-strength medium containing a glass bead, and this subculture was incubated for 20 h at 27 °C with constant shaking. One millilitre of the suspension obtained was pipetted into a tube containing 5 ml of sterile single-strength basal medium and mixed to give the inoculum culture.

7.3.4. PREPARATION OF THE BASAL MEDIUM

The basal medium contains all the nutritional factors necessary for the normal growth and metabolism of the assay organism, except the vitamin to be determined. It is formulated from highly purified natural products, synthetic vitamins and other reagent-grade compounds. An assay medium used for lactic acid bacteria must contain a fermentable carbohydrate, a variable assortment of essential amino acids, various vitamins and mineral salts, certain purine and pyrimidine bases, and an appropriate buffer system. Glucose is universally used as a source of carbon and energy; the amino acids are provided in the form of acid-hydrolysed casein plus tryptophan or a mixture of the specific amino acids; and the buffer salt is usually sodium acetate, which also has a stimulatory effect on growth. Dehydrated media for use with assays utilizing lactic acid bacteria and *S. carlsbergensis* are available from Difco Laboratories. The formulations of commonly used Difco basal media are presented in Tables 7.2 to 7.7. In traditional assay procedures, the assay media are prepared at double strength, either from commercial dehydrated formulations (if available) or from individual ingredients.

In addition to factors essential for bacterial growth, other substances which stimulate growth must be considered. Ideally, the medium should contain sufficient amounts of all growth factors and stimulatory substances so that the effects of these nutrients added with the hydrolysed food extract being assayed will be eliminated. In practice, the ideal is seldom achieved and the adequacy of a basal medium depends upon the experimental conditions (Snell, 1948). A basal medium which, when supplied with the missing vitamin, contains all of the nutrients essential for growth, but is lacking in one or more substances which markedly stimulate growth, may give satisfactory assays if the period of incubation is long enough to eliminate the effects

Table 7.2 Formulations of Difco dehydrated basal media for the determination of niacin, pantothenic acid and biotin using *L. plantarum*

Vitamin assayed	Niacin (0322)	Pantothenic acid (0604)	Biotin (0419)
Acid-hydrolysed casein	12 g	10 g	12 g
Glucose	40 g	40 g	40 g
Sodium acetate	20 g	20 g	20 g
L-Cystine	0.4 g	0.4 g	0.2 g
DL-Tryptophan	0.2 g	0.2 g	0.2 g
Adenine sulphate	20 mg	20 mg	20 mg
Guanine hydrochloride	20 mg	20 mg	20 mg
Uracil	20 mg	20 mg	20 mg
Thiamin hydrochloride	200 μg	200 μg	2 mg
Calcium pantothenate	200 μg	None	2 mg
Pyridoxine hydrochloride	400 μg	800 μg	2 mg
Riboflavin	400 μg	400 μg	2 mg
Nicotinic acid	None	1 mg	2 mg
p-Aminobenzoic acid	100 μg	200 μg	200 μg
Biotin	0.8 μg	0.8 μg	None
Dipotassium phosphate	1 g	1 g	1 g
Monopotassium phosphate	1 g	1 g	1 g
Magnesium sulphate heptahydrate	0.4 g	0.4 g	0.4 g
Sodium chloride	20 mg	20 mg	20 mg
Iron (II) sulphate heptahydrate	20 mg	20 mg	20 mg
Manganese sulphate tetrahydrate	20 mg	20 mg	20 mg

Difco code in parentheses.

Table 7.3 Formulation of Difco dehydrated basal medium (Code 0808) for the determination of thiamin using *L. viridescens*

Thiamin-free yeast extract	10 g	Sodium chloride	10 g
Tryptone	20 g	Magnesium sulphate	1.6 g
Glucose	20 g	Manganese chloride	0.28 g
Sodium citrate	10 g	Iron (II) sulphate	80 mg
Dipotassium phosphate	10 g	Sorbitan monooleate complex	2 g

Table 7.4 Formulation of Difco dehydrated basal medium (Code 0325) for the determination of riboflavin using *L. casei*

Photolysed peptone	22 g	Dipotassium phosphate	1 g
Yeast supplement	2 g	Magnesium sulphate	0.4 g
Glucose	20 g	Sodium chloride	20 mg
Sodium acetate	1.8 g	Iron (II) sulphate	20 mg
L-Cystine	0.2 g	Manganese sulphate	20 mg
Monopotassium phosphate	1 g		

Table 7.5 Formulation of Difco dehydrated basal medium (Code 0951) for the determination of vitamin B_6 using *S. carlsbergensis*

Asparagine	4 g	Inositol	5 mg
L-Histidine hydrochloride	20 mg	Boric acid	200 μg
DL-Methionine	40 mg	Monopotassium phosphate	3 g
DL-Tryptophan	40 mg	Magnesium sulphate	1 g
DL-Isoleucine	40 mg	Ammonium sulphate	4 g
DL-Valine	40 mg	Calcium chloride	0.49 g
Glucose	40 g	Potassium iodide	200 μg
Thiamin hydrochloride	400 μg	Ammonium molybdate	40 μg
Calcium pantothenate	400 μg	Manganese sulphate	80 μg
Nicotinic acid	400 μg	Copper (II) sulphate	90 μg
Biotin salt	8 mg	Zinc sulphate	80 μg
Riboflavin	20 mg	Iron (II) sulphate	500 μg

Table 7.6 Formulation of Difco dehydrated basal medium (Code 0822) for the determination of total folate using *L. casei*

Acid-hydrolysed casein (charcoal-treated)	10 g	Sorbitan monooleate complex	0.1 g
		Glutathione (reduced)	5 mg
Glucose	40 g	Magnesium sulphate	0.4 g
Sodium acetate	40 g	Sodium chloride	20 mg
Dipotassium phosphate	1 g	Iron (II) sulphate	20 mg
Monopotassium phosphate	1 g	Manganese sulphate	15 mg
DL-Tryptophan	0.2 g	Riboflavin	1 mg
L-Asparagine	0.6 g	P-Aminobenzoic acid	2 mg
L-Cysteine hydrochloride	0.5 g	Pyridoxine hydrochloride	4 mg
Adenine sulphate	10 mg	Thiamin hydrochloride	400 μg
Guanine hydrochloride	10 mg	Calcium pantothenate	800 μg
Uracil	10 mg	Nicotinic acid	800 μg
Xanthine	20 mg	Biotin	20 μg

Table 7.7 Formulation of Difco dehydrated basal medium (Code 0360) for the determination of vitamin B_{12} using *L. delbrueckii* (ATCC No. 4797)

Acid-hydrolysed casein	12 g	Niacin	2 mg
Glucose	40 g	*p*-Aminobenzoic acid	200 μg
Sodium acetate	20 g	Calcium pantothenate	200 μg
L-Cystine	0.2 g	Pyridoxine hydrochloride	4 mg
DL-Tryptophan	0.2 g	Folic acid	100 μg
Adenine sulphate	20 mg	Monopotassium phosphate	1 g
Guanine hydrochloride	20 mg	Dipotassium phosphate	1 g
Uracil	20 mg	Magnesium sulphate	0.4 g
Xanthine	1 mg	Sodium chloride	20 mg
Riboflavin	2 mg	Iron (II) sulphate	20 mg
Thiamin hydrochloride	2 mg	Manganese sulphate	20 mg
Biotin	10 μg	Sorbitan monooleate complex	2 g

of the nonessential growth stimulants. Such a medium will also be satisfactory for assaying samples which are rich in the vitamin to be determined, as the interfering material will be diluted out. Conversely, such a medium will tend to give erroneous results if used with a short incubation period, and with samples of low vitamin potency.

Fatty acids are notorious growth stimulants for a number of lactic acid bacteria (Williams, Broquist and Snell, 1947) but it is not customary to add these acids to the basal medium; rather they are removed from the food sample after the extraction step.

7.3.5 EXTRACTION OF THE VITAMIN FROM THE TEST MATERIAL

The vitamins are extracted from the food matrix in a form that can be utilized by the particular assay organism being used. This generally involves autoclaving the food sample in the presence of acid or, for acid-labile vitamins, digesting the sample with suitable enzymes. After precipitating the proteins at their isoelectric point (*c.* pH 4), the pH of the extract is adjusted to that of the basal medium (typically pH 6.8). This step is necessary to ensure that the pH of the medium is not altered by the addition of different amounts of the extract. The extract is then diluted to bring the concentration of the vitamin to be assayed within the range of the standard curve. Hopefully, the dilution factor is sufficiently high to dilute out any interfering substances that would cause drift and invalidate the assay. The minimum dilutions of foods necessary to avoid the inhibitory effects of food preservatives and neutralization salts have been calculated by Voigt, Eitenmiller and Ware (1979). Finally, the extracts are filtered to remove the precipitated protein and lipoidal material, and to obtain a clear solution for assay.

7.3.6 PREPARATION OF VITAMIN STANDARD SOLUTIONS

Methods for preparing stock standard solutions of the B-group vitamins (except for vitamin B_{12}) and their storage and usage conditions are summarized in Table 7.8.

To make up a vitamin B_{12} stock solution, weigh out 100 mg of cyanocobalamin crystals and allow them to dissolve in about 750 ml of water by stirring in the dark overnight. Make the volume up to 1 litre and mix to give a 100 μg/ml solution. Dilute 1 ml of this solution to 10 ml (in triplicate) and read the absorbances of these 10 μg/ml solutions at 361 nm. The $A_1{}^{1\%}_{\text{cm}}$ of cyanocobalamin at λ_{max} 361 nm is 207, so a solution of 10 μg/ml gives a theoretical absorbance of 0.207. If the mean absorbance reading is 0.228, for example, the corrected concentration of the original bulk solution will be 0.228/0.207 × 100 = 110.14 μg/ml.

Table 7.8 Preparation and storage of vitamin stock standard solutions (from Barton-Wright, 1967)

Vitamin	Concentration	Preparation	Storage	Usage
Thiamin	1 mg/ml	Dissolve 0.1 g thiamin hydrochloride in 100 ml 0.005 N HCl	Below 4 °C	Within 1 month of preparation
Riboflavin	50 μg/ml	Dissolve 50 mg riboflavin in glacial acetic acid and make up to 1 litre with water. **Protect from light**	Below 4 °C	Within 1 month of preparation
Nicotinic acid	1 mg/ml	Dissolve 0.1 g nicotinic acid in 100 ml water	Under sulphur-free toluene below 4 °C	Within 7 days of preparation
Pyridoxine	1 mg/ml	Dissolve 0.1 g pyridoxine hydrochloride in 100 ml water	Under sulphur-free toluene below, 4 °C	Within 7 days of preparation
Pantothenic acid	1 mg/ml	Dissolve 0.108 g calcium *d*-pantothenate in 100 ml water	Under sulphur-free toluene below 4 °C	Within 7 days of preparation
Biotin	20 μg/ml	Dissolve 20 mg biotin in a small quantity of water and make up to 1 litre with v/v ethanol	Below 4 °C 20%	Within 1 month of preparation
Folic acid	100 μg/ml	Dissolve 0.1 g folic acid in 50 ml water by the cautious addition of 0.05 N NaOH solution with constant mixing so that the pH of the solution does not rise above 7.0. Make up to 1 litre with 20% v/v ethanol.	Under sulphur-free toluene below 4 °C	Within 1 month of preparation

It is recommended that two independent vitamin standard solutions, prepared on separate occasions, are taken through the entire procedure. This will provide a check on the accuracy of the standard concentrations and indicate vitamin instability during the storage of the solutions. It is also advisable to include an internal standard by adding a suitable amount of the vitamin to the sample at the beginning of the extraction procedure. Comparison of the internal standard concentration at the end of the analysis with the conventional standard concentration taken through the entire procedure will give an indication of matrix effects upon the assay. Recovery data obtained from spiking the test material with the vitamin in question are not conclusive, as the free added vitamin often behaves differently to the indigenous bound vitamin during the extraction process.

7.3.7 SETTING UP THE ASSAY

At all stages during the assay procedure, the solutions must be protected from daylight.

Aliquots of the working standard vitamin solution are added in increasing volumes up to 5 ml to a duplicate series of tubes for the construction of a standard curve; duplicate blanks containing no vitamin are included. Similar volumes of the neutralized test extracts are added to a single series of tubes. A range of contentration levels of each test extract is assayed in the expectation that at least three will fall on the standard curve. Fresh glass-distilled water is added to all tubes to bring the volume in each tube to 5.0 ml, after which 5.0 ml of double-strength basal medium is added so that the total volume is 10 ml. The addition of basal medium to the extract and water gives better mixing of the two solutions than adding the extract and water to the medium. The entire rack of filled tubes is covered with a sheet of aluminium foil. Sterilization at 15 lb pressure (121 °C) according to Pearson (1967a) is based on lower levels of glucose used in earlier medium formulations and can lead to caramelization and darkening of the solutions. Barton-Wright (1952) recommended autoclaving under the milder conditions of 10 lb pressure for 10 min as a means of avoiding this problem. The tubes are removed immediately from the autoclave when atmospheric pressure is reached, and the tubes are cooled to below the subsequent incubation temperature. It is imperative that all tubes are cooled to the same temperature, because turbidity is a measure of the rate of growth rather than the extent of growth, and small differences in the temperature between tubes at the start of the incubation influence the growth rate. Temperature equilibration of the whole rack of tubes is best achieved using a water bath or convection incubator.

All tubes are inoculated with one drop of freshly prepared inoculum culture using a sterile pipette or a 10 ml syringe fitted with a 20-gauge needle. If the plunger is removed from the syringe barrel after starting the inoculation through the needle, uniform drops will continue to fall from the needle. It is not necessary to flame the tubes during inoculation. The inclusion of a control run, which is not inoculated but is otherwise treated identically, is advisable to check the sterility of the basal medium. For turbidimetric assays using lactic acid bacteria or yeasts, the tubes are incubated for 22–24 h at a constant temperature near the optimum for these organisms. Suitable temperatures are 37 °C for *L. casei, L. plantarum* and *L. delbrueckii*; 30 °C for *L. viridescens*; and 28 °C (with constant shaking) for *S. carlsbergensis* and *Kloeckera apiculata*. Acidimetric assays require 72 h of incubation.

The setting-up procedure described by Bell (1974) involves less manipulations than the conventional procedure, owing to the volumes of standard or sample assay solutions being reduced from millilitre aliquots to microlitre aliquots ranging from 0 to 250 μl. The addition of such small volumes to 10 ml of assay medium has two advantages: (1) no significant volume change occurs so that single-strength medium can be used; and (2) the need for adjustment of the pH value of samples extracted with acids is greatly reduced. For example, no pH adjustment is required when acids less than 0.1 N are used, and for strongly acid hydrolysates the solution need only be adjusted to pH 1–2.

7.3.8 QUANTIFICATION

At the end of the incubation period, the cells are uniformly suspended by shaking the tubes, and time is allowed for the air bubbles to disperse before measurement. The turbidities of all tubes are measured in a nephelometer using a neutral filter, colorimeter with a filter in the region of 640 nm (Association of Vitamin Chemists, Inc., 1966) or spectrophotometer at 540–660-nm wavelength (Difco Laboratories, 1985). The turbidity may be expressed as an extinction, as a transmittance (in $\%T$), as a difference $100 - T$ (in %) or simply as a galvanometer reading. The arithmetic means of the replicates are calculated, and the means for the standard solutions are plotted on semilogarithmic graph paper with the turbidity values as ordinates (linear scale) and concentrations in ng/ml as abscissae (logarithmic scale). The calibration curve is drawn through these points (Figure 7.2). The vitamin contents of the sample tubes are read off from the calibration curve and the values for the original samples are calculated from simple dilution factors. Values for the vitamin content of a given sample calculated from at least three dilutions should check within the limits of error of the assay, which is usually considered to be ±10–15% (Association of Vitamin Chemists, Inc., 1966); that is, they should not differ by more than 15% from their common

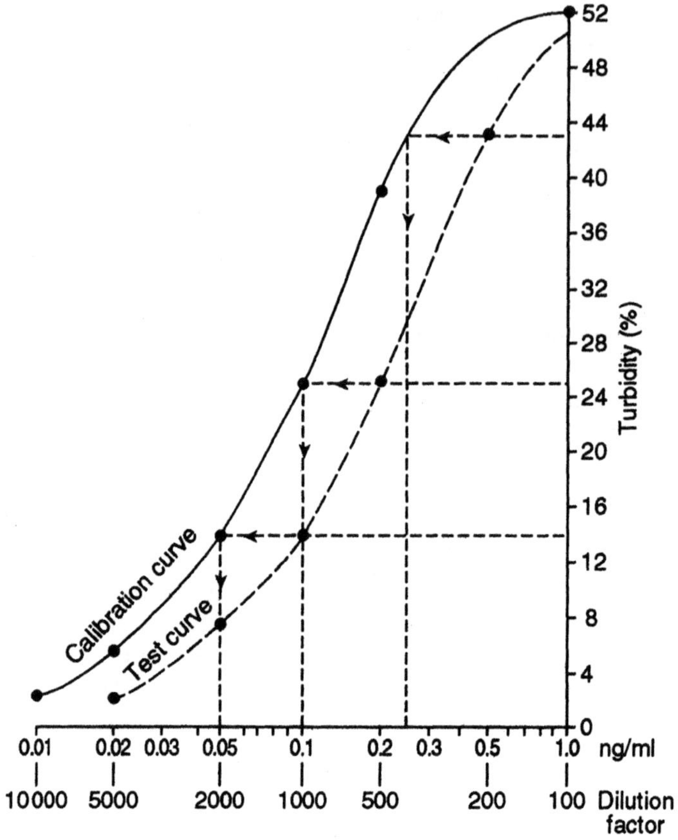

Figure 7.2 Example of a typical calibration curve and an ideal test curve. Ordinate: percentage turbidities (100 − 7) on the linear scale. Abscissa: vitamin concentrations of the calibration solutions in ng/ml and dilution factors of the test solutions on the logarithmic scale. (From Strohecker and Henning, 1966.)

mean. If this condition is not fulfilled, the determination must be repeated.

The reliability of a determination can be assessed by testing for the presence or absence of drift. This simply entails plotting on the calibration curve the mean turbidity values for the sample dilutions against the corresponding dilution factors. In the example given in Figure 7.2, three dilutions, 1 : 200, 1 : 500 and 1 : 1000, give mean percentage turbidities of 43%, 25% and 14%, respectively. Joining the points together gives a check curve which is roughly parallel to the calibration curve, signifying the absence of drift. Drift is manifested by a check curve that deviates widely from the calibration curve, either increasing or decreasing with concentration of the sample as shown in

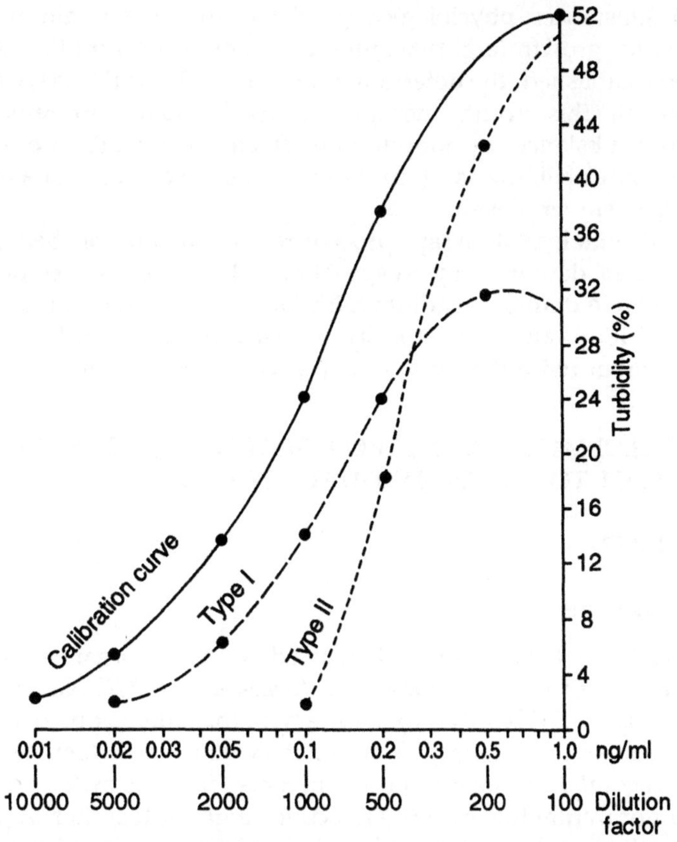

Figure 7.3 Examples of the anomalous curves known as 'drift'. Type I: test curve exhibiting a regressive course due to inhibiting factors that become effective at higher concentrations. Type II: test curve exhibiting a regressive course due to inhibiting factors that influence growth only at low concentrations. (From Strohecker and Henning 1966.)

Figure 7.3. The occurrence of drift in assay values is evidence for the presence of interfering materials in the test solution presented for assay. Snell (1948) recognized three general causes of drift: (1) a substance chemically unrelated to the vitamin may stimulate or inhibit the response of the assay organism to suboptimal levels of the vitamin (e.g. free fatty acids affect the response of *L. casei* to riboflavin and *L. plantarum* to pantothenic acid); (2) substances chemically related to the vitamin may replace the vitamin in the nutrition of the test organism, but the dose–response curve to the vitamin and the related compound may be completely different (e.g. polyglutamyl folates with 4–7 glutamate residues cause positive drift in folate assays using *L. casei*);

and (3) substances physiologically related to the vitamin may also replace it for growth (e.g. D-alanine may replace vitamin B_6). If a drift has been established, the determination is invalid and the assay must be repeated. In this event, measures must be taken to remove the interfering substances by adopting an effective extraction procedure. If these measures fail, the assay conditions must be changed or a different assay organism employed.

The microbiological assay procedure is capable of being semi-automated as described by Keagy (1986). Using a microcomputer to control sample dilution, medium addition, turbidity determination and data acquisition, an assay capacity of 600 tubes/day can be achieved, which is about twice that of a comparative manual assay.

7.4 DEVELOPMENTS IN MICROBIOLOGICAL ASSAYS WITH RESPECT TO THE INDIVIDUAL VITAMINS

7.4.1 THIAMIN

Assay organisms

Two *Lactobacilli* have been widely used as assay organisms for the determination of thiamin, namely *L. fermentum* (ATCC No. 9338) and *L. viridescens* (ATCC No. 12706). Of the two, the latter is preferred as it is less susceptible to inhibitory or stimulatory substances (Scholes, 1960). *L. viridescens* requires the intact thiamin molecule for growth; neither the thiazole nor pyrimidine moiety are active singly or together. Equimolar concentrations of thiamin pyrophosphate (TPP) are approximately 60% as active as thiamin (Deibel, Evans and Niven, 1957). Pearson (1967b) encountered a mutant strain of *L. viridescens* that did not respond to TPP. The *L. viridescens* assay was compared with manual and semi-automated fluorimetric methods in terms of their ability to recover added thiamin hydrochloride from commercially processed foods whose natural thiamin content was destroyed with thiaminase (Defibaugh, Smith and Weeks, 1977). The microbiological method gave the best results for eight products tested, with a recovery of 99.9 ± 1.03%.

Extraction

In order to ensure the complete utilization of total thiamin by *L. viridescens*, the extraction procedure involves hot acid digestion, followed by enzymatic hydrolysis as a means of liberating free thiamin from all bound forms. The enzyme treatment is omitted for the analysis of grain products and milk, and for the determination of the added thiamin hydrochloride in fortified foods.

In a procedure recommended by Pearson (1967b), a suitable weight of the finely ground or homogenized material is suspended or dissolved in at least 15 times its weight of 0.1 N HCl. The mixture is autoclaved for 15 min at 121 °C or steamed in an autoclave for 30 min. A lower autoclaving temperature of 108–109 °C is required for the digestion of grain products, which contain mostly nonphosphorylated thiamin. Distinctly acid conditions (pH 1.0–1.5) must be maintained during the digestion. The mixture is then cooled to room temperature and adjusted to pH 4.0–4.5 with 2.5 M sodium acetate solution. A 5-ml quantity of a freshly prepared 6% solution of Takadiastase (or other diastatic enzyme preparation) in 2.5 M sodium acetate is added, and the mixture is incubated for 3 h at 45–50 °C or overnight at 37 °C. If overnight incubation is used, the mixture must be protected from bacterial action with a layer of toluene. After incubation, the extract is steamed in an autoclave for 20 min to deactivate the enzyme, cooled, adjusted to pH 6.5–6.6, and diluted to give an appropriate thiamin concentration for the assay. If the extract is cloudy at this point, it may be filtered through Whatman No. 1 filter paper. A reagent blank is taken through the same procedure.

7.4.2 RIBOFLAVIN

Assay organisms

The organism traditionally used for determining riboflavin is *Lactobacillus casei* subsp. *rhamnosus* (ATCC No. 7469). The original basal medium developed by Snell and Strong (1939) was later modified to give a faster assay (Roberts and Snell, 1946). Results obtained turbidimetrically at 16 h were in agreement with those obtained acidimetrically at 72 h. Lactic acid bacteria cannot utilize FAD, and the growth response of *L. casei*, measured turbidimetrically, differs significantly between riboflavin and FMN (Langer and Charoensiri, 1966) (Figure 7.4). As most of the vitamin B_2 activity is present in food sources as FMN after acid extraction, it would be more accurate to use FMN as the standard in the microbiological assay instead of riboflavin. *L. casei* is stimulated by starch (Andrews, Boyd and Terry, 1942), and either stimulated or inhibited by long-chain free fatty acids (e.g. palmitic, stearic, oleic and linoleic acids) and other lipids, including lecithin (Bauernfeind, Sotier and Boruff, 1942; Strong and Carpenter, 1942; Kodicek and Worden, 1945). Theoretically, the interference from fatty materials could be avoided by incorporating them into the basal medium. Unfortunately, this is not feasible in practice, owing to the diversity of such compounds, and the conflicting action between different concentrations of a given lipid and between different lipids, as well as their insolubility in water.

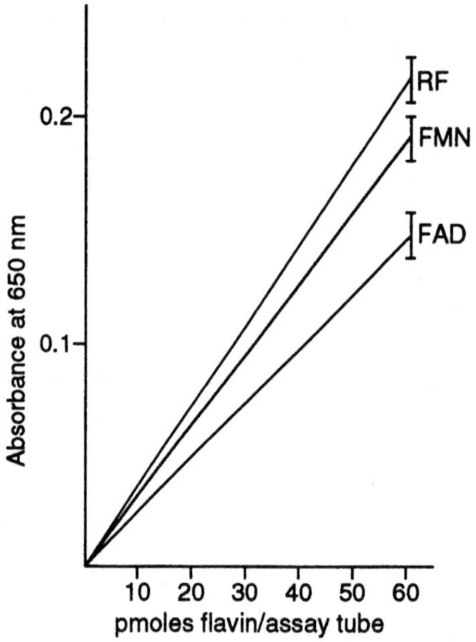

Figure 7.4 Growth response of *L. casei* to riboflavin (RF), FMN and FAD. (From Langer and Charoensiri, 1966.)

Kornberg, Langdon and Cheldelin (1948) proposed the use of *Enterococcus faecalis* (ATCC No. 10100) which, with a sensitivity to 0.1 ng riboflavin/ml (Barton-Wright, 1952), is 50 times more sensitive compared with *L. casei*. *E. faecalis* is also stimulated by lipids, but its higher sensitivity allows samples to be prepared for assay at a higher dilution, resulting in negligible amounts of interfering lipids and other extraneous matter in the assay tubes. Barton-Wright (1967) used a basal medium that contained tryptone solution, yeast supplement, glucose, several amino acids, purines and pyrimidines, vitamins and salts; this medium is more synthetic in composition than the original medium used by Kornberg, Langdon and Cheldelin (1948). Comparative assay values using *E. faecalis* and *L. casei* (Table 7.9) show excellent agreement for many of the foods tested. The higher value of 0.33 μg/g obtained for white flour using *L. casei* is apparently due to the stimulatory effect of lipids, as a prior ether extraction lowered this value to 0.20 μg/g, making it comparable to the value of 0.21 μg/g using *E. faecalis*. The same ether treatment produced no lowering of the *E. faecalis* assay value. *E. faecalis*, being practically unaffected by lipids and other substances, is preferred to *L. casei* as an assay organism (Barton-Wright, 1967). Bell (1971) pointed out that there are no dehydrated media available for this assay, and media have to be prepared from the ingredients.

Table 7.9 Comparative assay values using *E. faecalis* and *L. casei*

Material	Riboflavin (μg/g)	
	E. faecalis	*L. casei*
Yeast	45	45
Navy beans	2.6	2.5
Green pea soup (dehydrated)	1.00	1.01
Pea puree	0.90	1.05
Sweet potato	0.95	0.94
Tomato juice	0.32	0.35
Carrots	1.68	1.83
Carrot puree	0.16	0.22
White potatoes	0.36	0.52
White flour (non-enriched)	0.21	0.33

Extraction

The flavins are released from their intimate association with proteins by autoclaving the sample at 121 °C for 15 min in the presence of 0.1 N HCl. For cooked wheaten products, such as bread, the autoclaving time must be increased to 30 min (Barton-Wright and Booth, 1943). As a result of the acid digestion, FAD, which cannot be utilized by lactic acid bacteria, is completely degraded to FMN and riboflavin, and some of the FMN is also degraded to riboflavin. The autoclaving of food samples with 0.1 N HCl hydrolyses the starch, but it also liberates sufficient amounts of free fatty acids to cause an interference in the *L. casei* assay.

The use of Takadiastase has been suggested as a means of hydrolysing starch (Scott, Randall and Hessel, 1941), but Barton-Wright and Booth (1943) reported that various commercial preparations of this enzyme complex showed a marked stimulatory action over other hydrolysing agents (ptyalin, HCl and H_2SO_4). In any case, the use of enzymes tends to complicate the analysis, because most crude enzyme preparations used for such purposes contain variable amounts of vitamins, which can lead to high and unpredictable blank values.

The general extraction procedure used in *L. casei* assays for analysing foods of very low fat content (such foods include many cereals) involves acid hydrolysis, followed by precipitation of the denatured proteins at pH 4.5 (near their isoelectric point). The precipitated proteins, together with the small amount of lipoidal material and any non-hydrolysed starch, is removed by simple filtration through paper. Omission of the filtration step produced a pronounced drift in riboflavin values for whole wheat flour, which was typical of cereal products in general (Strong and Carpenter, 1942). Ether extraction could be used to remove interfering lipids, but, for samples of negligible fat content, the filtration step results in a valid assay (i.e. free from drift), and is much simpler and quicker to accomplish. High-fat foodstuffs should be given a preliminary extraction with petroleum ether to remove the bulk of the lipids before the acid hydrolysis step. This initial extraction does not completely remove the stimulatory lipids (Wegner, Kemmerer and Fraps, 1942), and a further extraction with diethyl ether is necessary after filtering off the precipitated proteins. Milk should be separated by centrifugation, and the serum shaken in a separating funnel with diethyl ether. Petroleum ether is not a suitable fat solvent with milk, as the mixture tends to form an emulsion (Barton-Wright and Booth, 1943).

Working procedures for extracting the riboflavin from materials of low and high fat content are outlined below.

For the extraction of cereals and other dry materials of negligible fat content, the method of Strong and Carpenter (1942) has been found to be satisfactory (Kent-Jones and Meiklejohn, 1944; Barton-Wright, 1945, 1952). In this procedure a suitable weight (usually 5 g is sufficient) of the finely ground sample is suspended in 50 ml of 0.1 N HCl, and then autoclaved for 15 min at 121 °C. The volume of 0.1 N HCl in millilitres must be equal to at least 10 times the dry weight of the sample in grams. The hydrolysed extract must be protected from light as soon as it is removed from the autoclave. After cooling, 2 ml of 2.5 M sodium acetate solution is added and the pH is adjusted to 4.5 with 0.5 N NaOH using bromocresol green or bromophenol blue as external indicator. A heavy precipitate of proteinaceous material forms at this point. The volume is made up to 100 ml, and the extract is filtered (repeatedly, if necessary) through a fluted Whatman No. 42 filter paper until a clear filtrate is obtained. A 50-ml aliquot of the filtrate is adjusted to pH 6.8 with 0.5 N NaOH, using bromothymol blue as external indicator, and diluted to 100 ml. It may be necessary to filter this final extract before assay to remove any turbidity. A reagent blank is taken through the same procedure.

High-fat materials, such as wheat germ, maize, oats, soya bean, meat, cheese and mixed diets, require a preliminary extraction with petroleum ether (b.p. 40–60 °C) before hydrolysis to remove neutral fats. This involves extracting the dried, finely ground sample with petroleum ether for 16–18 h in a Soxhlet apparatus. The defatted material is autoclaved, adjusted to pH 4.5, diluted and filtered as described in the above procedure for the extraction of cereals. A 50-ml aliquot of the filtrate is shaken with two or three 30-ml portions of diethyl ether in a separating funnel. The combined ether layers are washed two or three times with water, and the washings are added to the bulked aqueous layers. Finally, the pH of the extract is adjusted to 6.8, and the extract is filtered, if necessary, and diluted to 100 ml (or other suitable volume) for direct assay (Barton-Wright, 1952).

The published extraction procedure using *E. faecalis* (Kornberg, Langdon and Cheldelin, 1948) entailed the addition of 20 ml of water and 3 ml of 1 N H_2SO_4 to 1 g of the dry material to be assayed, and autoclaving for 30 min. The pH was adjusted to 4.5–5.0, and the extract diluted to contain *c.* 0.001–0.002 μg riboflavin/ml.

7.4.3 NIACIN

Determination of total niacin

Microbiological techniques currently employed for determining total niacin are based on the assay method developed by Snell and Wright (1941) using *Lactobacillus plantarum* (ATCC No. 8014). *L. plantarum* responds equally well on a molar basis to nicotinic acid, nicotinamide, nicotinuric acid (an inactive metabolite) and the nicotinamide-containing coenzyme (NAD) without preliminary hydrolysis (Snell and Wright, 1941); hence this organism cannot be used to differentiate between nicotinic acid and nicotinamide. The growth of *L. plantarum* on a nicotinic acid-deficient basal medium is not affected by free fatty acids or phospholipids, apart from an inhibitory effect of linoleic acid at a relatively high concentration (Kodicek and Pepper, 1948a), so there are no problems of growth stimulation or inhibition due to lipids as encountered in the riboflavin assay using *L. casei*. Nevertheless, Barton-Wright (1945, 1952) recommended that high-fat samples be Soxhlet-extracted with light petroleum ether for 16–18 h before acid or alkaline hydrolysis, to prevent the formation of oily emulsions which may hinder complete extraction.

The extraction procedure recommended by the Association of Vitamin Chemists, Inc. (1966) for the microbiological determination of total niacin for all foodstuffs, including cereals and cereal products, entails autoclaving the sample at 121 °C for 30 min in the presence of 1 N H_2SO_4. This treatment liberates nicotinamide from its coenzyme forms and simultaneously hydrolyses it to nicotinic acid. The treatment does not completely liberate the bound nicotinic acid from cereal products; alkaline hydrolysis, as used in the AOAC colorimetric method (see Chapter 5), is necessary to achieve this. However, extraction of cereal products with 1 N H_2SO_4 yielded similar nicotinic acid values obtained microbiologically as did extraction with 1 N NaOH (Melnick, 1942), and microbiological values obtained on wheat bran, corn bran and rice bran were uniformly higher than chemical values when 1 N H_2SO_4 was used for extraction (Sweeney and Parrish, 1954). These findings support the experimental evidence presented by Krehl and Strong (1944) that the assay organism *L. plantarum* is able to utilize the bound nicotinic acid in cereals to a considerable extent. Although alkaline hydrolysis has been used to ensure the complete liberation of bound nicotinic acid in microbiological assays (Kodicek and Pepper, 1948b), the use of 1 N H_2SO_4 is preferred for practical reasons because alkaline extraction of fatty samples gives extracts that are difficult to clarify.

The extraction procedure described below is that recommended by the Association of Vitamin Chemists, Inc. (1966) and is based on the (AOAC, 1990a) microbiological method for determining total niacin.

A suitable weight (normally 2–10 g) of the comminuted sample judged to contain about 0.1 mg of nicotinic acid after hydrolysis is mixed with 100 ml of 1 N H_2SO_4 and autoclaved at 121 °C for 30 min. The volume of 1 N H_2SO_4 in millilitres must be greater than 10 times the dry weight of the sample in grams. For liquid samples, the pH of the sample is adjusted to 5.0–6.0 with dilute H_2SO_4 or NaOH solution, as appropriate, and diluted with water, if necessary, to give a solution containing less than 5 mg nicotinic acid/ml. An equivalent of 10 ml of 10 N H_2SO_4 is then added per 100 ml of liquid. The autoclaved extract is cooled, and the pH is adjusted to 6.0–6.5 by the addition of NaOH solution, and then immediately readjusted to pH 4.5 with dilute HCl, at which point the proteins in solution are precipitated. Alternatively, proteins can be precipitated by the addition of 2 ml of 2.5 M sodium acetate and adjustment to pH 4.5 with NaOH solution as performed by Strong and Carpenter (1942). The mixture is diluted to a measured volume with water and filtered through a suitable filter paper (e.g. Whatman No. 42 paper for fatty samples or No. 541 for non-fatty samples) (Bell, 1974). The first few millilitres of filtrate passing through the non-wetted filter paper will be turbid and should be discarded. An aliquot of the filtrate is adjusted with 1 N NaOH to pH 6.8 using a pH meter or bromothymol blue as external indicator, and diluted to a final measured volume containing as nearly as possible 50 ng of nicotinic acid/ml (range 20–100 ng/ml). A reagent blank is taken through the same procedure.

A radiometric–microbiological assay has been developed for the determination of total niacin in foods based upon the measurement of $^{14}CO_2$ generated from the metabolism of L-[1-^{14}C]methionine by *Kloeckera apiculata* (ATCC No. 9774; formerly called *K. brevis*) (Guilarte and Pravlik, 1983). Sample preparation entailed autoclaving with 1 N HCl for 90 min at 121 °C and, after cooling, pH adjustment to 4.5. Removal of precipitated debris was not necessary. Radiometric assay sensitivity, defined as the lowest concentration of vitamin producing a response of at least twice background (no vitamin), was 2 ng/vial (5.2 ml).

Determination of bound nicotinic acid

In cereals, most of the niacin present exists in the form of bound nicotinic acid, which is biologically unavailable to humans unless pretreated with alkali. The general approach to estimating the bound nicotinic acid content of a sample is to treat the sample with weak (0.1 N) acid, which extracts the free niacin but does not liberate nicotinic acid from the bound forms. This extract therefore contains both free and bound nicotinic acid, but yields only the free form when analysed microbiologically using a selective organism. A portion of the acid extract is subsequently treated with 1 N NaOH to liberate bound nicotinic acid, and the resultant solution is assayed for total niacin. The difference between the results obtained for total and free niacin is a measure of bound nicotinic acid. This approach depends upon the test organism being unresponsive to bound nicotinic acid, so the usual organism, *L. plantarum*, is unsuitable. The two methods described below utilize organisms that fulfil this requirement.

Samples weighing 2–4 g are extracted with 50 ml of 0.1 N HCl on a boiling water bath for 30 min. After cooling, the pH of the solution is adjusted to 3.5 with 0.1 N NaOH, with constant stirring to avoid localized alkalinity. The extract is made up to 100 ml and filtered, and a measured volume is washed with an equal volume of chloroform. An aliquot of the fat-free extract is heated with 1 N NaOH on a boiling water bath for 30 min to liberate the bound niacin. The alkali-treated solution and an untreated aliquot of the fat-free extract at pH 3.5 are adjusted to pH 6.5 and diluted to contain *c.* 30 ng of total or free niacin per ml, respectively. In order to avoid the liberation of bound nicotinic acid during the subsequent autoclaving of medium plus sample, aliquots of the alkali-untreated solution are added aseptically to previously autoclaved assay tubes containing the medium. The alkali-treated solution is dispensed into assay tubes before autoclaving in accordance with standard procedure. The difference between the results for total and free niacin, using *L. casei* as the test organism, represents the bound niacin content of the sample (Clegg, 1963).

A similar procedure for determining the bound nicotinic acid in natural materials was reported by Ghosh, Sarkar and Guha (1963), using *Leuconostoc mesenteroides* subsp. *mesenteroides* (ATCC No. 9135) as the test organism. In this procedure the homogenized sample was extracted with 0.1 N HCl in a boiling water bath for 45 min, and the extract was cooled and centrifuged. The residue was treated twice with 0.1 N HCl in the cold and then centrifuged. The combined centrifugate was used for the assay of free nicotinic acid, bound nicotinic acid and nicotinamide. Free nicotinic acid was determined by adjusting an aliquot of the acid extract to pH 6.2–6.4 and centrifuging off the precipitated material. The centrifugate was brought to pH 3.5, and then sterilized by steaming at atmospheric pressure for 15 min. It was found that a portion of the bound nicotinic acid was hydrolysed when the materials were sterilized at 10 lb/in^2 for 15 min at pH 6.2–6.4, but when the sterilization was effected at pH 3.5–4 by steaming, only traces of nicotinic acid were released from the bound form. Bound nicotinic acid, together with free nicotinic acid, was determined by treating a second aliquot of the extract with 0.5 N NaOH for 10 min at room temperature, and assaying the nicotinic acid content after removal of the material precipitated at pH 6.2–6.4. Nicotinamide, together with free and bound nicotinic acid, was estimated by hydrolysing the bound nicotinic acid with 0.5 N NaOH, and then hydrolysing the amide with 1 N HCl at 15 lb/in^2 for 1 h. The total nicotinic acid was assayed after removal of the material precipitated at pH 6.2–6.4. The difference in *Leuc. mesenteroides* assay results between the nicotinic acid content of the extract before and after alkaline hydrolysis represented the bound nicotinic acid content of the sample. The difference between the total nicotinic acid content and the nicotinic acid content obtained after alkaline hydrolysis represented the nicotinamide content of the sample.

Determination of added nicotinic acid

The nicotinic acid added to fresh meat can be determined directly using *Leuc. mesenteroides*. Gorin and Schütz (1970) suspended the minced meat sample in 0.2 M acetate buffer (pH 4.8) and shook the suspension for 10 min at room temperature. Nicotinic acid was extracted while the buffer flocculated the meat proteins. This mild extraction process does not convert nicotinamide to nicotinic acid. The results obtained were in good agreement with a spectrophotometric method.

7.4.4 VITAMIN B_6

The vitamin B_6 compounds known to occur naturally are pyridoxine (PN), pyridoxal (PL) and pyridoxamine (PM), the 5′-phosphate esters of the aldehyde and amine forms (PLP and PMP), and conjugates of PN. Animal sources of vitamin B_6 contain the vitamin mainly as protein-bound PLP, while plant sources contain mostly PN, a proportion of which may be glycosylated.

Assay organisms

The ideal assay organism for the microbiological determination of total vitamin B_6 should exhibit an equal growth response to PN, PL and PM, as these vitamers have equal biological activities in humans (Brin, 1978).

Lactic acid bacteria have no utility, because they do not respond to PN (Snell, 1981). The yeast *Saccharomyces carlsbergensis* (*uvarum*) (ATCC No. 9080) responds vigorously to all three free bases and is the most widely used test organism for vitamin B_6. The growth response of *S. carlsbergensis* to PL relative to that to PN is practically equal, or somewhat less, but the response to PM is markedly less than that to PN and is dose-dependent within the working concentration range of 2–10 ng molar equivalents of PN per tube (Guilarte, McIntyre and Tsan, 1980; Gregory, 1982). This unequal response leads to an under-estimation of the total vitamin B_6 content if the sample extract contains predominantly PM (e.g. a processed meat product), but is of little concern in plant-derived foods or foods that are substantially fortified with PN. Morris, Hughes and Mulder (1959) pointed out that cultures of *S. carlsbergensis* obtained from different sources, but reputed to be derived from the same parent strain, possess different nutritional requirements, particularly in their response to thiamin and vitamin B_6. It is therefore important to study the growth requirements of any strain of *S. carlsbergensis* before it is used as an assay organism.

The problem of differential response in the *S. carlsbergensis* assay can be overcome by separating PN, PL and PM chromatographically and assaying each vitamer relative to its own standard curve. Toepfer and Polansky (1970) reported the results of a collaborative study using such a technique, which was adopted as Final Action by the AOAC in 1975 (AOAC, 1990b). In this method, acid-hydrolysed food samples are adjusted to pH 4.5 with 6 N KOH, diluted with water to 250 ml and filtered. An aliquot of the filtrate is applied to an open column packed with Dowex AG 50W-X8 cation exchange resin, and PL, PN and PM are eluted successively with a sequence of boiling buffer solutions. For a number of animal products, total vitamin B_6 values, obtained by adding the results of the individual vitamers, were statistically higher than non-chromatographed values calculated using a PN standard curve (Polansky and Toepfer, 1969). An additional benefit of the chromatographic technique is the removal from high-starch plant products of acid-treated glucose compounds which would otherwise stimulate yeast growth (Toepfer and Polansky, 1964). Data obtained by the chromatographic procedure compared well with data obtained by rat growth assay for total vitamin B_6 in a few selected food samples (Toepfer *et al.*, 1963).

The open-column ion exchange chromatographic technique described above is laborious and requires care to ensure a clean separation of PL, PN and PM fractions. A more efficient and reproducible fractionation of B_6 vitamers can be obtained using HPLC as performed by Gregory, Manley and Kirk (1981).

Guilarte, McIntyre and Tsan (1980) compared *S. carlsbergensis* with another yeast, *Kloeckera apiculata* (ATCC No. 9774; formerly called *K. brevis*), for their ability to utilize PN, PL and PM in the concentration range needed for the measurement of vitamin B_6 in biological materials. The results showed that, unlike *S. carlsbergensis*, *K. apiculata* responded equally to all three vitamers at a concentration range of 2–10 ng molar equivalents of PN per tube. A practically equal response of *K. apiculata* to PN, PL and PM was previously reported by Barton-Wright (1971) and Daoud, Luh and Miller (1977). Guilarte, McIntyre and Tsan (1980) proposed that *K. apiculata* should be used instead of *S. carlsbergensis* as the standard turbidimetric microbiological assay for vitamin B_6 in biological materials. However, this proposal has not found acceptance in certain other laboratories. Gregory (1982) conducted a study under conditions comparable to those employed by Guilarte, McIntyre and Tsan (1980), and found that *K. apiculata* exhibited an even lower relative response to PM than that obtained with *S. carlsbergensis*. A similar disparity in the response to PM with *K. apiculata* was reported by Polansky (1981). These conflicting data (Gregory, 1983; Guilarte and Tsan, 1983) suggest that subtle environmental factors or culturing variables affect the specificity of *K. apiculata*. This as yet unresolved discrepancy between results from different laboratories illustrates the importance of checking the growth response to PN, PL and PM of any test organism before proceeding to routine determinations.

The growth response of *S. carlsbergensis* and *K. apiculata* is influenced by KCl and NaCl formed as a result of pH adjustment of acid-hydrolysed food samples with 6 N KOH or NaOH (Guilarte, 1984). This potential source of interference can be reduced or eliminated by treating the standard in a similar fashion as the food sample to be assayed.

Barton-Wright (1971) encountered the occasional problem of excessive growth in the blanks using *K. apiculata*, which could not be reduced using the PN-depletion technique of Gare (1968). The problem was overcome by maintaining the organism in liquid stock culture containing PN.HCl instead of on the conventional malt agar slope. The basal medium was modified in several respects, notably by substituting a 10% charcoal-treated malt extract solution for vitamin-free casein hydrolysate, which often proved difficult to free completely from vitamin B_6.

A radiometric–microbiological assay developed for the determination of total vitamin B_6 in foods, and based upon the measurement of $^{14}CO_2$ generated from the metabolism of L-[1-^{14}C]valine by *K. apiculata* (Guilarte, Shane and McIntyre 1981; Guilarte, 1983, 1986), gave an assay sensitivity of 0.25 ng of PN, PL or PM per vial (3.2 ml total volume). The method described is subject to the same controversy encountered in the turbidimetric assay with regard to the specificity of *K. apiculata* towards PN, PL and PM.

Extraction

The bound and phosphorylated forms of vitamin B_6 cannot be utilized for growth by the yeasts and bacteria used as microbiological assay organisms, and food samples must be subjected to vigorous acid hydrolysis to free the PN, PL and PM vitamers from their association with phosphate and from all bound forms prior to assay. Unfortunately, there is no single hydrolytic procedure which gives optimal results with all types of food.

In the AOAC microbiological method for determining vitamin B_6 in food extracts (AOAC, 1990b), the weighted sample (1–2 g for dry products and up to 20 g for fresh products) is placed in a wide-mouthed conical flask and mixed with 200 ml of 0.44 N HCl or 0.055 N HCl for plant and animal products, respectively. The mixtures are autoclaved at 121 °C for 2 h (plant products) or 5 h (animal products). Polansky, Reynolds and Vanderslice (1985) suggested that food composites be mixed with 200 ml of 0.2 N HCl and autoclaved for 5 h at 121 °C. For milk-based infant formula, 10-g samples are mixed with 200 ml of 0.05 N HCl and autoclaved for 5 h at 121 °C (AOAC, 1990c). The autoclaved extracts are cooled to room temperature, adjusted to pH 4.5 with 6 N KOH solution (to precipitate the denatured proteins at their isoelectric point), diluted with water to 250 ml, and filtered through Whatman No. 40 filter paper. In the AOAC (1990b) procedure, 40–200 ml of the filtrate is passed through an ion exchange column to obtain the PN, PL and PM fractions, which are then assayed individually. The chromatographic step is deemed necessary because the growth response of the assay organism, *S. carlsbergensis*, to PM is markedly less than that to PN. For routine purposes, the chromatographic step is omitted, and aliquots of the filtrate are diluted according to the expected vitamin B_6 content (1 ml to 20 ml in the case of milk-based infant formula) before addition to the assay tubes.

Guilarte (1984) used a modified version of the AOAC (1990b) procedure in which 200 ml of 0.5 N HCl or 0.05 N HCl, for plant and animal products respectively, was added to 1–2 g of the dry product, and the mixtures were autoclaved for 90 min at 121 °C. The cooled extracts were adjusted to pH 4.5 using 6 N NaOH, diluted to 250 ml with water, centrifuged or filtered, and finally diluted to the appropriate concentration for turbidimetric assay.

7.4.5 PANTOTHENIC ACID

Assay organism

Lactobacillus plantarum (ATCC No. 8014) is the usual assay organism and has been deployed in the AOAC (1990d) procedure for the determination of free pantothenate. The medium is based on that originally developed by Snell and Wright (1941) for the determination of nicotinic acid, except that pantothenic acid instead of nicotinic acid is the limiting factor. Fatty acids are stimulatory in the presence of suboptimal amounts of pantothenic acid (Skeggs and Wright, 1944), so an ether extraction step may be included in the procedure.

A radiometric–microbiological assay for pantothenic acid in human blood and milk based on the metabolism of L-[1-^{14}C]methionine or L-[1-^{14}C]valine by *Kloeckera apiculata* (ATCC No. 9774) was reported by Guilarte (1989). Assay sensitivity was 1 ng/vial (5 ml) with either radioactive substrate. None of the analogues tested (pantetheine, panthenol and pantoyl lactone) generated a response or interfered with the analysis of pantothenic acid.

Extraction

Neither acid nor alkaline hydrolysis can be used to liberate the pantothenic acid from coenzyme A and other bound forms, since the vitamin is degraded by such treatments. The only practicable alternative is enzymatic hydrolysis, which is accomplished through the simultaneous action of intestinal alkaline phosphatase and an avian liver enzyme.

Both intestinal alkaline phosphatase and avian liver enzyme preparations are available commercially as powdered extracts. Liver enzyme preparations contain a relatively high amount of coenzyme A, which is converted to pantothenate during the incubation period, thus creating an unacceptably high blank value. Purification of the liver preparation by treatment with Dowex-1 anion exchange resin reduces the blank value to a very low level without appreciable loss of coenzyme A-splitting activity (Novelli and Schmetz, 1951). Intestinal phosphatase preparations contain negligible amounts of coenzyme A and do not require purification.

The following procedure can be applied to the purification of commercial preparations (Sigma Chemicals) of either pigeon or chicken acetone-dried liver powder. The procedure is based on the original method of Novelli and Schmetz (1951) as modified by Toepfer, Zook and Richardson (1954), Clegg (1958) and Bell (1974).

One hundred grams of Dowex 1-X4 strongly basic anion exchange resin, 200–400 mesh (Bio-Rad Laboratories), is washed twice by stirring with 10 volumes of 1 N HCl and filtering with suction, followed by 8–10 washings with 10 volumes of water until the pH is 5. The acid-washed resin is left as a slurry and is adjusted to pH 8 just before use by adding a few drops of 1 M tris-(hydroxymethyl)-methylamine buffer, pH 8.3. The liver powder (typically 2 g) is stirred with 10 times its weight of ice-cold freshly prepared 0.02 M sodium bicarbonate solution to give a smooth suspension, and then centrifuged at 2 °C for 20 min at 4000**g**. The reddish-brown supernatant is poured into an equal volume of the ice-cold slurry of pH-adjusted Dowex resin, and the suspension is stirred for 15 min in an ice-bath and centrifuged at 2 °C. The supernatant is treated in a similar manner with another equal volume of resin, and the resultant supernatant containing the purified enzyme is dispensed in 5-ml portions into specimen tubes for storage at −20 °C. The Dowex-treated enzyme solution is prepared every month, and each tube is thawed immediately before use.

Methods of extracting the bound pantothenic acid from food samples are based upon the original enzymatic procedure of Novelli and Schmetz (1951), but there is no standardized treatment of samples with the enzymes. Toepfer, Zook and Richardson (1954) used the hydrolytic procedure in a standardized microbiological assay and obtained pantothenic acid values for whole egg powder, kale, peanuts, pig liver and brewer's yeast that did not differ significantly from values obtained on the same samples using a rat bioassay. The microbiological results for carrots were significantly lower than the bioassay results. The use of a commercially purified hog kidney extract instead of Dowex-treated avian liver yielded similar results within laboratories in a collaborative study of the standardized microbiological procedure (Toepfer, 1957). However, considerable variation was found among the data reported by collaborators. Loss of activity of the enzyme preparations showed a need for establishing the activity of the enzymes before they could be relied upon for use in an official assay procedure (Toepfer, 1960). Measurement of enzyme activity requires a stable standard of bound pantothenic acid, but such a standard has yet to be found. Coenzyme A did not prove satisfactory because only minute quantities of enzymes could release most of the bound pantothenate. The present AOAC microbiological method (AOAC, 1990d) is confined to the determination of free pantothenate in vitamin preparations; this method omits enzymatic hydrolysis.

In the procedure employed by Bell (1974), the test material is homogenized with 10 ml of 0.2 M tris-(hydroxymethyl)-methylamine buffer (pH 8.0) at 70 °C, and then autoclaved for 15 min at 121 °C. After mixing and cooling to room temperature, 1.0 ml of 2% w/v alkaline phosphatase (Sigma) in Tris buffer and 0.5 ml of Dowex-treated pigeon liver enzyme solution are added, and the mixture is incubated at 37 °C overnight. On the following day, the extracts are steamed in an autoclave for 5 min to destroy any remaining enzyme activity, cooled to room temperature and diluted to a suitable volume with Tris buffer. The extracts are centrifuged at 15 000**g** for 20 min (additional step used by

Finglas *et al.*, 1988), and then filtered through Whatman No. 42 (or, if non-fatty, through Whatman No. 541) filter paper into polythene bottles for storage at −20 °C pending analysis. For conventional assay procedures using double-strength media, the filtrates are adjusted to pH 6.8 with NaOH solution and diluted to place them in the range of the standard curve. A reagent blank is taken through the same procedure.

Walsh, Wyse and Hansen (1979) omitted the filtration step, which was reported to be slow and troublesome, and used dialysis to isolate the liberated pantothenate from the large amount of protein in the food digest. This entailed transferring the extract to a short length of 1-cm dialysis tubing with water washings, tying both ends of the tube to form a sac, and immersing the sac in a conical flask containing 60–150 ml of distilled water. Each flask was stirred continuously in the cold (5 °C) for at least 8 h. Following dialysis, the tubing and its contents were discarded and the remaining clear water extract was used for the assay.

7.4.6 BIOTIN

Assay organisms

Among the several organisms that have been used for the microbiological determination of biotin (Achuta Murthy and Mistry, 1977), *Lactobacillus plantarum* (ATCC No. 8014) is currently the most widely used. This organism shows a high specificity towards free *d*-biotin and does not respond to biocytin or other bound forms. Biotin-*d*-sulphoxide elicits an equal growth response to that of *d*-biotin, while biotin sulphone is inhibitory (Langer and György, 1968). However, these oxidation products are not likely to be present in food samples in sufficient concentration to cause significant interference. The growth requirements of *L. plantarum* are less complex than those of *L. casei*, but both organisms are stimulated by non-esterified unsaturated fatty acids and other lipids when biotin is present in suboptimal amounts (Williams and Fieger, 1945; Williams, 1945; Broquist and Snell, 1951). The high sensitivity of the biotin assay (0.1–1.0 ng/assay tube; Dakshinamurti *et al.*, 1974) necessitates a high sample dilution, which will reduce this growth stimulation. A practical advantage of using *L. plantarum* is that the basal medium used for nicotinic acid and pantothenic acid can be used with the exclusion of the relevant vitamin (in this case biotin) from the formulation. The use of the same organism for assaying the three vitamins also eliminates the need for preparing separate stock cultures.

Guilarte (1985) applied a radiometric-microbiological assay to the determination of biotin in numerous foods based on the metabolism of L-[1-^{14}C] methionine by *Kloeckera apiculata* (ATCC No. 9774) and compared the results with those obtained using the conventional turbidimetric *L. plantarum* assay. With the exception of cereals, there was good agreement between the two assays. In cereals, the *L. plantarum* assay gave lower biotin levels, and this was attributed to the removal of biotin during filtering in the extraction procedure.

Extraction

It has been recommended to remove lipid material by adjusting the pH of the acid hydrolysate to 4.5 and filtering through paper (Skeggs, 1963b; Strohecker and Henning, 1966). (Note: Guilarte (1985) reported a possible loss of biotin during filtration.) This procedure might not be adequate for materials with a high fat content (e.g. wheat germ, meat, eggs), which should be defatted by a preliminary Soxhlet extraction with light petroleum (Barton-Wright, 1952). The following extraction procedure for all types of foodstuff is based upon that of Barton-Wright (1952).

A 2–10-g amount of finely comminuted sample is homogenized with 20 ml of 3 N H_2SO_4 and autoclaved for 30 min at 121 °C. The pH of the cooled extract is adjusted to 4.5 with NaOH solution, and the extract is diluted with water to a suitable volume and then filtered through Whatman No. 42 filter paper. An aliquot from the filtrate is adjusted to pH 6.8 with NaOH solution, and then further diluted with water to give the optimum concentration for assay. The reagent blank is taken through the same procedure.

7.4.7 FOLATE

Assay organisms

Three organisms, *Lactobacillus casei* subsp. *rhamnosus* (ATCC No. 7469), *Enterococcus hirae* (ATCC No. 8043) and *Pediococcus acidilactici* (ATCC No. 8081), have been routinely employed in folate assays because they respond specifically to certain metabolic forms of folate, and therefore can be used to distinguish between the different forms present in the assay material. The growth responses of the assay organism to representative folates are presented in Table 7.10. *L. casei* can utilize for growth the widest spectrum of folates, and these constitute the mono-, di- and triglutamates of folic acid (pteroylglutamic acid, PteGlu) and their di- and tetrahydro reduced forms, regardless of the single carbon substituent. *E. hirae* responds to all mono- and diglutamyl folates, except those with a methyl group at the N-5 position. It also responds to pteroic acid and its 5- and 10-formyl derivatives, which are metabolically inactive for animals and humans. *P. acidilactici* is the most specialized in its requirements, being able to utilize only the mono, di- and

Table 7.10 Growth-supporting activity of representative folates for three test organisms

	Activity for test organism		
Compound	*L. casei*	*E. hirae*	*P. acidilactici*
PteGlu (folic acid)	+ (100%)	+	−
H_2PteGlu (dihydrofolic acid)	+	+	−
H_4PteGlu (tetrahydrofolic acid)	+	+	+
10-CHO-PteGlu	+	+	−
10-CHO-H_2PteGlu	+	+	−
10-CHO-H_4PteGlu	+	+	+
5-CHO-H_4PteGlu	+	+	+
5-CH_3-H_4PteGlu	+	−	−
5-CH_3-H_4PteGlu$_2$	+	−	−
5-CHO-H_4PteGlu$_3$	+	−	+
PteGlu$_2$	+ (100%)	+	−
PteGlu$_3$	+ (100%)	−	−
PteGlu$_4$	+ (65%)	−	−
PteGlu$_5$	+ (20%)	−	−
PteGlu$_6$	+ (3.6%)	−	−
PteGlu$_7$	+ (2.4%)	−	−
5-CHO-H_4PteGlu$_n$[a]	−	−	−
5-CH_3-H_4PteGlu$_n$[a]	−	−	−
10-CHO-H_4PteGlu$_n$[a]	−	−	−
Pteroic acid	−	+	−

[a] The *n* unspecified; probably >5.

From Krumdieck, Tamura and Eto (1983). *Vitamins and Hormones*, Vol. 40, 45–104. By permission of Academic Press.

triglutamates of tetrahydro reduced folates, with the exception of 5-methyl analogues.

The above three organisms have been used with a single medium in a differential microbiological folate assay carried out before and after treatment of the sample with conjugase (Bird, McGlohon and Vaitkus, 1969). An increase in growth-supporting activity after conjugase treatment reveals the presence of pteroylpolyglutamates with more than three glutamate residues if *L. casei* is the assay organism used, and conjugates with more than two glutamate residues if *E. hirae* is used. Increased activity after conjugase using *P. acidilactici* reveals the presence of tetrahydropolyglutamates longer than H_4PteGlu$_3$. The difference between *L. casei* and *E. hirae* activity indicates the amount of 5-methyl folate present. If *E. hirae* activity is greater than *P. acidilactici* activity, the presence of dihydro reduced folates and/or pteroic acid is indicated.

Tamura *et al.* (1972) demonstrated that, contrary to earlier beliefs, *L. casei* exhibits a growth response to $PteGlu_n$ (n = 4–7; see Table 7.10), the response curves showing progressively steeper slopes. The consequence of this is that serial dilutions of sample extracts containing significant amounts of the longer polyglutamates, when read against a calibration curve prepared with a monoglutamate standard, will give falsely high results with increasing amounts of assay material. This disproportionate response to serial dilutions of an extract is known as 'positive drift'. The *L. casei* activity of the longer polyglutamates was also shown to be sensitive to the length of incubation of the assay. These variations in response to different pteroylpolyglutamates must be considered in evaluating the values of 'free folate' in foods as assayed by *L. casei*. Note: Goli and Vanderslice (1992) reported that, contrary to the general belief that *L. casei* responds equally to pteroylmono-, di- and triglutamates, the relative responses of the di- and triglutamates are approximately 90% and 60%, respectively, of the response of the monoglutamate.

For routine food analysis purposes, the chain length of folate polyglutamates is not required, and the combined monoglutamate folate activity (total folate) is determined using *L. casei* after enzymatic deconjugation. The basic premise using this approach is that all active monoglutamyl folates have identical equimolar growth-support activities for *L. casei*, under the conditions of the assay. This assumption is, however, a subject of controversy. While some investigators (O'Broin *et al.*, 1975; Shane, Tamura and Stokstad, 1980) reported that various monoglutamates gave essentially the same response, others (Bird, McGlohon and Vaitkus 1969; Ruddick, Vanderstoep and Richards, 1978; Reingold and Picciano, 1982; Phillips and Wright, 1982; Goli and Vanderslice, 1989) have demonstrated different responses.

Phillips and Wright (1982) observed a concentration-dependent reduced response of *L. casei* to 5-methyl-THF in sample extracts relative to folic acid and 5-formyl-THF standards using the assay procedure of Bell (1974). The resultant underestimation of total folate caused by this positive drift effect could be rectified by increasing the buffering capacity of the medium, and using an initial pH of 6.2 instead of 6.8 (Phillips and Wright, 1982, 1983; Wright and Phillips, 1985). These authors further modified the Bell (1974) method by adding the standards later by aseptic addition, instead of autoclaving them, and by increasing the ascorbate concentration from 0.25 to 1 g/litre in the standard solutions and in the incubation medium. These changes were made to ensure that the folate did not deteriorate due to heat or by atmospheric oxidation. It was also important to conduct the assay within the linear response range of 0–1 ng/10 ml.

Microbiological assays for folate have been reported using 96-well microtitration plates combined with an automatic plate reader interfaced with a data management system (Newman and Tsai, 1986; Horne and Patterson, 1988). Chen, Hill and McIntyre (1983) applied the radiometric–microbiological assay by measuring the $^{14}CO_2$ generated from the metabolism of [1-^{14}C]gluconate by *L. casei*, while Goli and Vanderslice (1989) measured nonspecific metabolic CO_2 using an infrared CO_2 analyser.

Extraction

The extraction procedure has the dual requirement of liberating protein-bound folate and deconjugating polyglutamyl folates to mono- or diglutamate forms. The commonly used sources for the conjugase enzymes are hog kidney, producing monoglutamates, and chicken pancreas, which produces diglutamates. It is widely assumed that the *L. casei* response to both forms of the enzyme is similar. However, Phillips and Wright (1983) reported that total folate values of vegetables measured after deconjugation with hog kidney enzyme were at least 50% higher than values obtained using chicken pancreas enzyme. These authors pointed out that mono- and diglutamyl forms of PteGlu, which are generally believed to elicit identical responses in *L. casei*, are actively transported in this organism, whilst the uptake of the tri- to octapolyglutamates for 5-methyl-THF is not subject to this process. If, in addition, the diglutamate of 5-methyl-THF is not actively transported, its uptake could be a rate-limiting step in the growth of *L. casei*, resulting in the observed lower growth response compared with the PteGlu standard using chicken pancreas enzyme. The total folate value for yeast extract obtained using hog kidney enzyme was nearly double that obtained using chicken pancreas enzyme. This large discrepancy could be explained by inhibition of the chicken pancreas enzyme by folate breakdown products that do not affect hog kidney enzyme. On the basis of these observations, Phillips and Wright (1983) recommended the use of hog kidney enzyme rather than chicken pancreas enzyme.

The following extraction and assay procedures are based on those of Phillips and Wright (1983).

Preparation of hog kidney enzyme solution

Ten grams of hog kidney acetone powder (Sigma Chemical Co.) are homogenized with 100 ml of L-cysteine hydrochloride (10 g/litre) which has been adjusted to pH 4.6 with NaOH. The homogenate is incubated for 4 h at 37 °C, and then centrifuged at 40 000**g** for 30 min. To the supernatant fraction is added 20 ml of activated charcoal–dextran mixture prepared by adding 1 g of dextran (molecular weight 40 000; Sigma) to 10 g of Darco G-60 charcoal and adding distilled water to a final volume of 100 ml. After 30 min at room temperature, the mixture is centrifuged, and the supernatant fraction is made up to 100 ml with L-cysteine hydrochloride solution (10 g/litre) at pH 4.6, and stored at −20 °C.

Folate extraction and deconjugation

The accurately weighed diced food sample (*c.* 10 g) is dropped into a 250-ml conical flask containing 60 ml of 57 mM ascorbic acid solution (10 g/litre adjusted to pH 4.6 with 1 M NaOH) at >90 °C. The flask contents are maintained above 90 °C for 5 min to inactivate all enzyme activity before cooling to room temperature. The mixture is homogenized, made up to 100 ml with further ascorbic acid solution, mixed, and centrifuged at 18 000***g*** for 20 min at 5 °C. A 5-ml aliquot of the supernatant is transferred by pipette to a 10-ml plastic test tube, which is capped and stored at −20 °C until required for deconjugation.

To 0.1–1.0 ml of food extract is added 1.0 ml of the hog kidney enzyme solution and sufficient ascorbic acid solution (pH 4.6) to give a final volume of 5 ml. This deconjugation system is incubated for a maximim of 6 h at 37 °C and then centrifuged at 2500***g*** for 5 min to pellet any material precipitated from solution during the incubation. The supernatant is taken directly for assay or stored at −20 °C in plastic tubes pending analysis.

Assay procedure

Bacto Folic Acid Casei Medium (Difco Code 0822) is prepared at single strength with added 5.7 mM ascorbic acid, and the pH of the medium is adjusted to 6.2 before dispensing 10 ml per assay tube, and autoclaving for 5 min at 121 °C. Deconjugated food extracts and deconjugase enzyme blanks are added aseptically to triplicate tubes of assay medium to a maximum addition of 250 μl. Each assay tube is inoculated with 100 μl of diluted inoculum culture (*L. casei*), and the tubes are incubated for 24 h at 37 °C. Folic acid standards, 0–1 ng/10-ml assay tube, are run simultaneously with each group of samples.

Results should be expressed as units of folate activity for the specific organisms, e.g. 'each gram of this material contains 100 ng folate activity for *L. casei*.'

7.4.8 VITAMIN B_{12}

Assay organisms

Most current procedures for the microbiological determination of vitamin B_{12} in foods use *Lactobacillus delbrueckii* subsp. *lactis* (formerly called *L. leichmannii*) (ATCC No. 4797), which gives a response range of 1–10 pg/ml assay medium (Skeggs, 1967). Either *L. delbrueckii* (ATCC No. 4797) or the 313 strain (ATCC No. 7830) may be used, although the latter requires a shorter time to reach nearly maximum growth (20 h versus 48 h) (Hoffmann *et al.*, 1949). *L. delbrueckii* does not respond specifically to vitamin B_{12}; clinically inactive analogues, in which the 5,6-dimethylbenzimidazole moiety is replaced by a purine base or a purine derivative, can replace the vitamin as a growth factor (Shaw and Bessell, 1960). Such analogues are found mainly in natural material that has undergone microbial fermentation, and they do not occur to any significant extent in foods for human consumption. Examples of potentially interfering analogues include so-called pseudovitamin B_{12} and factor A, in which the base substituents are adenine, and 2-methyladenine, respectively. DNA, deoxyribonucleotide and deoxyribonucleosides can also replace vitamin B_{12} for the growth of *L. delbrueckii* (Kitay, McNutt and Snell, 1949). The nucleotides and nucleosides are less active than vitamin B_{12} by a factor of 10^4, while DNA is less active by a factor of 10^6 (Hoff-Jørgensen, 1954). The activity attributable to deoxyribonucleosides can be determined by *L. delbrueckii* assay after the cobalamins have been destroyed by heating to 100 °C at pH 11 for 30 min (Hoffmann *et al.*, 1949). Deoxyribonucleosides do not occur in usual foods at levels likely to constitute a significant interference (Rosenthal, 1968), and they only substitute for B_{12} at concentrations above 1 μg/ml of assay solution (Skeggs, 1963a). Any such interference can therefore be eliminated by simply diluting to an inactive concentration.

Ford (1953) developed an assay using the protozoan *Ochromonas malhamensis* (ATCC No. 11532), which is as sensitive as the *L. delbrueckii* assay, but is more specific in that it responds only slightly, if at all, to clinically inactive cobalamins. A disadvantage of the *O. malhamensis* assay is the long incubation period of 72 h, during which the culture must be shaken continuously in the dark. A comparative study between the *O. malhamensis* and *L. delbrueckii* methods applied to a cross-section of 27 different foods did not reveal any problems of interference with the latter method. On the contrary, the *O. malhamensis* results were statistically higher at the 5% level of significance than the *L. delbrueckii* results, suggesting the presence in certain foods of unknown non-cobalamin substances which stimulate the growth of the protozoan (Lichtenstein, Beloian and Reynolds, 1959). Ford's method has been recommended for the determination of vitamin B_{12} in animal feedstuffs (Analytical Methods Committee, 1964), although Shrimpton (1956) reported that *O. malhamensis* was no better than *L. delbrueckii* in predicting the vitamin B_{12} activity of feeding stuffs for chicks.

Chen and McIntyre (1979) applied the radiometric–microbiological assay to the determination of vitamin B_{12} in foods by measuring the $^{14}CO_2$ generated from the metabolism of L-[guanido-^{14}C)arginine by *L. delbrueckii*. The assay allowed immediate inoculation with previously lyophilized cultures of *L. delbrueckii,* thus eliminating the routine subculturing required in the standard maintenance procedure.

Extraction

The extraction procedure employed in the AOAC microbiological method for determining vitamin B_{12} activity in vitamin preparations (AOAC, 1990e) is also applicable to foods, having been found satisfactory by interlaboratory collaborative analysis of a crude liver paste, condensed fish solubles and a crude vitamin B_{12} fermentation product (Krieger, 1954). The procedure entails homogenizing the sample with a 0.1 M phosphate-citrate buffer at pH 4.5 containing freshly prepared sodium metabisulphite ($Na_2S_2O_5$), and then autoclaving the mixture for 10 min at 121 °C. The metabisulphite converts the various cobalamins to the more stable sulphitocobalamin as soon as they are released from their association with proteins. For the determination of vitamin B_{12} activity in milk-based infant formula (AOAC, 1990f), protein is removed by filtration after adjustment of the autoclaved extract to the point of maximum precipitation (*c.* pH 4.5). Methods in which the sample is heated on a boiling water bath, rather than autoclaved, may not completely extract all of the bound vitamin (Casey *et al.*, 1982). Prior treatment with Takadiastase may be employed for starchy samples that yield turbid extracts after filtration or centrifugation (Analytical Methods Committee, 1956).

For the microbiological determination of vitamin B_{12} in bovine milk using *L. delbrueckii*, Gregory (1954) added 1 ml of 0.1 M sodium acetate buffer pH 4.6 and one drop of 1% w/v sodium cyanide to 1 ml of the test milk. The mixture was steamed for 30 min, and then cooled, diluted, readjusted to pH 4.6 and filtered. An acetate buffer cannot be used in the assay procedure published by the Analytical Methods Committee (1956), as the assay organism, *O. malhamensis,* is inhibited by the presence of acetate in the medium. In this procedure the test material is mixed with water and sodium cyanide, and the pH is adjusted to between 4.6 and 5.0 with 1 N HCl. The mixture is allowed to stand for 30 min at room temperature with occasional shaking, after which it is heated on a boiling water bath for 30 min. The cooled extract is diluted and then centrifuged. Starchy samples can be cleared by treatment with Takadiastase.

REFERENCES

Achuta Murthy, P.N. and Mistry, S.P. (1977) Biotin. *Prog. Fd Nutr. Sci.*, **2**, 405–55.

Analytical Methods Committee (1956) The estimation of vitamin B_{12} *Analyst, Lond.*, **81**, 132–6.

Analytical Methods Committee (1964) The determination of water-soluble vitamins in compound feeding stuffs. *Analyst. Lond.*, **89**, 1–6.

Andrews, J.S., Boyd, H.M. and Terry, D.E. (1942) Riboflavin analysis of cereals. Application of the microbiological method. *Ind. Engng Chem. Analyt. Edn*, **14**, 271–4.

AOAC (1990a) Niacin and niacinamide (nicotinic acid and nicotinamide) in vitamin preparations. Microbiological methods. Final action 1960. In *AOAC Official Methods of Analysis*, 15th edn (ed. K. Helrich), Association of Official Analytical Chemists, Inc., Arlington, VA, 944.13.

AOAC (1990b). Vitamin B_6 (pyridoxine, pyridoxal, pyridoxamine) in food extracts. Microbiological method. Final action 1975. In *AOAC Official Methods of Analysis*, 15th edn (ed. K. Helrich), Association of Official Analytical Chemists, Inc., Arlington, VA, 961.15.

AOAC (1990c) Vitamin B_6 (pyridoxine, pyridoxal, pyridoxamine) in ready-to-feed milk-based infant formula. Microbiological method. Final action 1988. In *AOAC Official Methods of Analysis*, 15th edn (ed. K. Helrich), Association of Official Analytical Chemists, Inc., Arlington, VA, 985.32.

AOAC (1990d) Pantothenic acid in vitamin preparations. Microbiological methods. Final action 1960. In *AOAC Official Methods of Analysis*, 15th edn (ed. K. Helrich), Association of Official Analytical Chemists, Inc., Arlington, VA, 954.74.

AOAC (1990e) Cobalamin (vitamin B_{12} activity) in vitamin preparations. Microbiological methods. Final action 1960. In *AOAC Official Methods of Analysis*, 15th edn (ed. K. Helrich), Association of Official Analytical Chemists, Inc., Arlington, VA, 952.20.

AOAC (1990f) Cobalamin (vitamin B_{12} activity) in milk-based infant formula. Turbidimetric method. Final action 1988. In *AOAC Official Methods of Analysis*, 15th edn (ed. K. Helrich), Association of Official Analytical Chemists, Inc., Arlington, VA, 986.23.

Association of Vitamin Chemists, Inc. (1966) *Methods of Vitamin Assay*, 3rd edn, Interscience Publishers, New York.

Barton-Wright, E.C. (1945) The theory and practice of the microbiological assay of the vitamin-B complex; together with the assay of selected amino acids and potassium. *Analyst, Lond.*, **70**, 283–94.

Barton-Wright, E.C. (1952) *The Microbiological Assay of the Vitamin B-Complex and Amino Acids*, Sir Isaac Pitman & Sons, Ltd, London.

Barton-Wright, E.C. (1967) The microbiological assay of certain vitamins in compound feeding stuffs. *J. Ass. Publ. Analysts*, **5**, 8–23.

Barton-Wright, E.C. (1971) The microbiological assay of the vitamin B_6 complex (pyridoxine, pyridoxal and pyridoxamine) with *Kloeckera brevis. Analyst. Lond.*, **96**, 314–18.

Barton-Wright, E.C. and Booth, R.G. (1943) The assay of riboflavin in cereals and other products. *Biochem. J.* **37**, 25–30.

Bauernfeind, J.C., Sotier, A.L. and Boruff, C.S. (1942) Growth stimulants in the microbiological assay for riboflavin and pantothenic acid. *Ind. Engng Chem. Analyt. Edn*, **14**, 666–71.

Bell, J.G. (1971) The microbiological assay of B-complex vitamins. In *Proceedings of the University of Nottingham Residential Seminar on Vitamins* (ed. M. Stein), Churchill Livingstone, Edinburgh and London, pp. 165–87.

Bell, J.G. (1974) Microbiological assay of vitamins of the B group in foodstuffs. *Lab. Pract.*, **23**, 235–42, 252.

Bird, O.D., McGlohon, V.M. and Vaitkus, J.W. (1969) A microbiological assay system for naturally occurring folates. *Can. J. Microbiol.*, **15**, 465–72.

Brin, M. (1978) Vitamin B_6: chemistry, absorption, metabolism, catabolism, and toxicity. In *Human Vitamin B_6 Requirements*, Food and Nutrition Board, National Research Council, National Academy of Sciences, Washington, D.C., pp. 1–20.

Broquist, H.P. and Snell, E.E. (1951) Biotin and bacterial growth. I. Relation to aspartate, oleate, and carbon dioxide. *J. Biol. Chem.*, **188**, 431–44.

Casey, P.J., Speckman, K.R., Ebert, F.J. and Hobbs, W.E. (1982) Radioisotope dilution technique for determination of vitamin B_{12} in foods. *J. Ass. Off. Analyt. Chem.*, **65**, 85–8.

Chen, M.F., Hill, J.W. and McIntyre, P.A. (1983) The folacin contents of foods as measured by a radiometric microbiologic method. *J. Nutr.*, **113**, 2192–6.

Chen, M. and McIntyre, P.A. (1979) Measurement of the trace amounts of vitamin B_{12} present in various foods by a new radiometric microbiologic technique. In *Trace Organic Analysis: a New Frontier in Analytical Chemistry* (eds H.S. Hertz and S.N. Chesler), National Bureau of Standards, Washington, DC pp. 257–65.

Clegg, K.M. (1958) The microbiological determination of pantothenic acid in wheaten flour. *J. Sci. Fd Agric.*, **9**, 366–70.

Clegg, K.M. (1963) Bound nicotinic acid in dietary wheaten products. *Br. J. Nutr.*, **17**, 325–9.

Dakshinamurti, K., Landman, A.D., Ramamurti, L. and Constable, R.J. (1974) Isotope dilution assay for biotin. *Analyt. Biochem.*, **61**, 225–31.

Daoud, H.N., Luh, B.S. and Miller, M.W. (1977) Effect of blanching, EDTA and $NaHSO_3$ on color and vitamin B_6 retention in canned garbanzo beans. *J. Fd Sci.*, **42**, 375–8.

Defibaugh, P.W., Smith, J.S. and Weeks, C.E. (1977) Assay of thiamin in foods, using manual and semiautomated fluorometric and microbiological methods. *J. Ass. Off. Analyt. Chem.*, **60**, 522–7.

Deibel, R.H., Evans, J.B. and Niven, C.F. (1957) Microbiological assay for thiamin using *Lactobacillus viridescens*. *J. Bact.*, **74**, 818–21.

Difco Laboratories (1985) Media for the microbiological assay of vitamins. In *Difco Manual*, 10th edn, Difco Laboratories, Detroit, MI, pp. 1055–1114.

Finglas, P.M., Faulks, R.M., Morris, H.C., Scott, K.J. and Morgan, M.R.A. (1988) The development of an enzyme-linked immunosorbent assay (ELISA) for the analysis of pantothenic acid and analogues, part II – determination of pantothenic acid in foods. *J. Micronutr. Anal.*, **4**, 47–59.

Ford, J.E. (1953) The microbiological assay of 'vitamin B_{12}'. The specificity of the requirement of *Ochromonas malhamensis* for cyanocobalamin. *Br. J. Nutr.*, **7**, 299–306.

Gare, L. (1968) The use of depleted cells as inocula in vitamin assays. *Analyst, Lond.*, **93**, 456–7.

Ghosh, H.P., Sarkar, P.K. and Guha, B.C. (1963) Distribution of the bound form of nicotinic acid in natural materials. *J. Nutr.*, **79**, 451–3.

Goli, D.M. and Vanderslice, J.T. (1989) Microbiological assays of folacin using a CO_2 analyzer system. *J. Micronutr. Anal.*, **6**, 19–33.

Goli, D.M. and Vanderslice, J.T. (1992) Investigation of the conjugase treatment procedure in the microbiological assay of folate. *Fd Chem.*, **43**, 57–64.

Gorin, N. and Schütz, G.P. (1970) Comparison of a microbiological and a spectrophotometric method for the determination of nicotinic acid in fresh meat. *J. Sci. Fd Agric.*, **21**, 423–5.

Gregory, J.F. (1982) Relative activity of the nonphosphorylated B-6 vitamers for *Saccharomyces uvarum* and *Kloeckera brevis* in vitamin B-6 microbiological assay. *J. Nutr.*, **112**, 1643–7.

Gregory, J.F. (1983) Response to Drs. Guilarte and Tsan letter. *J. Nutr.*, **113**, 722–4.

Gregory, J.F., Manley, D.B. and Kirk, J.R. (1981) Determination of vitamin B-6 in animal tissues by reverse-phase high-performance liquid chromatography. *J. Agric. Fd Chem.*, **29**, 921–7.

Gregory, M.E. (1954) The microbiological assay of 'vitamin B_{12}' in the milk of different animal species. *Br. J. Nutr.*, **8**, 340–7.

Guilarte, T.R. (1983) Radiometric microbiological assay of vitamin B_6: assay simplification and sensitivity study. *J. Ass. Off. Analyt. Chem.*, **66**, 58–61.

Guilarte, T.R. (1984) Effect of sodium chloride and potassium chloride on growth response of yeasts *Saccharomyces uvarum* and *Kloeckera brevis* to free vitamin B_6. *J. Ass. Off. Analyt. Chem.*, **67**, 617–20.

Guilarte, T.R. (1985) Analysis of biotin levels in selected foods using a radiometric-microbiological method. *Nutr. Rep. Int.*, **32**, 837–45.

Guilarte, T.R. (1986) Radiometric-microbiological assay of vitamin B_6 and derivatives. In *Vitamin B_6. Pyridoxal phosphate. Chemical, Biochemical, and Medical Aspects*, part A (eds D. Dolphin, R. Poulson and O. Avramovic), John Wiley & Sons, New York, pp. 595–627.

Guilarte, T.R. (1989) A radiometric microbiological assay for pantothenic acid in biological fluids. *Analyt. Biochem.*, **178**, 63–6.

Guilarte, T.R. (1991a) Radiometric microbiological assay of B vitamins. Part 1: assay procedure. *J. Nutr. Biochem.*, **2**, 334–8.

Guilarte, T.R. (1991b) Radiometric microbiological assay of B vitamins. Part 2: extraction methods. *J. Nutr. Biochem.*, **2**, 399–402.

Guilarte, T., McIntyre, P.A. and Tsan, M.-F. (1980) Growth response of the yeasts *Saccharomyces uvarum* and *Kloeckera brevis* to the free biologically active forms of vitamin B-6. *J. Nutr.*, **110**, 954–8.

Guilarte, T.R. and Pravlik, K. (1983) Radiometric-microbiologic assay of niacin using *Kloeckera brevis*: analysis of human blood and food. *J. Nutr.*, **113**, 2587–94.

Guilarte, T., Shane, B. and McIntyre, P.A. (1981) Radiometric-microbiologic assay of vitamin B-6: application to food analysis. *J. Nutr.*, **111**, 1869–75.

Guilarte, T.R. and Tsan, M.-F. (1983) Microbiological assays of total vitamin B-6 using the yeasts *Saccharomyces uvarum* and *Kloeckera brevis*. *J. Nutr.*, **113**, 721–2.

Hoff-Jørgensen, E. (1954) Microbiological assay of vitamin B_{12}. In *Methods of Biochemical Analysis*, Vol. I (ed. D. Glick), Interscience Publishers, Inc., New York, pp. 81–113.

Hoffmann, C.E., Stokstad, E.L.R., Hutchings, B.L., Dornbush, A.C. and Jukes, T.H. (1949) The microbiological assay of vitamin B_{12} with *Lactobacillus leichmannii*. *J. Biol. Chem.*, **181**, 635–44.

Horne, D.W. and Patterson, D. (1988) *Lactobacillus casei* microbiological assay of folic acid derivatives in 96-well microtitre plates. *Clin. Chem.*, **34**, 2357–9.

Keagy, P.M. (1986) Computerized semiautomated microbiological assay of folacin. *J. Ass. Off. Analyt. Chem.*, **69**, 773–7.

Kent-Jones, D.W. and Meiklejohn, M. (1944) Some experiences of microbiological assays of riboflavin, nicotinic acid and other nutrient factors. *Analyst, Lond.*, **69**, 330–6.

Kitay, E., McNutt, W.S. and Snell, E.E. (1949) The non-specificity of thymidine as a growth factor for lactic acid bacteria. *J. Biol. Chem.*, **177**, 993–4.

Kodicek, E. and Pepper, C.R. (1948a) A critical study of factors influencing the microbiological assay of nicotinic acid. *J. Gen. Microbiol.*, **2**, 292–305.

Kodicek, E. and Pepper, C.R. (1948b) The microbiological estimation of nicotinic acid and comparison with a chemical method. *J. Gen. Microbiol.*, **2**, 306–14.

Kodicek, E. and Worden, A.N. (1945) The effect of unsaturated fatty acids on *Lactobacillus helveticus* and other Gram-positive micro-organisms. *Biochem. J.*, **39**, 78–85.

Kornberg, H.A., Langdon, R.S. and Cheldelin, V.H. (1948) Microbiological assay for riboflavin. *Analyt. Chem.*, **20**, 81–3.

Krehl, W.A. and Strong, F.M. (1944) Studies on the distribution, properties, and isolation of a naturally occurring precursor of nicotinic acid. *J. Biol. Chem.*, **156**, 1–12.

Krieger, C.H. (1954) Report on vitamin B_{12}. Microbiological method. *J. Ass. Off. Agric. Chem.*, **37**, 781–92.

Krumdieck, C.L., Tamura, T. and Eto, I. (1983) Synthesis and analysis of the pteroylpolyglutamates. *Vitams Horm.*, **40**, 45–104.

Langer, B.W. Jr and Charoensiri, S. (1966) Growth response of *Lactobacillus casei* (ATCC 7469) to riboflavin, FMN, and FAD. *Proc. Soc. Exp. Biol. Med.*, **122**, 151–2.

Langer, B.W. Jr and György, P. (1968) Biotin, VIII. Active compounds and antagonists. In *The Vitamins. Chemistry, Physiology, Pathology, Methods*, 2nd edn, Vol. II (eds W.H. Sebrell, Jr and R.S. Harris), Academic Press, New York, pp. 294–322.

Lichtenstein, H., Beloian, A. and Reynolds, H. (1959) Comparative vitamin B_{12} assay of foods of animal origin by *Lactobacillus leichmannii* and *Ochromonas malhamensis*. *J. Agric. Fd Chem.*, **7**, 771–4.

Melnick, D. (1942) Collaborative study of the applicability of microbiological and chemical methods to the determination of niacin (nicotinic acid) in cereal products. *Cereal Chem.*, **19**, 553–67.

Morris, J.G., Hughes, D.T.D. and Mulder, C. (1959) Observations on the assay of vitamin B_6 with *Saccharomyces carlsbergensis* 4228. *J. Gen. Microbiol.*, **20**, 566–75.

Newman, E.M. and Tsai, J.F. (1986) Microbiological analysis of 5-formyltetrahydrofolic acid and other folates using an automated 96-well plate reader. *Analyt. Biochem.*, **154**, 509–15.

Novelli, G.D. and Schmetz, F.J. Jr (1951) An improved method for the determination of pantothenic acid in tissues. *J. Biol. Chem.*, **192**, 181–5.

O'Broin, J.D., Temperley, I.J., Brown, J.P. and Scott, J.M. (1975) Nutritional stability of various naturally occurring monoglutamate derivatives of folic acid. *Am. J. Clin. Nutr.*, **28**, 438–44.

Pearson, W.N. (1967a) Principles of microbiological assay. In *The Vitamins. Chemistry, Physiology, Pathology, Methods*, 2nd edn, Vol. VII (eds P. György and W.N. Pearson), Academic Press, New York, pp. 1–26.

Pearson, W.N. (1967b) Thiamine. In *The Vitamins. Chemistry, Physiology, Pathology, Methods*, 2nd edn, Vol. VII (eds P. György and W.N. Pearson), Academic Press, New York, pp. 53–94.

Phillips, D.R. and Wright, A.J.A. (1982) Studies on the response of *Lactobacillus casei* to different folate monoglutamates. *Br. J. Nutr.*, **47**, 183–9.

Phillips, D.R. and Wright, A.J.A. (1983) Studies on the response of *Lactobacillus casei* to folate vitamin in foods. *Br. J. Nutr.*, **49**, 181–6.

Polansky, M.M. (1981) Microbiological assay of vitamin B-6 in foods. In *Methods in Vitamin B-6 Nutrition. Analysis and Status Assessment* (eds J.E. Leklem and R.D. Reynolds), Plenum Press, New York, pp. 21–44.

Polansky, M.M., Reynolds, R.D. and Vanderslice, J.T. (1985) Vitamin B_6. In *Methods of Vitamin Assay*, 4th edn (eds J. Augustin, B.P. Klein, D. Becker and P.B. Venugopal), John Wiley & Sons, New York, pp. 417–43.

Polansky, M.M. and Toepfer, E.W. (1969) Vitamin B_6 components in some meats, fish, dairy products, and commercial infant formulas. *J. Agric. Fd Chem.*, **17**, 1394–7.

Reingold, R.N. and Picciano, M.F. (1982) Two improved high-performance liquid chromatographic separations of biologically significant forms of folate. *J. Chromat.*, **234**, 171–9.

Roberts, E.C. and Snell, E.E. (1946) An improved medium for microbiological assays with *Lactobacillus casei*. *J. Biol. Chem.*, **163**, 499–509.

Rosenthal, H.L. (1968) Vitamin B_{12}. IV. Estimation in foods and food supplements. In *The Vitamins. Chemistry, Physiology, Pathology, Methods*, 2nd edn, Vol. II (eds W.H. Sebrell, Jr and R.S. Harris), Academic Press, New York, pp. 145–70.

Ruddick, J.E., Vanderstoep, J. and Richards, J.F. (1978) Folate levels in food – a comparison of microbiological assay and radioassay methods for measuring folate. *J. Fd Sci.*, **43**, 1238–41.

Scheiner, J. and De Ritter, E. (1975) Biotin content of feedstuffs. *J. Agric. Fd Chem.*, **23**, 1157–62.

Scholes, P.M. (1960) The microbiological assay of thiamine. Two methods modified for use with small amounts of test material. *Analyst, Lond.*, **85**, 883–9.

Scott, M.L., Randall, F.E. and Hessel, F.H. (1941) A modification of the Snell and Strong microbiological method for determining riboflavin. *J. Biol. Chem.*, **141**, 325–6.

Shane, B., Tamura, T. and Stokstad, E.L.R. (1980) Folate assay: a comparison of radioassay and microbiological methods. *Clin. Chim. Acta*, **100**, 13–19.

Shaw, W.H.C. and Bessell, C.J. (1960) The determination of vitamin B_{12}. A critical review. *Analyst, Lond.*, **85**, 389–409.

Shrimpton, D.H. (1956) The estimation of vitamin-B_{12} activity in feeding stuffs with *Lactobacillus leichmannii* and *Ochromonas malhamensis*. *Analyst, Lond.*, **81**, 94–9.

Skeggs, H.R. (1963a) *Lactobacillus leichmannii* assay for vitamin B_{12}. In *Analytical*

Microbiology (ed. F. Kavanagh), Academic Press, New York, pp. 551–65.

Skeggs, H.R. (1963b) Biotin. In *Analytical Microbiology* (ed. F. Kavanagh), Academic Press, New York, pp. 421–30.

Skeggs, H.R. (1967) Vitamin B_{12}. In *The Vitamins. Chemistry, Physiology, Pathology, Methods*, 2nd edn, Vol. VII (eds P. György and W.N. Pearson), Academic Press, New York, pp. 277–93.

Skeggs, H.R. and Wright, L.D. (1944) The use of *Lactobacillus arabinosus* in the microbiological determination of pantothenic acid. *J. Biol. Chem.*, **156**, 21–6.

Snell, E.E. (1948) Use of microorganisms for assay of vitamins. *Physiol. Rev.*, **28**, 255–82.

Snell, E.E. (1950) Microbiological methods in vitamin research. In *Vitamin Methods*, Vol. I (ed. P. György), Academic Press, New York, pp. 327–505.

Snell, E.E. (1981) Vitamin B-6 analysis: some historical aspects. In *Methods in Vitamin B-6 Nutrition. Analysis and Status Assessment* (eds J.E. Leklem and R.D. Reynolds), Plenum Press, New York, pp. 1–19.

Snell, E.E. and Strong, F.M. (1939) A microbiological assay for riboflavin. *Ind. Engng Chem. Analyt. Edn*, **11**, 346–50.

Snell, E.E. and Wright, L.D. (1941) A microbiological method for the determination of nicotinic acid. *J. Biol. Chem.*, **139**, 675–86.

Strohecker, R. and Henning, H.M. (1966) *Vitamin Assay. Tested Methods*, Verlag Chemie, Weinheim.

Strong, F.M. and Carpenter, L.E. (1942) Preparation of samples for microbiological determination of riboflavin. *Ind. Engng Chem. Analyt. Edn*, **14**, 909–13.

Sweeney, J.P. and Parrish, W.P. (1954) Report on the extraction of nicotinic acid from naturally-occurring materials. *J. Ass. Off. Agric. Chem.*, **37**, 771–7.

Tamura, T., Shin, Y.S., Williams, M.A. and Stokstad, E.L.R. (1972) *Lactobacillus casei* response to pteroylpolyglutamates. *Analyt. Biochem.*, **49**, 517–21.

Toepfer, E.W. (1957) Report on pantothenic acid. Assay for total pantothenic acid: 1956. Collaborative study. *J. Ass. Off. Agric. Chem.*, **40**, 853–5.

Toepfer, E.W. (1960) Microbiological assay for total pantothenic acid. *J. Ass. Off. Analyt. Chem.*, **43**, 28–9.

Toepfer, E.W. and Polansky, M.M. (1964) Recent developments in the analysis for vitamin B_6 in foods. *Vitams Horm.*, **22**, 825–32.

Toepfer, E.W. and Polansky, M.M. (1970) Microbiological assay of vitamin B_6 and its components. *J. Ass. Off. Analyt. Chem.*, **53**, 546–50.

Toepfer, E.W., Zook, E.G. and Richardson, L.R. (1954) Microbiological procedure for the assay of pantothenic acid in foods: results compared with those by bioassay. *J. Ass. Off. Agric. Chem.*, **37**, 182–90.

Toepfer, E.W., Polansky, M.M., Richardson, L.R. and Wilkes, S. (1963) Comparison of vitamin B_6 values of selected food samples by bioassay and microbiological assay. *J. Agric. Fd Chem.*, **11**, 523–5.

Voigt, M.N. and Eitenmiller, R.R. (1978) Comparative review of the thiochrome, microbial and protozoan analyses of B-vitamins. *J. Fd Protection*, **41**, 730–8.

Voigt, M.N., Eitenmiller, R.R. and Ware, G.O. (1979) Vitamin analysis by microbial and protozoan organisms: response to food preservatives and neutralization salts. *J. Fd Sci.*, **44**, 723–8, 737.

Walsh, J.H., Wyse, B.W. and Hansen, R.G. (1979) A comparison of microbiological and radioimmunoassay methods for the determination of pantothenic acid in foods. *J. Fd Biochem.*, **3**, 175–89.

Wegner, M.I., Kemmerer, A.R. and Fraps, G.S. (1942) Influence of the method of preparation of sample on microbiological assay for riboflavin. *J. Biol. Chem.*, **146**, 547–51.

Williams, V.R. (1945) Growth stimulants in the *Lactobacillus arabinosus* biotin assay. *J. Biol. Chem.*, **159**, 237–8.

Williams, V.R. and Fieger, E.A. (1945) Growth stimulants for microbiological biotin assay. *Ind. Engng Chem., Analyt. Edn*, **17**, 127–30.

Williams, W.L., Broquist, H.P. and Snell, E.E. (1947) Oleic acid and related compounds as growth factors for lactic acid bacteria. *J. Biol. Chem.*, **170**, 619–30.

Wright, A.J.A. and Phillips, D.R. (1985) The threshold growth response of *Lactobacillus casei* to 5-methyl-tetrahydrofolic acid: implications for folate assays. *Br. J. Nutr.*, **53**, 569–73.

Biospecific methods for the determination of water-soluble vitamins

8

8.1 INTRODUCTION

Biospecific methods of analysis for selected vitamins of the B group can be broadly classified as immunoassays and protein-binding assays. Enzymatic assays have been developed for vitamin C. Immunoassays are based on the specific interaction of an antibody with its antigen, and are represented by the radioimmunoassay and the ELISA. Protein-binding assays utilize natural vitamin-binding proteins and are represented by the radioassay and the non-isotopic competitive protein-binding assay. Biospecific assays can be performed on complex biological matrices, so they require minimal sample clean-up. The analytical stages of immunoassays and protein-binding assays can be automated using equipment that is commercially available, but the methods can only be described as semi-automated, as it is necessary to liberate the vitamins from their bound forms using manual extraction procedures.

8.2 THE ANTIGEN–ANTIBODY RELATIONSHIP

If a rabbit, for instance, is given repeated small injections of a 'foreign' protein (antigen), then a specific antibody against the foreign protein is produced by the rabbit and circulates in its bloodstream. When the serum of the rabbit (referred to now as antiserum) is added *in vitro* to a solution containing the antigen, the antigen binds to specific sites on the surface of the antibody as it did *in vivo*.

The following terms encountered in immunoassays are taken from Morris, Clifford and Jackman (1988).

Antibody. A binding protein (immunoglobulin) which is synthesized by the immune system of an animal in response to either the invasion of a foreign organism or the injection of an immunogen.
Antigen. A substance that will react with its specific antibody.
Immunogen. A foreign substance that, when injected into a suitable animal, stimulates the production of antibody or antibodies that can combine with the same substance as an antigen.
Antigenic determinant. Structural feature of an antigen which defines the recognition pattern of an antibody.
Hapten. A compound which is unable to act alone as an immunogen because of its low molecular weight (<1000) but which can be made

immunogenic by covalently binding it to a suitable macromolecule, usually a protein.
Antiserum. Serum containing polyclonal antibodies to an antigen.
Polyclonal antibodies. Antibodies to a given antigen which are present in an antiserum and which are derived from several clones of lymphocyte produced in a single animal as the result of an injection of immunogen.
Monoclonal antibodies. Antibodies derived from a single clone of lymphocytes and produced in cell culture by hybridoma cells, which are formed by the fusion of lymphocytes with myeloma cells (cancerous lymphocytes) from an immunized animal donor. The antibody molecules are chemically identical and exhibit identical binding properties.
Cross-reactivity. Ability of substances, other than the antigen, to bind to the antibody, and the ability of substances other than the antibody to bind the antigen. Cross-reactants may be substances that carry on their surface a molecular configuration similar to the antigenic determinants on the antigen being measured.
Affinity. The energy with which the combining sites of an antibody bind its specific antigen. It is analogous to the association constant (K_A) in physical chemistry and has the dimensions of moles/litre.
Avidity. There are several populations of antibodies with different affinities in a polyclonal antiserum, the mean affinity being referred to as its avidity. The high-affinity antibodies dictate the sensitivity of an immunoassay.

The production of monoclonal antibodies (Galfré and Milstein, 1981) is more costly, labour intensive and time-consuming than the production of polyclonal antiserum. However, the provision of potentially unlimited amounts of a homogeneous reagent is a major advantage in the development of commercial assay kits. The higher specificity compared with polyclonal antibodies is another advantage. On the demerit side, monoclonal antibodies rarely exhibit such a high affinity for the antigen as do polyclonal antibodies, and this can result in a less sensitive assay. The affinity is less important for the sensitivity of an excess reagent assay than it is for a competitive assay.

8.3 RADIOASSAY METHODS FOR THE DETERMINATION OF BIOTIN, FOLATE AND VITAMIN B_{12}

8.3.1 GENERAL PROCEDURE

The radioassays which have been applied to the determination of vitamins in biological materials are more precisely termed radiometric competitive protein-binding assays. They are based on the radioisotope-dilution principle, whereby the unknown quantity of the vitamin in the test material, after first being liberated from bound materials, is used to dilute the radioactivity of an added measured quantity of tracer (radioactively labelled vitamin). The analysis usually involves an initial heating step to denature indigenous binding proteins. The radioassay procedure is carried out as follows. Into a centrifuge tube are placed measured volumes of a suitable buffer solution, the test extract or unlabelled vitamin standard, and the tracer. The labelled vitamin is available commercially in powdered form or in solution, and can be standardized against the unlabelled vitamin standard by the isotopic dilution method of Lau *et al.* (1965). The standardization technique allows the actual quantity of labelled vitamin to be calculated for any percentage change in the binding capacity of the protein for the labelled vitamin. A soluble natural vitamin-binding protein is then added in a predetermined quantity that has a maximal capacity to bind only some of the labelled vitamin present. Typical binding capacities are 80–90% for biotin assays (Hood, 1979), 50–60% for folate assays (Waxman, Schreiber and Herbert, 1971), and 60–80% for vitamin B_{12} assays (Lau *et al.*, 1965). The binding protein has a high affinity and specificity for the vitamin in question, but it does not discriminate between labelled and unlabelled vitamin. The tubes are stored at ambient temperature in the dark for a prescribed period. During this time, unlabelled and labelled vitamin will compete stoichiometrically for the limited number of binding sites on the protein molecule. The amount of labelled vitamin that is subsequently bound is inversely related to the amount of indigenous vitamin present. Activated charcoal coated with haemoglobin, albumin or dextran is added and the tube contents are mixed thoroughly. The charcoal coating acts as a molecular sieve, allowing the unbound vitamin to pass through and be adsorbed onto the charcoal, but excluding the protein-bound vitamin. The unbound vitamin is separated from bound vitamin by centrifugation. The specific radioactivity in the supernatant fluid (bound fraction) or in the pellet (unbound fraction) is measured as counts per minute (cpm) in a liquid scintillation counter for β-emitters such as ^{3}H or ^{14}C isotopes or in a gamma counter for γ-emitters such as ^{125}I, ^{75}Se or ^{57}Co isotopes. Included in the assay procedure is a control tube which contains only the tracer and coated charcoal (plus buffer solution to make up the volume). The control represents the amount of radioactivity that is not bound to the charcoal and is due to radioactive degradation products of the tracer. The cpm for the control is subtracted from those for the unknown and the standards in order to obtain net counts. All cpm data must be corrected for counting efficiency if significant differences in efficiency are observed between samples and standards due to quenching effects.

Quantification is achieved by assaying a range of unlabelled vitamin standards of known concentration. Let B represent the amount of bound tracer (net cpm) corresponding to each concentration of standard, and B_M represent the amount of bound tracer (net cpm) corresponding to a zero amount of standard (i.e. the maximal binding capacity of the fixed amount of protein). A linear calibration curve is obtained on logit–log paper (1 × 3 cycle log–log paper) by plotting the percentage of tracer bound at each concentration of standard ($B/B_M \times 100$) as the logit function (ordinate) versus the log concentration (abscissa) or standard in ng/ml. Alternatively, the reciprocal of the percentage of tracer bound versus concentration can be plotted as a straight line on nonlogarithmic graph paper (Dakshinamurti *et al.*, 1974). The concentration of vitamin in the assay solution can be obtained from the standard curve by interpolation of the percentage of tracer binding found or by calculation from the regression equation of the standard curve (Hood, 1977).

8.3.2 DETERMINATION OF BIOTIN

Radioassay techniques for determining biotin are based on the high affinity of the glycoprotein avidin for the functional ureido group of the biotin molecule. Early methods used [^{14}C]biotin, which has a specific radioactivity of 45 mCi/mmol, but a higher sensitivity can be obtained using [^{3}H]biotin of specific activity 2.5 Ci/mmol (Hood, 1979). In a procedure described by Hood (1975), samples of pelleted poultry feeds and wheat were autoclaved with 2 N H_2SO_4 for 1 h at 121 °C, and then neutralized with 20% NaOH. The filtered extracts were incubated with [^{14}C]biotin and the avidin–biotin complex was precipitated with 2% zinc sulphate solution. The method was capable of measuring biotin levels down to 5 μg/kg of biological material and was more than adequate for wheat and poultry feeds, which contained from 68 to 341 μg/kg. Results obtained by radioassay and microbiological (*Lactobacillus plantarum*) assay were similar for poultry feeds, but the radioassay values for two wheat samples were approximately 20% and 55% higher than the microbiological assay values.

Technical difficulties are encountered when acid hydrolysis is used to extract the biotin from biological materials. Firstly, there is the problem of achieving maximum liberation of biotin from bound forms without incurring loss of the vitamin. This requires autoclaving with 6 N H_2SO_4 for animal tissues and 2 N or 3 N H_2SO_4 for plant tissues. Secondly, a large amount of salt is produced on neutralization of the acid extracts, and it is necessary to lower the salt concentration by further dilution.

Bitsch, Salz and Hötzel (1986, 1989) released protein-bound biotin from food samples by means of papain digestion after treatment with liquid nitrogen and homogenization. This enzymatic extraction was used instead of acid hydrolysis. [^{3}H]Biotin was used as the tracer, and non-bound biotin was removed by adsorption on dextran-coated charcoal. The method was applied to samples of meat, offal, cereal products, milk, vegetables and bananas. Results by this method generally agreed well with data from food composition tables, although these literature data vary considerably in some cases. Values for biotin level in cabbage and bananas by the radioassay technique were higher than literature data.

8.3.3 DETERMINATION OF FOLATE

The reported presence of folate-binding activity in cow's milk (Ghitis, 1967; Ghitis, Mandelbaum-Shavit and Grossowicz, 1969), and the association of this binding activity with a minor whey protein isolated from the *β*-lactoglobulin fraction of milk (Ford, Salter and Scott, 1969), led to the development of a radiometric competitive binding assay for measuring folate levels in blood serum (Waxman, Schreiber, and Herbert, 1971). Subsequently, many variations of this technique have been applied to the measurement of folate levels in serum, plasma or red blood cells, and a large number of radioassay kits are commercially available for such analyses. Sources of folate-binding protein (FBP) used in radioassays have included non-fat dry milk, skim milk and whey protein concentrate (Gregory, 1985) as well as crystalline bovine *β*-lactoglobulin (Waxman and Schreiber, 1980). At the physiological pH range of 7.3–7.6, milk FBP shows a greater affinity for binding PGA than for 5-methyl-THF, whereas at pH 9.3 FBP exhibits a similar binding capacity for these folates (Gregory, 1989). The presence of at least one glutamate residue is required for binding to take place as shown by the nonbinding of pteroic acid (Ghitis, Mandelbaum-Shavit and Grossowicz, 1969). Pterin-6-carboxylic acid and *p*-aminobenzoylglutamic acid exhibit little or no affinity for FBP, indicating that these folate degradation products would not significantly interfere with the accuracy of the radioassay (Gregory, Day and Ristow, 1982). Tritiated folic acid, [^{3}H]PGA, labelled in the 3′-, 5′-, 7- and 9-positions, is commercially available in high specific activity (43 Ci/mmol) (Gregory, 1985). The use of ^{125}I- and ^{75}Se-labelled PGA simplifies the assay procedure by eliminating liquid scintillation counting, but these γ-emitters are available only as components of radioassay kits (Waxman and Schreiber, 1980).

In contrast to blood plasma or serum, in which monoglutamyl 5-methyl-THF is virtually the sole folate present (Herbert, Larrabee and Buchanan, 1962), the naturally occurring folates in foodstuffs comprise a variety of polyglutamyl forms, chiefly THF, 5-methyl-THF and 10-formyl-THF (Gregory, 1984). Shane, Tamura and Stokstad (1980) reported that the molar response of different folate compounds in radioassay procedures varied considerably, depending upon the stereochemical form, the reduction state of the pteridine nucleus, the nature of the one-carbon substituent and the number of glutamate residues. This observation appears to rule out the application of radiometric assays for accurately determining the naturally occurring folates in foods. Several studies have been conducted in which the results of the pH 9.3 radioassay have been compared with those of the *L. casei* assay for the determination of total folate in foods (Ruddick, Vanderstoep and Richards, 1978; Graham, Roe and Ostertag, 1980; Klein and Kuo, 1981; Gregory, Day and Ristow, 1982; Österdahl and Johansson, 1989). Ruddick, Vanderstoep and Richards (1978) concluded that the radioassay is suitable only for measuring the particular folate compound used to construct the standard curve for the assay. Another problem is that FBP does not exhibit significant affinity for 5-formyl-THF in the pH 9.3 radioassay (Gregory, Day and Ristow, 1982). Although a minor folate vitamer in most tissues, 5-formyl-THF can be formed extensively from 10-formyl-THF during thermal extraction or food processing, leading to an underestimate of folate activity (Gregory, 1989).

8.3.4 DETERMINATION OF VITAMIN B_{12}

Published radioassay techniques for determining vitamin B_{12} in foods (Richardson *et al.*, 1978; Beck, 1979; Casey *et al.*, 1982; Österdahl *et al.*, 1986; Andersson, Lundqvist and Öste, 1990) are based on the original method of Lau *et al.* (1965), which was developed for measurement of serum B_{12}. Food extracts prepared for radioassay contain 200–1000 pg vitamin B_{12}/ml, which is well within the 50–2000 pg/ml range of commercially available assay kits. A preliminary extraction step is necessary to release the cobalamins from their bound forms and convert them to a single, stable form, cyanocobalamin or sulphitocobalamin. The radioassay utilizes [^{57}Co]cyanocobalamin as the tracer, and intrinsic factor as the binding protein.

In one of two commercial assay kits evaluated by Richardson *et al.* (1978), the binding agent is supplied in the form of a Sephadex (dextran)–intrinsic factor complex, which simplifies the analysis and was found to function more satisfactorily with food extracts than the separate use of intrinsic factor and albumin-coated charcoal.

Ellenbogen (1984) stressed the importance of using purified intrinsic factor for the assay of serum vitamin B_{12} to avoid the binding of inactive non-cobalamin corrinoids to extraneous proteins. As a result of earlier reports of unreliable results, the United States Committee for Clinical Laboratory Standards published a standard, which was ratified by the Food and Drug Administration in 1980, recommending that all radioassay kits for vitamin B_{12} should contain purified intrinsic factor as the vitamin-binding protein.

The extraction techniques employed for the determination of serum vitamin B_{12} are not sufficiently rigorous to liberate the more tightly bound cobalamins present in many foods (Newmark *et al.*, 1976), and it is necessary in food analysis to implement a more rigorous extraction step prior to the radioassay. Beck (1979) developed an extraction procedure that was compatible with radioassay techniques for the determination of cyanocobalamin in seafoods. Homogenized tissue was mixed with sodium nitrite and sodium cyanide, adjusted to pH 4.0 with hydrochloric acid, and boiled for 1 h. The extract was cooled and the coagulated protein was removed by suction filtration. The filtrates from oily fish were extracted with petroleum ether. The extracts were purified and concentrated by extracting the cyanocobalamin into benzyl alcohol, followed by re-extraction into water after the addition of chloroform. Richardson *et al.* (1978) extracted the cobalamins from various foods using pH 4.6 acetate buffer containing sodium cyanide and heating in a boiling water bath for 30 min. Results obtained by radioassay were found to be somewhat lower than comparative results obtained by microbiological assay using *Lactobacillus delbrueckii*. The differences between the two sets of results were postulated to be caused by the extraction not releasing all of the vitamin B_{12} in a form capable of binding to intrinsic factor, although it was usable by the micro-organism. On the other hand, Österdahl *et al.* (1986), using a similar extraction procedure to that of Richardson *et al.* (1978), obtained a very high correlation ($r = 0.987$) between the results from the radioassay method and the microbiological method for the determination of vitamin B_{12} in gruel. Gruel is an infant food based mainly on dry milk and cereals, and its vitamin B_{12} content is mainly derived from the dried milk component. Some gruel products are also fortified with vitamin B_{12}, so these free and bound forms are apparently readily extractable by the method employed. Casey *et al.* (1982) mixed ground food samples with 1.3% w/v anhydrous sodium phosphate dibasic (Na_2HPO_4), 1.2% w/v citric acid and 1.0% w/v sodium metabisulphite ($Na_2S_2O_5$), and then autoclaved the mixture for 10 min at 121 °C according to the extraction procedure described in the AOAC (1990) microbiological method for determining vitamin B_{12} in vitamin preparations. The problems of incomplete extraction reported by Richardson *et al.* (1978) were not encountered, probably because of the more rigorous heat treatment employed, and the results compared quite favourably with results obtained by the AOAC microbiological method. The purification step involving partitioning into benzyl alcohol (Beck, 1979) was not necessary, as the increased specificity of the highly purified intrinsic factor effectively eliminated interference by other biochemical compounds.

Andersson, Lundqvist and Öste (1990) established, by statistical analysis of experimental data, the optimal extraction conditions (cyanide concentration, buffer concentration, pH, method of heating and heating time) for the determination of total vitamin B_{12} in milk by radioassay. The optimized procedure entailed mixing 2 ml of milk with 5 ml of sodium acetate buffer (0.4 M, pH 4.5) and sodium cyanide (2000 ppm), and autoclaving at 121 °C for 25 min. When the optimized extraction technique was used in the *L. delbrueckii* assay there was no significant difference as compared with the radioassay technique. However, the radioassay had a better reproducibility than the microbiological assay. It was shown that autoclaving gave a significantly higher yield than a boiling water bath.

8.4 RADIOIMMUNOASSAY METHOD FOR THE DETERMINATION OF PANTOTHENIC ACID

8.4.1 GENERAL PROCEDURE

The radioimmunoassay is a variation of the radioassay and is based on the competition for a fixed, but limited, number of antibody binding sites by antigen (the vitamin analyte) and a trace amount of radiolabelled antigen added to the sample extract. The amount of tracer that subsequently becomes bound to the antibody is inversely proportional to the amount of analyte initially present. The free and antibody-bound fractions are separated by adsorption or precipitation, followed by centrifugation, and the radioactivity in the supernatant or precipitate is measured. The concentration of vitamin in the assay solution is obtained by reference to a standard curve.

8.4.2 DETERMINATION OF PANTOTHENIC ACID

Walsh, Wyse and Hansen (1979) compared a radioimmunoassay method with the microbiological (*Lactobacillus plantarum*) method for the determination of pantothenic acid in 75 processed and cooked foods. Samples were homogenized in distilled water and stored frozen at −10 °C until analysed. The pantothenic acid was released by autoclaving at 121 °C for 10 min, followed by treatment with a double enzyme system (alkaline phosphatase and pigeon liver enzyme), and the protein was removed by dialysis. Antibody was prepared by injecting rabbits with a pantothenic acid–bovine serum albumin conjugate, and the resulting antiserum was diluted 100-fold with a solution of rabbit albumin. Each assay tube contained 0.5 ml of the diluted antiserum, 0.50 ml of standard or sample, and 50 μl of [^{3}H]sodium *d*-pantothenate. After incubation at room temperature for 15 min, neutral saturated ammonium sulphate was added to achieve a 50% saturation, and the suspension was centrifuged. The precipitate was washed with 0.5 ml of half-saturated ammonium sulphate and recentrifuged. The washed precipitate, containing antibody-bound pantothenic acid, was dissolved in 0.5 ml of tissue solubilizer and transferred quantitatively to vials containing 12 ml of scintillation fluid. The radioactivity results (cpm) were read on a 5–150 ng (per 0.5 ml) standard curve. An enzyme blank value was subtracted from each sample value. Although the results from the radioimmunoassay and microbiological assay were highly correlated ($r = 0.94$), the microbiological assay produced a higher average result for the food types meats, fruits and vegetables, and breads and cereals. It was postulated that bacterial enzymes in the assay organism promote further breakdown of bound vitamin, or nonenzymatic breakdown occurs during the long microbiological incubation period. The results of the individual foods analysed by the radioimmunoassay method have been reported by Walsh, Wyse and Hansen (1981).

8.5 ELISA METHODS FOR THE DETERMINATION OF PANTOTHENIC ACID AND VITAMIN B_6

8.5.1 GENERAL PROCEDURE

An ELISA is an enzyme-linked immunoassay in which one of the reactants is immobilized by physical adsorption onto the surface of a solid phase. In its simplest form, as used in food analysis applications, the solid phase is provided by the plastic surface of a 96-well microtitration plate. The ELISA can be performed manually, with the aid of push-button dispensers, or it can be totally automated, complete with computer for calculation of standard curves, statistical analysis of results and data storage.

There are many variants of the ELISA, but in a discussion of basic principles they fall into two main types, namely competitive and noncompetitive (reagent excess) immunoassays.

In the direct competitive ELISA the analyte vitamin molecules and added enzyme–vitamin conjugate compete for a limited number of binding sites on the immobilized antibody. The proportion of added enzyme–vitamin conjugate present in either the free or bound phases after equilibrium has been reached is dependent upon the amount of analyte initially present. The phases are separated by emptying the well contents and washing the plate. The amount of bound enzyme is then determined by addition of substrate and spectrophotometric measurement of the coloured product. A variation of this format is the indirect competitive ELISA, in which the analyte and immobilized analyte compete for a limited number of binding sites on the enzyme-labelled antibody. The characteristic feature of competitive ELISAs is that the higher the optical density, the lower is the amount of analyte.

The generally preferred ELISA format for vitamin assays in food analysis is a two-site noncompetitive assay used in the indirect mode. This format employs two antibodies: a primary anti-vitamin antibody raised against a hapten–protein conjugate, and an enzyme-labelled, species-specific second antibody, which binds specifically to the primary antibody. The scheme for performing such an ELISA is depicted in Figure 8.1. A protein conjugate of the vitamin is immobilized to the well surface of the microtitration plate, the attached protein being different to that used for the immunogen. The protein adsorbs passively and strongly to the plastic and, once coated, plates can usually be stored for several months. To perform the assay, the sample or standard is added to the well, followed by a limited amount of primary antibody. After incubation, the antibody becomes distributed between immobilized vitamin and free vitamin according to the amount of analyte initially present. After phase separation, achieved by well emptying and washing, the second antibody is added in excess, and the plate is incubated for a second time. Excess unbound material is removed and

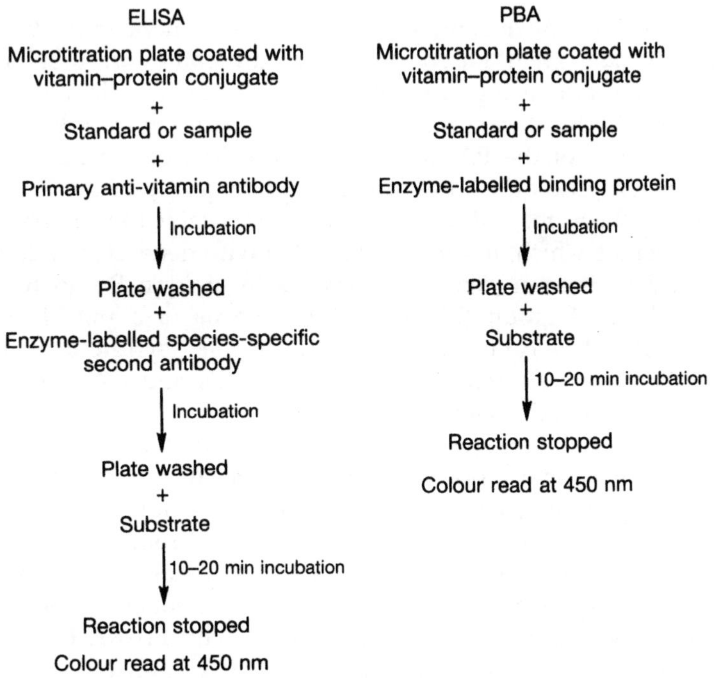

Figure 8.1 Comparison of methodologies for the two-site noncompetitive ELISA (indirect mode) and the competitive PBA (indirect mode) (from Lee *et al.*, 1990).

substrate is added. Optical densities are measured after a suitable time, and unknown samples are quantified by reference to the behaviour of vitamin standards.

In contrast to the competitive ELISA, the noncompetitive assay uses an excess of antibody, so that the optical densities increase with increasing amount of analyte. Although the competitive assay produces its greatest signal (optical density) for low concentrations of analyte, the noncompetitive assay gives lower detection limits. It is also more specific, since the two antibodies recognize separate antigenic determinants on the analyte. Two other advantages of the noncompetitive assay are that the affinity of the primary antibody is less important than in the competitive assay, since excess antibody is used, and the accuracy of pipetting the primary antibody is less critical, since it is no longer a limiting factor (Gould, 1988). Enzyme-labelled second antibodies are widely available commercially, active against different species, and labelled with a variety of enzymes. In summary, noncompetitive assays are more reliable and more rugged than competitive assays, with the added advantages of improved sensitivity and specificity.

8.5.2 DETERMINATION OF PANTOTHENIC ACID

With the aim of developing an indirect two-site noncompetitive ELISA, Morris *et al.* (1988) raised polyclonal antibodies in rabbits against pantothenic acid using two different pantothenic acid–bovine serum albumin (PA–BSA) immunogens, each prepared by coupling at one of the two ends of the PA molecule. In the first of the hapten–protein conjugation procedures, the primary alcohol group of the PA molecule (Figure 8.2) was reacted with bromoacetyl bromide to form bromoacetyl pantothenate which, in turn, was reacted with denatured reduced BSA. The second immunogen was prepared by linking PA to BSA at the carboxylic acid group (Figure 8.2) by means of a mixed anhydride procedure. Purification of the immunogens synthesized by each procedure was effected by extensive dialysis and column chromatography on Sephadex G-25.

Two ELISAs were set up with the different antisera, using two pantothenic acid–keyhole limpet haemocyanin (PA–KLH) protein conjugates for plate coating. ELISA system 1 employed the antiserum raised against immunogen prepared by the bromoacetyl method in association with PA-KLH prepared in a similar manner. ELISA system 2 employed the antiserum raised against immunogen prepared by the mixed anhydride procedure in association with PA-KLH produced by reaction with carbodiimide. Both systems utilized commercially available anti-rabbit immunoglobulin–alkaline phosphatase conjugate as the enzyme-labelled second antibody.

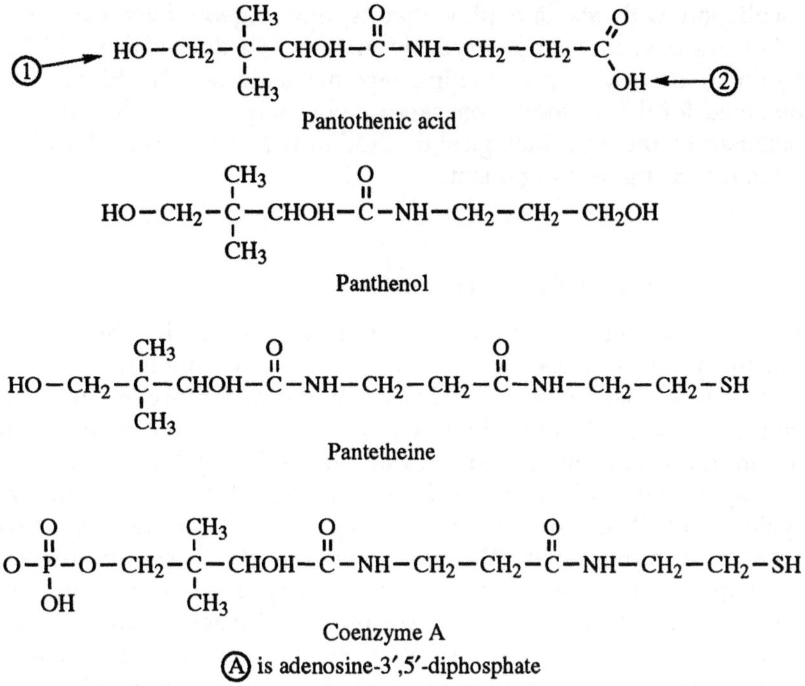

Figure 8.2 Structures of pantothenic acid and related compounds. The coupling of pantothenic acid to protein (BSA) is indicated by (1) for bromoacetyl derivatization and conjugation and (2) for mixed anhydride procedure.

ELISA system 1, using the primary alcohol group for hapten–protein coupling, was very specific for PA, and did not recognize the analogues panthenol or pantetheine. In contrast, ELISA system 2, using the carboxylic acid group for coupling, gave high cross-reactions with panthenol and pantetheine. These analogues differ structurally from PA at the carboxyl end of the molecule (Figure 8.2), and the observations illustrate that antibodies exhibit the greatest specificity for functional groups on the hapten molecule that are distal to the point of coupling. Neither ELISA system recognized coenzyme A, the major bound form of PA in foods, because this compound contains PA derivatized at both ends of the molecule (Figure 8.2).

ELISA system 1, rather than system 2, was selected for application because of its greater specificity and lower limit of detection (0.5 ng/well versus 5 ng/well). The validation and application of ELISA system 1 for the analysis of six foods representing major sources of PA in the UK diet was reported by Finglas *et al.* (1988a). Sample preparation entailed autoclaving at 121 °C for 15 min, homogenization, and overnight incubation with alkaline phosphatase and pigeon liver extract. The following day, the sample hydrolysates were autoclaved at 121 °C for 5 min to destroy any remaining enzyme activity. The ELISA values obtained for the six foods compared favourably ($r = 0.999$) with values obtained by the microbiological method of Bell (1974) using *Lactobacillus plantarum* as the test organism.

8.5.3 DETERMINATION OF VITAMIN B_6

The ideal biospecific assay for vitamin B_6 is one which exhibits a broad specificity and provides a value for the total B_6 content, but no such assay has yet been reported. Alcock, Finglas and Morgan (1990) raised polyclonal antibodies in rabbits using a purified PL–BSA conjugate as the immunogen, but the antisera all showed a preference for PM. A corresponding preference for PMP was reported for antisera raised against PLP–BSA using polyclonal (Córdoba, Gonzalez and Rivera, 1966) and monoclonal (Viceps-Madore *et al.*, 1983) immunization techniques. The general preference displayed for the amine forms probably reflects the fact that the protein linkage to the 4-carbonyl groups is an ε-amino group of a lysine residue, and hence the conjugate is an amine derivative most resembling PM or PMP.

Alcock, Finglas and Morgan (1990) set up an indirect two-site noncompetitive ELISA procedure using a PM-specific antiserum preparation and anti-rabbit immunoglobulin horseradish peroxidase conjugate as the enzyme-labelled second antibody. The microtitration plates were coated with a PL–KLH conjugate. The assay limit of detection was 7 pg of PM per well. Food samples were autoclaved with 0.2 N H_2SO_4 at 121 °C for 20 min, cooled, homogenized, adjusted to pH 4.5, centrifuged and filtered.

PM measurement alone by ELISA is of little practical use in food analysis as, after acid hydrolysis, PL and PN frequently predominate in animal- and plant-derived foods, respectively. One of the antiserum preparations, which exhibited 80% cross-reactivity with PN with a detection limit of 100 pg/well, would be useful for the determination of added PN in fortified foods. There are two possible approaches towards developing an ELISA for determining total vitamin B_6. Experiments with different conjugation procedures might produce an antibody that could recognize vitamin B_6 irrespective of the functional group at the C-4 position, although such an antibody would probably also recognize the non-active metabolite, 4-pyridoxic acid. Alternatively, antisera or monoclonal antibodies specific for each nonphosphorylated B_6 vitamer could be produced, and mixed to allow the determination of total B_6 after acid hydrolysis, or used separately to determine the individual vitamers.

8.6 NON-ISOTOPIC PROTEIN-BINDING ASSAY METHODS FOR THE DETERMINATION OF BIOTIN, FOLATE AND VITAMIN B_{12}

8.6.1 GENERAL PROCEDURE

A non-isotopic competitive protein-binding assay (PBA) in the indirect mode has been developed for food analysis applications using the 96-well microtitration plate as the solid phase. Individual methods have been reported for the determination of biotin, folate and vitamin B_{12} using avidin, milk FBP and R-protein as the respective vitamin-specific binding proteins. The principle of the assay is based on the competition between immobilized vitamin and free vitamin (analyte) in the assay solution for a limited number of binding sites on the enzyme-linked vitamin-binding protein. The amount of protein bound to the well surface is inversely proportional to the concentration of free vitamin in the assay solution and is determined, after plate washing, by measuring the enzyme activity. The scheme for performing such an assay is compared with an ELISA format in Figure 8.1.

8.6.2 DETERMINATION OF BIOTIN

In a protein-binding assay for the determination of biotin in fresh lamb's liver (Finglas, Faulks and Morgan, 1986), biotin–KLH conjugate was synthesized by the carbodiimide method and used to form the immobilized phase. The binding protein–enzyme conjugate was avidin–horseradish peroxidase, which is commercially available, and the substrate was 2,2′-azino-bis-(3-ethylbenzthiazoline sulphonic acid) (ABTS). The extraction of liver samples entailed autoclaving with 6 N H_2SO_4 at 121 °C for 30 min, followed by neutralization to pH 7.0, filtration, and dilution with phosphate-buffered saline (pH 7.4) containing 0.05% Tween 20. The value obtained for biotin in the pooled liver sample was 37.0 μg per 100 g fresh weight, which compared favourably with the microbiological assay value of 41 μg per 100 g fresh weight of lamb's liver quoted by Paul and Southgate (1978). From a biotin standard curve, the detection limit was calculated to be 10 pg/well.

8.6.3 DETERMINATION OF FOLATE

In a protein-binding assay developed for folate determination in foods (Finglas, Faulks and Morgan, 1988), the immobilized phase was PGA–KLH, the enzyme–protein conjugate was peroxidase–FPB, and the substrate was ABTS. Based on the interpretation of cross-reactivity data, the assay has no utility for the simultaneous determination of PGA, 5-formyl-THF and 5-methyl-THF in foods. However, the assay, using a PGA standard, would be applicable for determining added PGA in fortified food, with cross-reactions of less than 10% for the two THF derivatives and a detection limit of 6 pg PGA per well. The requirement for analysing non-fortified foods is to determine 5-formyl-THF and 5-methyl-THF, since these two compounds represent the major naturally occurring folates in food samples subjected to prolonged heat treatment during extraction (Gregory, 1989). Using the more stable 5-formyl-THF as the standard, the cross-reaction with 5-methyl-THF was 87%, which implies that the method would be suitable for estimating naturally occurring folate at detection limits of 34 and 36 pg per well for the two respective THF derivatives. Experiments using 5-formyl-THF–KLH-coated plates were unsuccessful in obtaining similar responses for the three folate compounds.

The assay procedure developed by Finglas, Faulks and Morgan (1988) has been applied to the determination of folate in raw and cooked vegetables (Finglas *et al.*, 1988b). Samples were also analysed by the microbiological assay procedure of Phillips and Wright (1982), using *Lactobacillus casei* as the test organism. The results from the two assays were compared using regression analysis. The data gave a linear relationship over the range 0–400 μg/100 g with a correlation coefficient, *r*, of 0.939, which signified good agreement. The folate values obtained using both assays were significantly higher than values reported in food composition tables, which were obtained using the *L. casei* method of Bell (1974). The underestimation of folate values using the method of Bell has been previously discussed (see section 7.4.7).

8.6.4 DETERMINATION OF VITAMIN B_{12}

In a protein-binding assay for the determination of cyanocobalamin in fortified breakfast cereals (Alcock, Finglas and Morgan, 1992), the immobilized phase was cyanocobalamin–KLH, the enzyme–protein conjugate was peroxidase–R-protein, and the substrate was 3,3′,5,5′-tetramethylbenzidine. The immobilized phase was prepared by the bromoacetyl bromide coupling procedure using the primary alcohol group on the ribose 3-phosphate moiety. This method of synthesis gave improved assay sensitivity compared to methods in which the conjugate was synthesized using the carboxylamide groups on the corrin ring structure (Olesen, Hippe and Haber, 1971; Van de Weil, Goedemans and Woldring, 1974). The binding protein–enzyme conjugate was prepared by reacting a dialysate of periodate-activated horseradish peroxidase with R-protein in pH 9.2 buffer. Sodium borohydride solution was added to the reaction mixture, and the mixture was stirred for 1 h before overnight dialysis against phosphate-buffered saline (pH 7.4) at 4 °C. The conjugate was purified on a Superose 6 column and stored in glycerol/water (1 : 1, v/v) at −20 °C. R-protein was used in preference to intrinsic factor because of its lower cost. R-protein binds all corrinoids (cobalamins and non-active analogues), whereas intrinsic factor binds only cobalamins. However, for application to fortified foods, where a single vitamin B_{12} form (cyanocobalamin) predominates, the lack of absolute specificity is of no practical significance.

The extraction step in the sample preparation was designed to be compatible with the maintenance of protein-binding activity. Finely ground samples of breakfast cereals (10 g) were shaken with 40 ml of buffered (pH 7.0) methanol/water (1 : 1, v/v) containing sodium nitrate, and then centrifuged. The pellet was twice further extracted with 25 ml and then 15 ml of extraction buffer, and the combined supernatants were made up to 100 ml with buffer. The lack of matrix interference was demonstrated by comparing standard curves prepared in extracts of non-fortified cereals and in assay buffer, and observing correlation coefficients of 0.971 and 0.972 for two different cereals. The assay exhibited a detection limit of 9 pg of cyanocobalamin standard per well, which was not sufficiently sensitive to measure the levels of naturally occurring vitamin B_{12} in foods.

8.7 ENZYMATIC METHODS FOR THE DETERMINATION OF VITAMIN C

Enzymatic assays have been reported for the quantitative determination of the coenzyme forms of most of the B-group vitamins. Among these is an assay for PLP based on the measurement of $^{14}CO_2$ evolved during the decarboxylation of L-[1-^{14}C]tyrosine by PLP-dependent tyrosine apo-decarboxylase (Chabner and Livingston, 1970). The use of such assays is limited to clinical analysis since, for food analysis, it is necessary to determine total vitamin activity, which requires the conversion of all vitamers to a coenzymatically active form. One exception is biotin, which exists as a single vitamer. One particular enzymatic method for determining biotin is based on the enzymatic binding of biotin *in situ* to the pyruvate carboxylase apoprotein of biotin-deficient bakers' yeast, and the subsequent estimation of the pyruvate carboxylase activity by a $^{14}CO_2$-fixation method (Haarasilta, 1978).

Enzymatic methods for determining ascorbic acid in foodstuffs have been reported. These are based on the enzymatic oxidation of ascorbic acid, and are inherently simpler than methods based on coenzymatic activity.

8.7.1 DETERMINATION OF VITAMIN C

The following enzymatic reactions have been utilized for determining ascorbic acid in biological materials.

$$\text{(1) L-ascorbic acid} + \tfrac{1}{2}O_2 \xrightarrow{\text{ascorbate oxidase}} \text{dehydroascorbic acid} + H_2O$$

Ascorbate oxidase is specific for substrates that possess an enediol function adjacent to a carbonyl group (Doner, 1984).

$$\text{(2) L-ascorbic acid} + H_2O_2 \xrightarrow{\text{ascorbate peroxidase}} \text{dehydroascorbic acid} + 2H_2O$$

Marchesini *et al.* (1974) determined ascorbic acid in fresh and canned spinach by monitoring the oxygen consumed during reaction (1) using a Clark oxygen electrode. A disadvantage of this technique is that the oxygen electrode needs repeated and very precise calibration at constant temperature (±0.01 °C), which limits the widespread applicability of the method for routine analysis.

Casella *et al.* (1989) utilized reaction (2) in a spectrophotometric method to determine ascorbic acid in fruits and vegetables using the dye 1,4-diaminobenzene as a synthetic substrate. Ascorbate peroxidase catalyses the oxidation of ascorbic acid at a much higher rate than it does 1,4-diaminobenzene, and therefore when a mixture of these compounds is treated with catalytic amounts of the enzyme in the presence of hydrogen peroxide, the appearance of the highly coloured products of oxidation of 1,4-diaminobenzene can be taken as the end-point for the oxidation of ascorbic acid. The procedure entailed placing an aliquot of the sample extract (previously adjusted to pH 5.3) into the optical cell, adding buffered enzyme and dye solution, and mixing. The reaction was initiated by addition of hydrogen peroxide, with constant stirring, and the time course of the reaction was monitored by reading the absorbance at 320 nm. Total vitamin C was determined by prior treatment of the sample extracts with homocysteine to reduce dehydro-ascorbic acid to ascorbic acid. The absence of interference by biological compounds was demonstrated by oxidizing the indigenous ascorbic acid by treatment of sample extracts with ascorbate oxidase, followed by addition of acid to deactivate the enzyme. Known amounts of ascorbic acid were then added to the treated extracts to determine the specificity of the peroxidase method.

The samples analysed by the peroxidase method were also analysed by the AOAC 2,6-dichlorophenolindophenol titration method and by the oxidase method of Marchesini *et al.* (1974). No significant difference was observed between the results obtained using the two enzymatic methods, but the results of the titration method were significantly higher, particularly for heat-treated (blanched) vegetables. The loss of accuracy of the titration method in these conditions was attributable to interference by some reducing substances produced during the heat treatment (Association of Vitamin Chemists, Inc., 1966). The peroxidase method represents an improvement upon the method using ascorbate oxidase, because it is more flexible, easier to handle, and does not require expensive instrumentation. In addition, the peroxidase enzyme is of relatively low cost and is available commercially in purified form.

REFERENCES

Alcock, S.C., Finglas, P.M. and Morgan, M.R.A. (1990) An enzyme-linked immunosorbent assay for pyridoxamine and its comparison with alternative analytical procedures. *Fd Agric. Immunol.* **2**, 197–204.

Alcock, S.C., Finglas, P.M. and Morgan, M.R.A. (1992) Production and purification of an R-protein–enzyme conjugate for use in a microtitration plate protein-binding assay for vitamin B_{12} in fortified food. *Fd Chem.*, **45**, 199–203.

Andersson, I., Lundqvist, R. and Öste, R. (1990) Analysis of vitamin B_{12} in milk by a radioisotope dilution assay. *Milchwissenschaft*, **45**, 507–9.

AOAC (1990) Cobalamin (vitamin B_{12} activity) in vitamin preparations. Microbiological methods. Final action 1960. In *AOAC Official Methods of Analysis*, 15th edn (ed. K. Helrich), Association of Official Analytical Chemists, Inc., Arlington, VA, 952.20.

Association of Vitamin Chemists, Inc. (1966) *Methods of Vitamin Assay*, 3rd edn, Interscience Publishers, New York.

Beck, R.A. (1979) Comparison of two radioassay methods for cyanocobalamin in seafoods. *J. Fd Sci.*, **44**, 1077–9.

Bell, J.G. (1974) Microbiological assay of vitamins of the B group in foodstuffs. *Lab. Pract.*, **23**, 235–42, 252.

Bitsch, R., Salz, I. and Hötzel, D. (1986) Determination of biotin in foods by a protein binding assay. *Deutsche Lebensmittel-Rundschau* **82**, 80–3.

Bitsch, R., Salz, I. and Hötzel, D. (1989) Biotin assessment in foods and body fluids by a protein binding assay (PBA). *Int. J. Vitam. Nutr. Res.*, **59**, 59–64.

Casella, L., Gullotti, M., Marchesini, A. and Petrarulo, M. (1989) Rapid enzymatic method for vitamin C assay in fruits and vegetables using peroxidase. *J. Fd Sci.*, **54**, 374–5, 378.

Casey, P.J., Speckman, K.R., Ebert, F.J. and Hobbs, W.E. (1982) Radioisotope dilution technique for determination of vitamin B_{12} in foods. *J. Ass. Off. Analyt. Chem.*, **65**, 85–8.

Chabner, B. and Livingston, D. (1970) A simple enzymic assay for pyridoxal phosphate. *Analyt. Biochem.*, **34**, 413–23.

Córdoba, F., Gonzalez, C. and Rivera, P. (1966) Antibodies against pyridoxal 5′-phosphate and pyridoxamine 5′-phosphate. *Biochim. Biophys. Acta*, **127**, 151–8.

Dakshinamurti, K., Landman, A.D., Ramamurti, L. and Constable, R.J. (1974) Isotope dilution assay for biotin. *Analyt. Biochem.*, **61**, 225–31.

Doner, L.W. (1984) Analysis of ascorbic acid and related compounds in fluids and tissues. In *Trace Analysis*, Vol. 3 (ed. J.F. Lawrence), Academic Press, Inc., New York, pp. 113–38.

Ellenbogen, L. (1984) Vitamin B_{12}. In *Handbook of Vitamins. Nutritional, Biochemical, and Clinical Aspects* (ed. L.J. Machlin), Marcel Dekker, Inc., New York, pp. 497–547.

Finglas, P.M., Faulks, R.M. and Morgan, M.R.A. (1986) The analysis of biotin in liver using a protein-binding assay. *J. Micronutr. Anal.*, **2**, 247–57.

Finglas, P.M., Faulks, R.M. and Morgan, M.R.A. (1988) The development and characterisation of a protein-binding assay for the determination of folate – potential use in food analysis. *J. Micronutr. Anal.*, **4**, 295–308.

Finglas, P.M., Faulks, R.M., Morris, H.C., Scott, K.J. and Morgan, M.R.A. (1988a) The development of an enzyme-linked immunosorbent assay (ELISA) for the analysis of pantothenic acid and analogues. Part II – Determination of pantothenic acid in foods. *J. Micronutr. Anal.*, **4**, 47–59.

Finglas, P.M., Kwiatkowska, C., Faulks, R.M. and Morgan, M.R.A. (1988b) Comparison of a non-isotopic, microtitration plate folate-binding protein assay and a microbiological method for the determination of folate in raw and cooked vegetables. *J. Micronutr. Anal.*, **4**, 309–22.

Ford, J.E., Salter, D.N. and Scott, K.J. (1969) The folate-binding protein in milk. *J. Dairy Res.*, **36**, 435–46.

Galfré, G. and Milstein, C. (1981) Preparation of monoclonal antibodies: strategies and procedures. *Methods Enzymol.*, **73B**, 3–46.

Ghitis, J. (1967) The folate binding in milk. *Am. J. Clin. Nutr.*, **20**, 1–4.

Ghitis, J., Mandelbaum-Shavit, F. and Grossowicz, N. (1969) Binding of folic acid and derivatives by milk. *Am. J. Clin. Nutr.*, **22**, 156–62.

Gould, B.J. (1988) The use of enzymes in ultrasensitive immunoassays. In *Immunoassays for Veterinary and Food Analysis – 1* (eds B.A. Morris, M.N. Clifford and R. Jackman), Elsevier Applied Science, London and New York, pp. 53–65.

Graham, D.C., Roe, D.A. and Ostertag, S.G. (1980) Radiometric determination and chick bioassay of folacin in fortified and unfortified frozen foods. *J. Fd Sci.*, **45**, 47–51.

Gregory, J.F. (1984) Determination of folacin in foods and other biological materials. *J. Ass. Off. Analyt. Chem.*, **67**, 1015–19.

Gregory, J.F. (1985) Folacin. Chromatographic and radiometric assays. In *Methods of Vitamin Assay*, 4th edn (eds J. Augustin, B.P. Klein, D. Becker and P.B. Venugopal), John Wiley & Sons, New York, pp. 473–96.

Gregory, J.F. (1989) Chemical and nutritional aspects of folate research: analytical procedures, methods of folate synthesis, stability, and bioavailability of dietary folates. *Adv. Fd Nutr. Res.*, **33**, 1–101.

Gregory, J.F., Day, B.P.F. and Ristow, K.A. (1982) Comparison of high performance liquid chromatographic, radiometric, and *Lactobacillus casei* methods for the determination of folacin in selected foods. *J. Fd Sci.*, **47**, 1568–71.

Haarasilta, S. (1978) Enzymatic determination of biotin. *Analyt. Biochem.*, **87**, 306–15.

Herbert, V., Larrabee, A.R. and Buchanan, J.M. (1962) Studies on the identification of a folate compound of human serum. *J. Clin. Invest.*, **41**, 1134–8.

Hood, R.L. (1975) A radiochemical assay for biotin in biological materials. *J. Sci. Fd Agric*, **26**, 1847–52.

Hood, R.L. (1977) The use of linear regression analysis in the isotope dilution assay of biotin. *Analyt. Biochem.*, **79**, 635–8.

Hood, R.L. (1979) Isotopic dilution assay for biotin: use of [^{14}C]biotin. *Methods Enzymol.*, **62D**, 279–83.

Klein, B.P. and Kuo, C.H.Y. (1981) Comparison of microbiological and radiometric assays for determining total folacin in spinach. *J. Fd Sci.*, **46**, 552–4.

Lau, K.-S., Gottlieb, C., Wasserman, L.R. and Herbert, V. (1965) Measurement of serum vitamin B_{12} level using radioisotope dilution and coated charcoal. *Blood*, **26**, 202–14.

Lee, H.A., Mills, E.N.C., Finglas, P.M. and Morgan, M.R.A. (1990) Rapid biospecific methods of vitamin analysis. *J. Micronutr. Anal.*, **7**, 261–70.

Marchesini, A., Montuori, F., Muffato, D. and Maestri, D. (1974) Application and advantages of the enzymatic method for the assay of ascorbic and dehydroascorbic acids and reductones. Determination in fresh and canned spinach. *J. Fd Sci.*, **39**, 568–71.

Morris, B.A., Clifford, M.N. and Jackman, R. (eds) (1988) *Immunoassays for Veterinary and Food Analysis – 1*, Elsevier Applied Science, London and New York.

Morris, H.C., Finglas, P.M., Faulks, R.M. and Morgan, M.R.A. (1988) The development of an enzyme-linked immunosorbent assay (ELISA) for the analysis of pantothenic acid and analogues. Part I – Production of antibodies and establishment of ELISA systems. *J. Micronutr. Anal.*, **4**, 33–45.

Newmark, H.L., Scheiner, J., Marcus, M. and Prabhudesai, M. (1976) Stability of vitamin B_{12} in the presence of ascorbic acid. *Am. J. Clin. Nutr.*, **29**, 645–9.

Olesen, H., Hippe, E. and Haber, E. (1971) Nature of vitamin B_{12} binding. 1. Covalent coupling of hydroxocobalamin to soluble and insoluble carriers. *Biochim. Biophys. Acta*, **243**, 66–74.

Österdahl, B.-G. and Johansson, E. (1989) Comparison of radiometric and microbiological assays for the determination of folate in fortified gruel and porridge. *Int. J. Vitam. Nutr. Res.*, **59**, 147–50.

Österdahl, B.-G., Janné, K., Johansson, E. and Johnsson, H. (1986) Determination of vitamin B_{12} in gruel by a radioisotope dilution assay. *Int. J. Vitam. Nutr. Res.*, **56**, 95–9.

Paul, A.A. and Southgate, D.A.T. (1978) *McCance and Widdowson's The Composition of Foods*, 4th edn, HM Stationery Office, London.

Phillips, D.R. and Wright, A.J.A. (1982) Studies on the response of *Lactobacillus casei* to different folate monoglutamates. *Br. J. Nutr.*, **47**, 183–9.

Richardson, P.J., Favell, D.J., Gidley, G.C. and Jones, G.H. (1978) Application of a commercial radioassay test kit to the determination of vitamin B_{12} in food. *Analyst, Lond.*, **103**, 865–8.

Ruddick, J.E., Vanderstoep, J. and Richards, J.F. (1978) Folate levels in food – a comparison of microbiological assay and radioassay methods for measuring folate. *J. Fd Sci.*, **43**, 1238–41.

Shane, B., Tamura, T. and Stokstad, E.L.R. (1980) Folate assay: a comparison of radioassay and microbiological methods. *Clin. Chim. Acta*, **100**, 13–19.

Van de Weil, D.F.M., Goedemans, W.T. and Woldring, M.G. (1974) Production and purification of antibody against protein–vitamin B_{12} conjugates for radioimmunoassay purposes. *Clin. Chim. Acta*, **56**, 143–9.

Viceps-Madore, D., Cidlowski, J.A., Kittler, J.M. and Thanassi, J.W. (1983) *J. Biol. Chem.*, **258**, 2689–96.

Walsh, J.H., Wyse, B.W. and Hansen, R.G. (1979) A comparison of microbiological and radioimunoassay methods for the determination of pantothenic acid in foods. *J. Fd Biochem.*, **3**, 175–89.

Walsh, J.H., Wyse, B.W. and Hansen, R.G. (1981) Pantothenic acid content of 75 processed and cooked foods. *J. Am. Dietetic Ass.*, **78**, 140–4.

Waxman, S. and Schreiber, C. (1980) Determination of folate by use of radioactive folate and binding proteins. *Methods Enzymol.*, **66**, 468–83.

Waxman, S., Schreiber, C. and Herbert, V. (1971) Radioisotopic assay for measurement of serum folate levels. *Blood*, **38**, 219–28.

Appraisal of analytical techniques 9

9.1 BIOLOGICAL ACTIVITY AND BIOAVAILABILITY

The nutritional value of a food commodity or diet with respect to a particular vitamin is related to the quantity of the vitamin present and its bioavailability. Bioavailability has been defined in the experimental context as the biological vitamin activity or potency (expressed as the sum concentration of biologically available forms of the vitamin) divided by the total concentration of the vitamin as determined by microbiological or physicochemical assay (Gregory, 1988). The biological activity can be determined directly by means of an animal bioassay, but it would be more practicable to use an *in vitro* method of analysis preceded by an appropriate extraction procedure. In most cases, the extraction procedures do not adequately model mammalian digestion and absorption processes, and an *in vitro* assay can only replace an animal bioassay if a statistical correlation (r = >0.95) can be demonstrated between the results of the two methods for a particular food sample.

9.2 PRINCIPAL ANALYTICAL TECHNIQUES

9.2.1 MICROBIOLOGICAL ASSAYS

Microbiological assays can be applied to all of the B-group vitamins, and have adequate sensitivity for measuring the levels of naturally occurring vitamins in those foods that are useful sources of the vitamin of interest. The assay organisms are selected on the basis of their specific requirement for vitamin forms that are biologically active in humans. Microbiological assays using lactic acid bacteria or yeasts require the chemical or enzymatic liberation of bound vitamin. Protozoa exhibit a more mammalian-like response to the various naturally occurring forms of the vitamins, but require longer incubation times than do lactic acid bacteria (3–5 days versus 24–48 h).

All of the B-group vitamins can be determined in a combined operation by means of the turbidimetric microbiological assay, and this is convenient for analytical surveys conducted in microbiological laboratories. The equipment, bacterial cultures and ready-made media are commercially available, and for most of the vitamins the assay procedure is standardized. Measurement of metabolic CO_2, instead of turbidimetric measurement, simplifies sample clean-up and can be accomplished, without the use of radioactivity, with the aid of an infrared CO_2 analyser.

Microbiological assays suffer from many disadvantages, such as their cumbersome nature, long incubation times, tedium and poor precision. Carefully standardized conditions and technical skill are required to obtain repeatable results but, even with good within-laboratory precision, reproducibility between laboratories can be difficult to achieve, especially with folate assays. Additional problems include stimulation or inhibition of growth by other compounds, nonlinear response (drift) for various volumes of food extract analysed, and unequal responses among vitamers of vitamin B_6 and folate. Ongoing research in microbial genetics may lead to the development of new strains of organisms that exhibit a more specific requirement for the vitamin analyte.

9.2.2 IMMUNOASSAYS AND PROTEIN-BINDING ASSAYS

Immunoassays and protein-binding assays are possible alternatives to microbiological assays, being at least as sensitive, but less prone to interference. ELISAs and non-isotopic protein-binding assays using microtitration plates allow the batchwise analysis of large numbers of sample extracts, without the problems of handling and disposal of radioactive material encountered with radioassays and radioimmunoassays. The high technology is built into the reagents, so the assays are simple to perform using either manual or automated operation. It is still necessary, however, to chemically or enzymatically extract the vitamins from the food matrix, as these biospecific techniques depend upon the vitamins being in their free forms. Biospecific techniques have not yet reached the stage of development where they can be applied routinely to food vitamin analysis. The routine use of microtitration plate techniques for vitamin assays will depend upon their successful applicability and validation, and commercial availability of standardized assay kits.

9.2.3 HPLC AND GLC

HPLC is undoubtedly the current method of choice for determining the added thiamin, riboflavin, nicotinamide and pyridoxine in fortified foods. Many food laboratories are equipped with HPLC, and combinations of these vitamins (certainly thiamin and riboflavin) can be analysed simultaneously. HPLC techniques using fluorimetric detection are more accurate than manual or semi-automated fluorimetric methods for determining thiamin and riboflavin, because their specificity depends upon chromatographic separation rather than a chemical reaction. The suitability of an HPLC method depends upon the use of appropriate extraction and clean-up procedures. The latter can often be achieved simply and efficiency using solid-phase extraction which, with selective elution, can also act as a concentration step.

The applicability of HPLC for the determination of naturally occurring vitamins is somewhat limited, and the technique lacks the required sensitivity to accurately measure the low levels of pantothenic acid, biotin and vitamin B_{12} in foods. It cannot be guaranteed that HPLC will account for all of the biologically active forms of a vitamin that would be measured by microbiological assay and, in this respect, the inherent specificity of HPLC may lead to an underestimation of vitamin content.

GLC has found only limited application in food vitamin analysis, but remains a powerful technique for separating, detecting and (with mass spectrometry) identifying vitamers and vitamin breakdown products in metabolic studies.

9.2.4 FLOW-INJECTION ANALYSIS

Flow-injection analysis is the most rapid analytical technique yet developed and could replace HPLC, at least for the analysis of fortified products. Unfortunately, the time-consuming preparation of sample extracts still remains, so the full capability of the automated technique cannot be fully exploited.

9.3 ASSAY TECHNIQUES FOR THE INDIVIDUAL VITAMINS

9.3.1 THIAMIN AND RIBOFLAVIN

The AOAC fluorimetric methods for determining thiamin and riboflavin have been semi-automated using continuous-flow techniques, with a resultant improvement in precision. Problems of low thiamin recovery (Pippen and Potter, 1975) or, conversely, non-removal of extraneous fluorescent material (Fellman *et al.*, 1982) have occurred when Decalso has been used as the cation exchanger in the manual fluorimetric purification step; however, the present procedure (AOAC, 1990a) uses Bio-Rex 70 instead of Decalso. Russell and Vanderslice (1992) have discussed problems that can occur with the AOAC manual and semi-automated methods for riboflavin, and showed by experimentation that the standard method does not appear to be suitable for use with samples containing large amounts of fat.

Several investigators have compared riboflavin values obtained by HPLC with those obtained by the AOAC manual fluorimetric method. Good or reasonable agreement has been reported for the determination of riboflavin in rice and rice products (Toma and Tabekhia, 1979), milk, eggs and dairy products (Ashoor *et al.*, 1983, 1985), infant formula products (Ayi, Yuhas and Deangelis, 1986) and various raw and processed foods (Fellman *et al.*, 1982; Wills, Wimalasiri and Greendfield, 1985; Reyes *et al.*, 1988; Ollilainen *et al.*, 1990). Dramatically higher riboflavin values using the AOAC method were reported for soy products due to interference from fluorescent impurities that were not removed by oxidation with permanganate (Fernando and Murphy, 1990). Evidence for this statement was that treatment of the samples with permanganate before HPLC analysis failed to eliminate all the non-vitamin peaks from the chromatogram. Similarly, higher riboflavin values have been reported for fortified cereal products using a semi-automated modification of the AOAC method (Wehling and Wetzel, 1984).

Favourable comparisons between HPLC and microbiological (*Lactobacillus casei*) assay for riboflavin determinations have been reported for the analysis of infant formula products (Ayi, Yuhas and Deangelis, 1986) and for a wide range of foods (Lumley and Wiggins, 1981; Johnsson and Branzell, 1987; Reyes *et al.*, 1988). For non-enriched flours and flours with a high rate of extraction, the HPLC values were as much as 25–50% lower than those found with the microbiological assay (Johnsson and Branzell, 1987). This discrepancy was considered to be caused by an underestimation of vitamin B_2 activity by the HPLC procedure, possibly due to the chromatographic separation and non-measurement of biologically active isomeric riboflavin monophosphates.

Thiamin is considered to be totally available in a wide variety of food products (Gregory and Kirk, 1978), and therefore a chemical assay, used in conjunction with an effective extraction procedure, can substitute for a biological assay as a measure of vitamin B_1 activity. This was illustrated in a study conducted by Gregory and Kirk (1978), in which a semi-automated fluorimetric method was compared with a rat bioassay for the determination of thiamin in green beans. Calculation of available thiamin using the various rat assay dose–response curves indicated a mean value of 7.30 ± 2.46 μg/g, as thiamin hydrochloride, which compared favourably with the mean chemically determined value of 7.46 ± 0.14 μg/g. The determination of riboflavin liberated from FMN and FAD also provides a good estimation of available vitamin B_2, although it has yet to be demonstrated if the covalently bound flavins, which are not extractable, contribute significantly to the total flavin content (Russell and Vanderslice, 1990).

HPLC methods are well suited for determining thiamin and riboflavin in fortified foods and foods containing appreciable amounts of these vitamins. The use of a common extraction procedure allows these vitamins to be assayed either simultaneously or successively with a high degree of precision. Recovery data have indicated that riboflavin remains stable during the oxidation of thiamin to thiochrome (Fellman *et al.*, 1982). Post-column chemistry eliminates any possible effect of the ferricyanide reaction upon riboflavin, and also eliminates the problem of reducing sugars (produced during acid hydrolysis) competing with thiamin for the oxidizing agent (Wehling and Wetzel, 1984).

The HPLC procedure proposed by Reyes and Subryan (1989) incorporates a number of desirable features designed to provide reliable results with high sensitivity, and to prolong the life of the analytical column. Simultaneous determination of thiamin and riboflavin is achieved through simple reversed-phase chromatography at neutral pH using a single fluorescence detector. Clean-up and concentration of the ferricyanide-treated sample extract is effected by solid-phase extraction, which provides a purified and neutralized solution for injection. Thiamin values obtained by the HPLC method for raw and processed foods were the same (within experimental error) as those obtained by the 1984 AOAC fluorimetric method, which uses Bio-Rex 70 in the purification step. The HPLC method was further validated by the good agreement obtained between HPLC values for both thiamin and riboflavin with certified values on three dry AACC (American Association of Cereal Chemists) check samples.

9.3.2 NIACIN

The determination of niacin is complicated by the various forms of the vitamin that occur in foods. In meat and milk, the niacin content is mainly in the form of free nicotinamide, which is also the form used in fortification. In mature cereal grains, most of the total niacin content exists as a chemically bound form of nicotinic acid, which is nutritionally unavailable unless released by prior treatment with alkali. Pulses and other non-cereal plant foods contain mainly free nicotinic acid. Until recently, it has been customary to determine the total niacin (i.e. free plus bound) content of the food sample using an alkaline or strong acid extraction procedure. However, this approach provides a gross overestimate of available niacin for several staple cereal-based foods. A better prediction of available niacin is to measure just the free niacin, yet this may result in a degree of undervaluation because of the apparent partial utilization of bound nicotinic acid (Carter and Carpenter, 1982a,b). Nevertheless, it is prudent to determine free niacin for cereal-based foods as a means of ensuring an adequate level of enrichment. Free niacin is frequently defined as the niacin extracted by autoclaving with 0.1 N acid (Gregory, 1985).

Food composition tables express niacin values in terms of niacin equivalents using data obtained from a chick growth assay. Apart from using an animal bioassay, or possibly a protozoan assay, an estimation of the niacin equivalent content would necessitate the determination of L-tryptophan in a separate assay. If the protein content of a particular food is known, the tryptophan content can be estimated on the basis that animal and vegetable proteins contain *c.* 1.4% and 1.0% tryptophan, respectively (Thompson, 1982).

The AOAC manual and semi-automated colorimetric methods for determining total niacin using externally generated cyanogen bromide produced analytical results that were not statistically different from results obtained by microbiological assay in a collaborative study (Egberg, 1979). The colorimetric method suffers from lack of specificity and often lacks the sensitivity required for low-potency samples; moreover, the use of toxic reagents is undesirable. The microbiological assay using *Lactobacillus plantarum* normally presents no problems (Favell, 1990), and allows cultures of the test organism to be used for biotin and pantothenic acid assays. The radiometric–microbiological assay using *Kloeckera apiculata* (Guilarte and Pravlik, 1983) is an alternative to the turbidimetric assay.

The use of nicotinic acid and nicotinamide as colour fixatives for meat and fish has been prohibited in many countries. HPLC techniques for the simultaneous determination of both vitamers, used in conjunction with mild extraction procedures that minimize hydrolysis, have been developed using strong cation exchange (Hamano *et al.*, 1988) and ion interaction (Tsunoda *et al.*, 1988) chromatography.

HPLC assays for naturally occurring niacin demand extensive clean-up of sample extracts; this was effectively achieved by Tyler and Genzale (1990) using solid-phase extraction. HPLC of 0.1 N acid-extracted samples would appear to provide a better estimate of free niacin than the *L. plantarum* assay using a similar extraction procedure, on the grounds that *L. plantarum* can partially utilize bound nicotinic acid (Krehl and Strong, 1944). However, it could be argued that the microbiological assay yields a better estimate of available niacin, as there is evidence that bound niacin is also partially utilized by humans (Carter and Carpenter, 1982a).

9.3.3 VITAMIN B_6

Microbiological assays are currently the most widely used and accepted method for the determination of total vitamin B_6 in biological materials. The standard turbidimetric method using the yeast *Saccharomyces carlsbergensis* underestimates the total vitamin B_6 content if the sample contains predominantly pyridoxamine (PM) (e.g. a processed meat product), as the growth response of *S. carlsbergensis* to this vitamer is markedly less than that to pyridoxal (PL) or pyridoxine (PN). This unequal response is of little concern in plant-derived foods or foods that are substantially fortified with PN.HCl. In the AOAC microbiological method (AOAC, 1990b), each dephosphorylated vitamer is assayed separately after fractionation of sample hydrolysates by open-column ion exchange chromatography. *Kloeckera apiculata* has been proposed as the assay organism in the standard turbidimetric (Guilarte, McIntyre and Tsan, 1980) and semi-automated radiometric–microbiological assay (Guilarte, Shane and McIntyre, 1981) on the basis of an equivalent growth response to all three vitamers. However, this proposal has not found acceptance in certain other laboratories, in which *K. apiculata* was found to exhibit an even lower relative response to PM than that obtained with *S. carlsbergensis* (Polansky, 1981; Gregory, 1982). This as yet unresolved discrepancy between different research groups is presumably due to subtle environmental factors or culturing variables that affect the specificity of *K. apiculata*.

A biospecific assay suitable for determining total vitamin B_6 has not as yet been reported. Antisera raised against PL respond mainly to PM, thus limiting the application of the ELISA to the determination of PN in fortified foods (Alcock, Finglas and Morgan, 1990).

The fluorimetric method based on the formation of 4-pyridoxic acid lactone (Gregory and Kirk, 1977) gave markedly higher values for vitamin B_6 than did microbiological (*S. carlsbergensis*) assay, rat bioassay and HPLC in model cereal systems and selected foods (Gregory and Kirk, 1981). This serious discrepancy underlined the unsuitability of the fluorimetric method, in its present form, for food analysis.

Owing to the high proportions of glycosylated vitamin B_6 (chiefly PN-glucoside) in many plant foods, there is no entirely satisfactory single set of conditions that can quantitatively extract vitamin B_6 from both plant and animal products. The AOAC microbiological method (AOAC, 1990b) advocates different extraction conditions for plant and animal products, but for composite foods and diets a compromise must be reached. Extraction of plant-derived foods by autoclaving with 0.44 N HCl for 2 h at 121 °C, whether it be for AOAC microbiological or HPLC assay, will lead to an overestimation of vitamin B_6 bioavailability. This is because the rigorous hydrolysis treatment completely liberates PN from PN-glucoside, and this conjugate, orally administered, is only 58 ± 10% available to humans relative to PN (Gregory *et al.*, 1991). Because the proportion of glycosylated B_6 is a determinant of the net availability of dietary B_6, the ability of an assay to differentiate between total and glycosylated B_6 is of value in the nutritional assessment of diets. This requirement is best fulfilled by means of HPLC used in conjunction with an extraction procedure (homogenization with sulphosalicylic acid) that preserves the integrity of the phosphorylated vitamers (Gregory and Ink, 1987; Addo and Augustin, 1988). The HPLC system utilizes ion interaction chromatography operated with gradient elution and post-column chemistry to enhance the fluorescence of PL and PLP. Additional information concerning bound forms of B_6 can be obtained by measurement of PN-glucoside and nonglycosylated forms before and after enzymatic and acid-catalysed hydrolysis techniques (Gregory and Sartain, 1991).

A more direct approach for estimating the biologically available vitamin B_6 content of foods is to employ extraction conditions that, as far as possible, simulate the human digestive process. The HPLC method of Ekanayake and Nelson (1988), used with an *in vitro* enzymatic digestion procedure, was validated as a true measure of available B_6 by comparing the ratio of available to total B_6 with the same ratio obtained by rat bioassay and microbiological assay taken from published data. The ratios were found to be statistically comparable for ground beef, non-fat dry milk and whole wheat flour.

A simplified reversed-phase HPLC procedure using isocratic elution and direct fluorescence detection can be used for determining the added PN in fortified foods (Gregory, 1980). Ion interaction HPLC with isocratic elution and a single fluorescence detector has been employed for the simultaneous determination of PN, PL and riboflavin in fortified infant formula products (Ayi, Yuhas and Deangelis, 1986); vitamin B_6 values compared well with values obtained using the AOAC microbiological method. The simultaneous determination of PN, riboflavin and thiamin in fortified cereal products (Wehling and Wetzel, 1984) and PN and nicotinamide in various fortified food products (Rees, 1989) has been accomplished using isocratic ion interaction chromatography and two fluorescence detectors.

9.3.4 PANTOTHENIC ACID

The 'free' (no enzyme treatment) or 'total' (after enzyme treatment) pantothenic acid content of a food is traditionally determined by microbiological assay with *L. plantarum*. Either the radioimmunoassay (RIA) or the ELISA can substitute for the microbiological assay in the determination of total pantothenic acid, as shown by the high correlations obtained for the analysis of foods using the same extract. In an extensive survey conducted by Walsh, Wyse and Hansen (1979), the microbiological results were 6.6% higher than those of the RIA for breads and cereals, 11.6% higher for fruits and vegetables, and 23.2% higher for meats (Table 9.1). A preliminary study (Finglas *et al.*, 1988a) showed good agreement between ELISA values and microbiological values for five important sources of pantothenic acid in the UK diet (Table 9.2). The detection limit of the ELISA was at least 10-fold lower than that of the microbiological assay. The inherent practical advantages of the ELISA over the RIA, and the better agreement with microbiological results, suggest that the ELISA could be the method of choice for determining pantothenic acid. The double enzyme extraction

Table 9.1 Comparison of radioimmunoassay (RIA) and microbiological (*L. plantarum*) assay (MBA) for the determination of pantothenic acid in various food groups (from Walsh, Wyse and Hansen, 1979)

		Pantothenic acid content (mg per 100 g)[a]	
Food group	*n*	RIA	MBA
All foods	75	0.43 ± 0.25	0.48 ± 0.25
Breads and cereals	40	0.39 ± 0.25	0.42 ± 0.28
Fruits and vegetables	17	0.25 ± 0.21	0.29 ± 0.24
Meats	16	0.71 ± 0.53	0.87 ± 0.70

[a] Mean (± standard deviation).

Table 9.2 Comparison of ELISA with microbiological (*L. plantarum*) assay (MBA) and food table data for the determination of pantothenic acid in selected foods (from Finglas *et al.*, 1988a)

	Pantothenic acid content (mg/100 g)[a]		
Food	ELISA[a]	MBA[b]	Food tables[c]
Milk	0.36 (0.32–0.43)	0.28 (0.27–0.30)	0.35
Potato	0.23 (0.18–0.30)	0.23 (0.22–0.24)	0.30
Bread	0.23 (0.21–0.30)	0.23 (0.21–0.24)	0.30
Eggs	1.74 (1.52–1.94)	1.46 (1.32–1.65)	1.80
Liver (lambs)	8.25 (7.50–9.38)	8.65 (8.25–9.13)	8.20
Lettuce	0.18 (0.14–0.20)	0.07 (0.05–0.09)	0.20

[a]Means of triplicate determinations for duplicate extracts of each sample with ranges in parentheses.
[b]Means of duplicate determinations for duplicate extracts of each sample with ranges in parentheses.
[c]Microbiological assay data from Paul and Southgate (1978).

procedure is the rate-limiting step in the batchwise analysis of large numbers of samples, and the need to establish the activity of the enzymes is an additional problem.

9.3.5 BIOTIN

The microbiological assay using *L. plantarum* is the standard method for determining biotin in foods, but the nutritional significance of the results obtained is largely dependent upon the extraction procedure employed. Maximum liberation of bound biotin from animal tissues requires autoclaving the sample with 6 N H_2SO_4 for 2 h at 121 °C, but these conditions promote losses of biotin in plant tissues, and a somewhat milder acid hydrolysis must be used for plant foods and food composites. Bitsch, Salz and Hötzel (1989) reported that treatment of samples with liquid nitrogen, followed by digestion with papain, was capable of quantitatively releasing bound biotin (including biotin from biocytin) from both plant and animal tissues.

The radiometric competitive protein-binding assay (radioassay) has been investigated as a possible alternative to the microbiological assay, and shown to have comparable sensitivity (Dakshinamurti and Allan, 1979). Hood (1975) extracted poultry feeds by autoclaving with 2 N H_2SO_4 for 1 h at 121 °C, and obtained radioassay values that were in good agreement with values obtained by microbiological assay. In the same study, radioassay values for two wheat samples were 20% and 55% higher than microbiological values. It appears that neither of the two assay techniques, using the stated extraction procedure, gives a reliable estimate of biological availability, as chick growth assays have shown the biotin content of wheat to be almost completely unavailable (Bonjour, 1984).

9.3.6 FOLATE

To date, the most widely used method for determining total folate in foods is the turbidimetric microbiological assay using *Lactobacillus casei*, because it allows measurement of total folate at the nanogram level, the typical physiological concentration. It has been generally assumed that polyglutamyl folates may be deconjugated either to monoglutamates with hog kidney enzyme or to diglutamates with chicken pancreas enzyme, on the grounds that *L. casei* responds equally well to pteroyl monoglutamates, diglutamates and triglutamates. However, Phillips and Wright (1982) found that the use of hog kidney conjugase resulted in folate values for vegetables that were at least 50% higher than values obtained using chicken pancreas conjugase. This discrepancy was attributed to the reduced bacterial growth response to diglutamyl 5-methyl-THF that predominated in the vegetable extracts following deconjugation with chicken pancreas enzyme. Phillips and Wright (1982) also observed a positive drift effect for monoglutamyl 5-methyl-THF using the standard assay procedure of Bell (1974). The resultant underestimation of total folate caused by this effect could be rectified by using an initial pH of 6.2 instead of 6.8. The implications of the Phillips and Wright study are that published food values based on the method of Bell (1974), which uses chicken pancreas enzyme and an initial incubation pH of 6.8, are underestimates.

Other research groups (Bird, McGlohon and Vaitkus 1969; Ruddick, Vanderstoep and Richards, 1978; Reingold and Picciano, 1982; Goli and Vanderslice, 1989) also reported different responses for various monoglutamyl folate vitamers, but some investigators (O'Broin *et al.*, 1975; Shane, Tamura and Stokstad, 1980; Wilson and Horne, 1984) have found a uniform molar response among monoglutamyl folates. Chen, Hill and McIntyre (1983) found that *L. casei* responded differently to changes in pH by the turbidimetric assay, and to changes in both pH and phosphate concentration by the radiometric–microbiological assay (RMA). Using a constant pH and the same concentration of phosphate throughout, the RMA gave a mean percentage recovery on 16 varied food samples of 99%, with a range of 71% (string beans) to 117% (spinach). The low recovery for string beans was obtained using both assay techniques, and was possibly due to folate binding by the insoluble components of this food. Goli and Vanderslice (1989) obtained the following growth responses of monoglutamyl folates relative to PGA: 93% for 5-methyl-THF, 115% for 5-formyl-THF, 80% for 10-formyl-THF, 81% for THF, and 45% for DHF. The responses were about the same when two different initial pH values (6.8 and 6.1) were used. These findings are at variance with those of Phillips and Wright (1982) and other investigators. The data show that determining folate levels from bacterial growth rates will lead to erroneously higher or lower values, depending on the folate vitamers present.

The overall picture reveals that the microbiological assay for folate is fragile, rather than robust. Careful control of pH and buffering capacity of the medium appear to be essential prerequisites. Food samples analysed by standard procedures using both hydrolysed vitamin-free casein and a mixture of crystalline amino acids, whose profile was identical to that in the casein, did not produce significantly different results in the two media, indicating that the casein did not contain factors that influence the growth of *L. casei* (Wilson, Clifford and Clifford, 1987). Even with its many unsolved problems, the microbiological assay remains the standard method at present, since other procedures, such as radioassay and HPLC, have their own inherent difficulties. In view of the contradictory findings regarding the response of different folate vitamers in *L. casei* assays, an investigation of vitamer response is warranted before the assay can be used.

Radioassay kits have clinical application (subject to prior testing) for the analysis of serum, in which monoglutamyl 5-methyl-THF is virtually the sole folate vitamer present (Cossins, 1984). However, radioassays do not, at present, give reliable data for foods because of variation of binding affinity among the various folates for the folate-binding protein commonly employed (Shane, Tamura and Stokstad, 1980). Another serious limitation is that the binding protein does not exhibit significant affinity for 5-formyl-THF, which is formed extensively from 10-formyl-THF during thermal processing (Gregory, 1989).

A non-isotopic microtitration plate protein-binding assay described by Finglas *et al.* (1988b) has potential application for the determination of either added PGA in fortified foods or naturally occurring folate in the form of 5-formyl-THF and 5-methyl-THF. It remains to be seen if the microtitration plate microbiological assays reported by Newman and Tsai (1986) and Horne and Patterson (1988) offer any significant advantages over the protein-binding assay.

It is evident from the foregoing that separation of the folate vitamers from one another and from interfering substances is an essential prerequisite for an accurate assay. HPLC procedures have been developed to meet this need. Reversed-phase HPLC with gradient elution and UV absorbance detection is adequate for determining the PGA content of fortified foods, following sample clean-up by DEAE cellulose chromatography (Hoppner and Lampi, 1982). Supplemental PGA can be determined without the need for preparative chromatography, using the post-column fluorogenic derivatization system developed by Day and Gregory (1981). For the determination of naturally occurring folate, reversed-phase HPLC with an acidic mobile phase and gradient elution permits the fluorimetric detection of the major vitamers, 5-methyl-THF, 5-formyl-THF (representing largely 10-formyl-THF) and THF after chromatographic clean-up on DEAE-Sephadex A-25 (Gregory, Sartain and Day, 1984). Folate values obtained by HPLC assay and by *L. casei* assay, using the same extract of each food for both assays, are given for fortified foods and selected biological materials in Tables 9.3 and 9.4. All samples tested, except infant formula, showed statistically significant differences between the results obtained by the two methods. For oat flakes, cabbage, orange juice and particularly whole wheat flour the *L. casei* assay yielded higher folate values, suggesting the influence of non-folate compounds on the bacterial growth response. The higher total folate content obtained by HPLC for liver could possibly be attributed to the high proportion of THF detected; this compound has been reported to elicit a relatively poor growth response in *L. casei*.

The use of electrochemical detection (White, 1990; White, Lee and Krüger, 1991) overcomes the need for an acidic (pH <3) mobile phase or post-column acidification when fluorimetric detection is utilized. Fluorimetric detection, although rather less sensitive than electrochemical detection, has the advantage of being more selective.

Even after chromatographic separation and detection of the major

Table 9.3 Comparison of assay procedures for the determination of folate in fortified foods

Procedure	Oat flakes (μg/g)	Infant formula (μg/ml)
L. casei	9.30 ± 0.36	0.189 ± 0.003
HPLC	6.19 ± 0.25	0.175 ± 0.002

Values (mean ± SD, $n = 3$) represent the concentration expressed as folic acid equivalents. Values for infant formula were not significantly different, $p < 0.05$.
Reprinted from Gregory, J.F. *et al.* (1982). *J. Fd Sci.* **47**, 1568–71. Copyright © Institute of Food Technologists.

folate vitamers, other biologically active folate compounds may escape quantification; furthermore, the individual vitamers may exhibit different potencies. There is also no guarantee that the extraction procedure does not incur loss of the vitamin. It appears that the animal bioassay remains the only valid method for estimating folate activity. Continuing bioavailability studies with human subjects are also warranted.

9.3.7 VITAMIN B_{12}

For many years the microbiological assay has been the only available method with adequate sensitivity and specificity to measure the low levels of vitamin B_{12} in foods. Using the conventional turbidimetric procedure, the maintenance of *Lactobacillus delbrueckii*, the preferred assay organism, requires special techniques to overcome problems of lack of growth in subcultures or loss of sensitivity to B_{12}. The radiometric–microbiological assay developed by Chen and McIntyre (1979) allows immediate inoculation with previously lyophilized cultures of *L. delbrueckii*, and hence does not suffer from the problems encountered in subculturing. *Ochromonas malhamensis* has been proposed as an alternative assay organism, on the grounds of its non-response to clinically inactive cobalamins. However, the long (3–4 days) growth requirement and the need for a large surface for growing are practical disadvantages for assays using protozoa.

Radioassays have been routinely used by clinical laboratories to monitor serum levels of B_{12}, and investigated for their possible application to food analysis. The investigations have led to the general conclusion that, provided the extraction technique is sufficiently rigorous to completely liberate the cobalamins from their bound forms, the radioassay yields B_{12} values that are comparable with those obtained using the *L. delbrueckii* assay. For example, Casey *et al.* (1982), using the extraction procedure of the AOAC microbiological method, analysed 8 various fortified and 12 various non-fortified food products, and obtained mean B_{12} contents of 8.01 and 7.54 μg/100 g by radioassay and AOAC (*L. delbrueckii*) assay, respectively. Reproducible results for B_{12} in sample extracts could be obtained at levels as low as 50 pg/ml, corresponding to 0.10 μg B_{12}/100 g (5-g sample weight). This compares well with the generally quoted detection limit of 0.12 μg/100 g for the AOAC method. In another comparative study, using optimized extraction conditions, Andersson, Lundqvist and Öste (1990) obtained mean B_{12} values ($n = 6$) for milk of 4.57 and 4.40 μg/litre for radioassay and *L. delbrueckii* assay, respectively. The radioassay was more precise than the microbiological assay, as indicated by a lower standard deviation (1.2% and 6%, respectively).

A non-isotopic microtitration plate competitive protein-binding assay has been developed which has potential commercial application for determining the added cyanocobalamin in fortified foods, but it lacks the sensitivity to determine naturally occurring vitamin B_{12} (Alcock, Finglas and Morgan, 1992).

9.3.8 VITAMIN C

Vitamin C activity is less of a problem to determine than that of the B-group vitamins, as it occurs mainly in unbound water-extractable form, and in milligram amounts per 100 g in fruits and vegetables. Ascorbic acid, and its immediate oxidation product, dehydroascorbic acid, possess equal biological activity and are readily interconvertible, thus permitting the measurement of only one compound.

The AOAC dye titration method is simple and rapid, but it only accounts for ascorbic acid. Moreover, the end-point is difficult to observe when sample extracts are coloured, and the method is subject to interference from sulphites and many naturally occurring reducing substances present in foods. The AOAC microfluorimetric method provides a value for total vitamin C activity and is supposedly less susceptible to interference, but it is a lengthy and tedious method. Other titrimetric methods and colorimetric methods have fallen into disuse, while spectrophotometric methods with background correction have found application for the determination of ascorbic acid in soft drinks, fruit juices and cordials. GLC permits the simultaneous determination of organic acids, including ascorbic acid, as their trimethylsilyl derivatives with excellent resolution and, in conjunction with the determination of sugars, is well suited to the routine multicomponent analysis of fruit juices (Heatherbell, 1974).

Many HPLC methods have been reported, reflecting the popularity of this technique for vitamin C analysis. HPLC is accurate and sensitive for the determination of ascorbic acid, but it is less than ideal for determining total vitamin C. The poor optical absorptivity of dehydroascorbic acid and its lack of electrochemical activity is a drawback, and necessitates the chemical reduction of this compound to ascorbic acid. Fluorescence detection can be used, but the lack of inherent fluorescence necessitates the chemical oxidation of ascorbic acid to dehydroascorbic acid, and subsequent derivatization. These chemical manipulations somewhat defeat the purpose of HPLC, as one of its principal advantages over GLC is that derivatization is not usually necessary.

Wills, Wimalasiri and Greenfield (1983) determined the vitamin C content of fresh fruit and vegetables by an HPLC method, which gave simultaneous separate values for ascorbic acid and dehydroascorbic acid, and by the AOAC methods of dye titration and microfluorimetry. The data presented in Table 9.5 show good general agreement between

Table 9.4 Folate concentration (nmol/g) and distribution in selected biological materials[a]

Sample	HPLC assay					
	THF	5-Methyl-THF	5-Formyl-THF	PGA	Total folate	*L. casei* assay
Whole cows' milk	ND	0.072 ± 0.005	ND	ND	0.072 ± 0.005	0.027 ± 0.005
Fresh cabbage	0.070 ± 0.005	0.112 ± 0.006	ND	ND	0.182 ± 0.008	0.293 ± 0.071
Frozen calf liver	48.1 ± 4.81	3.51 ± 0.95	1.91 ± 0.19	0.76 ± 0.33	54.3 ± 4.9	36.3 ± 10.9
Orange juice	ND	0.370 ± 0.026	ND	ND	0.370 ± 0.026	1.90 ± 0.73
Whole wheat flour	ND	ND	ND	ND	ND	1.59 ± 0.31

[a]Mean and standard deviation, triplicate analyses. ND, not detected.
From Gregory, J.F. *et al.* (1984) *J. Nutr.*, **114**, 341–53, © American Institute of Nutrition.

Table 9.5 Vitamin C content (mg/100 g) of fresh fruits and vegetables using the dichlorophenolindophenol (DCPIP) titration method, the microfluorimetric method and weak anion HPLC with $UV_{254\ nm}$ and $UV_{214\ nm}$ detection for ascorbic acid (AA) and dehydroascorbic acid (DHAA), respectively (from Wills, Wimalasiri and Greenfield, 1983)

			HPLC[a]		
Sample	DCPIP[a]	Fluorimetry[a]	AA	DHAA	Total vitamin C
Banana	10.4	11.9	9.6	3.1	12.7
Broccoli	67.8	80.5	66.0	2.3	68.3
Brussels sprouts	53.8	65.0	54.0	8.0	60.0
Cabbage	43.1	45.0	41.0	3.0	44.0
Capsicum	143.7	145.8	142.0	3.2	145.2
Cauliflower	46.5	54.0	47.1	2.6	49.7
Celery	7.0	7.8	5.2	2.0	7.2
Cucumber	7.6	8.5	7.4	1.6	9.0
Kiwi fruit	95.7	101.2	92.3	4.7	97.0
Lemon	49.0	52.0	49.7	0	49.7
Lime	30.2	33.5	32.0	0	32.0
Oranges	50.9	56.2	54.0	0	54.0
Parsley	131.0	140.5	130.6	4.1	134.7
Potatoes	10.8	12.7	10.2	2.0	12.2
Rock melon	60.2	63.6	62.0	0	62.0
Spinach	46.3	56.0	44.0	8.2	52.2
Strawberries	(56.0)[b]	50.7	46.0	5.3	51.3
Tomatoes	(13.5)[b]	10.9	10.2	0	10.2

[a]Average of duplicate determinations.
[b]End-point of titration difficult to determine because of coloured extract.

the ascorbic acid values obtained by the dye titration method and by HPLC. If ascorbic acid values only were required, the dye titration method would give adequate results for horticultural produce. Several products exhibit higher total vitamin C values by microfluorimetric assay than by HPLC assay. This could be due to an underestimation of dehydroascorbic acid by the HPLC assay, but the observation that the greatest discrepancies occur in green leafy vegetables (especially broccoli) suggests a pigment-related interference in the fluorescence measurement.

Chromatographic modes utilized in HPLC assays have included strong anion exchange, weak anion exchange using aminopropyl-bonded phases, ion exclusion partition, reversed-phase with ion suppression, and reversed-phase with an ion interaction agent. Of these, a reversed-phase column with ion suppression is convenient and easy to operate, but the need to use acidified mobile phases to achieve ion suppression reduces the life of silica-based column packings. Here, the use of polymeric packings comes to the fore because of their resistance to acidic conditions. An interesting application using reversed-phase chromatography with ion suppression is the method of Ziegler, Meier and Sticher (1987), in which ascorbic acid is separated from dehydroascorbic acid, and the latter is reduced to ascorbic acid in a post-column in-line reaction system. This technique enables the dehydro-ascorbic acid to be measured photometrically with the same sensitivity as ascorbic acid.

Despite the popularity of HPLC, the future of vitamin C analysis may lie in the application of enzymatic assays using ascorbate peroxidase. Enzymatic assays confer a high degree of specificity and, with homocysteine reduction, can measure total vitamin C. The use of immobilized enzyme in flow-injection systems with amperometric detection (Greenway and Ongomo, 1990) offers the opportunity for a precise, accurate and automated procedure using relatively simple apparatus.

REFERENCES

Addo, C. and Augustin, J. (1988) Changes in the vitamin B-6 content in potatoes during storage. *J. Fd Sci.*, **53**, 749–52.

Alcock, S.C., Finglas, P.M. and Morgan, M.R.A. (1990) An enzyme-linked immunosorbent assay for pyridoxamine and its comparison with alternative analytical procedures. *Fd Agric. Immunol.*, **2**, 197–204.

Alcock, S.C., Finglas, P.M. and Morgan, M.R.A. (1992) Production and purification of an R-protein–enzyme conjugate for use in a microtitration plate protein-binding assay for vitamin B_{12} in fortified food. *Fd Chem.*, **45**, 199–203.

Andersson, I., Lundqvist, R. and Öste, R. (1990) Analysis of vitamin B_{12} in milk by a radioisotope dilution assay. *Milchwissenschaft*, **45**, 507–9.

AOAC (1990a) Thiamin (vitamin B_1) in foods. Fluorometric method. Final action. In *AOAC Official Methods of Analysis*, 15th edn (ed. K. Helrich), Association of Official Analytical Chemists, Inc., Arlington, VA, 942.23.

AOAC (1990b) Vitamin B_6 (pyridoxine, pyridoxal, pyridoxamine) in food extracts. Microbiological method. Final action 1975. In *AOAC Official Methods of Analysis*, 15th edn (ed. K. Helrich), Association of Official Analytical Chemists, Inc., Arlington, VA, 961.15.

Ashoor, S.H., Seperich, G.J., Monte, W.C. and Welty, J. (1983) HPLC determination of riboflavin in eggs and dairy products. *J. Fd Sci.*, **48**, 92–4, 110.

Ashoor, S.H., Knox, M.J., Olsen, J.R. and Deger, D.A. (1985) Improved liquid chromatographic determination of riboflavin in milk and dairy products. *J. Ass. Off. Analyt. Chem.*, **68**, 693–6.

Ayi, B.K., Yuhas, D.A. and Deangelis, N.J. (1986) Simultaneous determination of vitamins B_2 (riboflavin) and B_6 (pyridoxine) in infant formula products by reverse phase liquid chromatography. *J. Ass. Off. Analyt. Chem.*, **69**, 56–9.

Bell, J.G. (1974) Microbiological assay of vitamins of the B group in foodstuffs. *Lab. Pract.*, **23**, 235–42, 252.

Bird, O.D., McGlohon, V.M. and Vaitkus, J.W. (1969) A microbiological assay system for naturally occurring folates. *Can. J. Microbiol.*, **15**, 465–72.

Bitsch, R., Salz, I. and Hötzel, D. (1989) Biotin assessment in foods and body fluids by a protein binding assay (PBA). *Int. J. Vitam. Nutr. Res.*, **59**, 59–64.

Bonjour, J.-P. (1984) Biotin. In *Handbook of Vitamins. Nutritional, Biochemical, and Clinical Aspects* (ed. L.J. Machlin), Marcel Dekker, Inc., New York, pp. 403–35.

Carter, E.G.A. and Carpenter, K.J. (1982a) The bioavailability for humans of bound niacin from wheat bran. *Am. J. Clin. Nutr.*, **36**, 855–61.

Carter, E.G.A. and Carpenter, K.J. (1982b) The available niacin values of foods for rats and their relation to analytical values. *J. Nutr.*, **112**, 2091–103.

Casey, P.J., Speckman, K.R., Ebert, F.J. and Hobbs, W.E. (1982) Radioisotope dilution technique for determination of vitamin B_{12} in foods. *J. Ass. Off. Analyt. Chem.*, **65**, 85–8.

Chen, M.F., Hill, J.W. and McIntyre, P.A. (1983) The folacin contents of foods as measured by a radiometric microbiological method. *J. Nutr.*, **113**, 2192–6.

Chen, M. and McIntyre, P.A. (1979) Measurement of the trace amounts of vitamin B_{12} present in various foods by a new radiometric microbiological technique. In *Trace Organic Analysis: a New Frontier in Analytical Chemistry* (eds H.S. Hertz and S.N. Chesler), National Bureau of Standards, Washington, DC, pp. 257–65.

Cossins, E.A. (1984) Folates in biological materials. In *Folates and Pterins*, Vol. 1. *Chemistry and Biochemistry of Folates* (eds R.L. Blakley and S.J. Benkovic), John Wiley & Sons, New York, pp. 1–59.

Dakshinamurti, K. and Allan, L. (1979) Isotope dilution assay for biotin: use of [^{3}H]biotin. *Methods Enzymol.*, **62D**, 284–7.

Day, B.P. and Gregory, J.F. (1981) Determination of folacin derivatives in selected foods by high-performance liquid chromatography. *J. Agric. Fd Chem.*, **29**, 374–7.

Egberg, D.C. (1979) Semiautomated method for niacin and niacinamide in food products: collaborative study. *J. Ass. Off. Analyt. Chem.*, **62**, 1027–30.

Eitenmiller, R.R. (1990) Strengths and weaknesses of assessing vitamin content of foods. *J. Fd Quality*, **13**, 7–20.

Ekanayake, A. and Nelson, P.E. (1988) Applicability of an *in vitro* method for the estimation of vitamin B_6 biological availability. *J. Micronutr. Anal.*, **4**, 1–15.

Favell, D.J. (1990) Vitamin analysis – microbiological methods. *J. Micronutr. Anal.*, **7**, 237–46.

Fellman, J.K., Artz, W.E., Tassinari, P.D., Cole, C.L. and Augustin, J. (1982) Simultaneous determination of thiamin and riboflavin in selected foods by high-performance liquid chromatography. *J. Fd Sci.*, **47**, 2048–50, 2067.

Fernando, S.M. and Murphy, P.A. (1990) HPLC determination of thiamin and riboflavin in soybeans and tofu. *J. Agric. Fd Chem.*, **38**, 163–7.

Finglas, P.M., Faulks, R.M., Morris, H.C., Scott, K.J. and Morgan, M.R.A. (1988a) The development of an enzyme-linked immunosorbent assay (ELISA) for the analysis of pantothenic acid and analogues. Part II – Determination of pantothenic acid in foods. *J. Micronutr. Anal.*, **4**, 47–59.

Finglas, P.M., Kwiatkowska, C., Faulks, R.M. and Morgan, M.R.A. (1988b)

Comparison of a non-isotopic, microtitration plate folate-binding protein assay and a microbiological method for the determination of folate in raw and cooked vegetables. *J. Micronutr. Anal.*, **4**, 309–22.

Goli, D.M. and Vanderslice, J.T. (1989) Microbiological assays of folacin using a CO_2 analyzer system. *J. Micronutr. Anal.*, **6**, 19–33.

Greenway, G.M. and Ongomo, P. (1990) Determination of L-ascorbic acid in fruit and vegetable juices by flow injection with immobilised ascorbate oxidase. *Analyst, Lond.*, **115**, 1297–9.

Gregory, J.F. (1980) Comparison of high-performance liquid chromatographic and *Saccharomyces uvarum* methods for the determination of vitamin B_6 in fortified breakfast cereals. *J. Agric. Fd Chem.*, **28**, 486–9.

Gregory, J.F. (1982) Relative activity of the nonphosphorylated B-6 vitamers for *Saccharomyces uvarum* and *Kloeckera brevis* in vitamin B-6 microbiological assay. *J. Nutr.*, **112**, 1643–7.

Gregory, J.F. (1985) Chemical changes of vitamins during food processing. In *Chemical Changes of Food during Processing* (eds T. Richardson and J.W. Finley), Van Nostrand Reinhold Co., New York, pp. 373–408.

Gregory, J.F. (1988) Methodology for nutrient analysis. In *Nutritional Evaluation of Food Processing* (eds E. Karmas and R.S. Harris), Van Nostrand Reinhold Company Inc., New York, pp. 719–43.

Gregory, J.F. (1989) Chemical and nutritional aspects of folate research: analytical procedures, methods of folate synthesis, stability, and bioavailability of dietary folates. *Adv. Fd Nutr. Res.*, **33**, 1–101.

Gregory, J.F., Day, B.P.F. and Ristow, K.A. (1982) Comparison of high performance liquid chromatographic, radiometric, and *Lactobacillus casei* methods for the determination of folacin in selected foods. *J. Fd Sci.*, **47**, 1568–71.

Gregory, J.F. and Ink, S.L. (1987) Identification and quantification of pyridoxine-β-glucoside as a major form of vitamin B_6 in plant-derived foods. *J. Agric. Fd Chem.*, **35**, 76–82.

Gregory, J.F. and Kirk, J.R. (1977) Improved chromatographic separation and fluorometric determination of vitamin B_6 compounds in foods. *J. Fd Sci.*, **42**, 1073–6.

Gregory, J.F. and Kirk, J.R. (1978) Comparison of chemical and biological methods for determination of thiamin in foods. *J. Agric. Fd Chem.*, **26**, 338–41.

Gregory, J.F. and Kirk, J.R. (1981) Determination of vitamin B-6 compounds by semiautomated continuous flow and chromatographic methods. In *Methods in Vitamin B-6 Nutrition. Analysis and Status Assessment* (eds J.E. Leklem and R.D. Reynolds), Plenum Press, New York, pp. 149–70.

Gregory, J.F. and Sartain, D.B. (1991) Improved chromatographic determination of free and glycosylated forms of vitamin B_6 in foods. *J. Agric. Fd Chem.*, **39**, 899–905.

Gregory, J.F., Sartain, D.B. and Day, B.P.F. (1984) Fluorometric determination of folacin in biological materials using high performance liquid chromatography. *J. Nutr.*, **114**, 341–53.

Gregory, J.F., Trumbo, P.R., Bailey, L.B. *et al.* (1991) Bioavailability of pyridoxine-5′-β-D-glucoside determined in humans by stable-isotopic methods. *J. Nutr.*, **121**, 177–86.

Guilarte, T., McIntyre, P.A. and Tsan, M.-F. (1980) Growth response of the yeasts *Saccharomyes uvarum* and *Kloeckera brevis* to the free biologically active forms of vitamin B-6. *J. Nutr.*, **110**, 954–8.

Guilarte, T.R. and Pravlik, K. (1983) Radiometric-microbiologic assay of niacin using *Kloeckera brevis*: analysis of human blood and food. *J. Nutr.*, **113**, 2587–94.

Guilarte, T., Shane, B., and McIntyre, P.A. (1981) Radiometric-microbiologic assay of vitamin B-6: application to food analysis. *J. Nutr.*, **111**, 1869–75.

Hamano, T., Mitsuhashi, Y., Aoki, N. and Yamamoto, S. (1988) Simultaneous determination of niacin and niacinamide in meats by high-performance liquid chromatography. *J. Chromat.*, **457**, 403–8.

Heatherbell, D.A. (1974) Rapid concurrent analysis of fruit sugars and acids by gas-liquid chromatography. *J. Sci. Fd Agric.*, **25**, 1095–107.

Hood, R.L. (1975) A radiochemical assay for biotin in biological materials. *J. Sci. Fd Agric.*, **26**, 1847–52.

Hoppner, K. and Lampi, B. (1982) The determination of folic acid (pteroylmonoglutamic acid) in fortified products by reversed phase high pressure liquid chromatography. *J. Liquid Chromat.*, **5**, 953–66.

Horne, D.W. and Patterson, D. (1988) *Lactobacillus casei* microbiological assay of folic acid derivatives in 96-well microtitre plates. *Clin. Chem.*, **34**, 2357–9.

Johnsson, H. and Branzell, C. (1987) High performance liquid chromatographic determination of riboflavin in food – a comparison with a microbiological method. *Int. J. Vitam. Nutr. Res*, **57**, 53–8.

Krehl, W.A. and Strong, F.M. (1944). Studies on the distribution, properties, and isolation of a naturally occurring precursor of nicotinic acid. *J. Biol. Chem.*, **156**, 1–12.

Lumley, I.D. and Wiggins, R.A. (1981) Determination of riboflavin and flavin mononucleotide in foodstuffs using high-performance liquid chromatography and a column-enrichment technique. *Analyst, Lond.*, **106**, 1103–8.

Newman, E.M. and Tsai, J.F. (1986) Microbiological analysis of 5-formyltetrahydrofolic acid and other folates using an automatic 96-well plate reader. *Analyt. Biochem.*, **154**, 509–15.

O'Broin, J.D., Temperley, I.J., Brown, J.P. and Scott, J.M. (1975) Nutritional stability of various naturally occurring monoglutamate derivatives of folic acid. *Am. J. Clin. Nutr.*, **28**, 438–44.

Ollilainen, V., Mattila, P., Varo, P., Koivistoinen, P. and Huttunen, J. (1990) The HPLC determination of total riboflavin in foods. *J. Micronutr. Anal.*, **8**, 199–207.

Paul, A.A. and Southgate, D.A.T. (1978) *McCance and Widdowson's The Composition of Foods*, 4th edn, HM Stationery Office, London.

Phillips, D.R. and Wright, A.J.A. (1982) Studies on the response of *Lactobacillus casei* to different folate monoglutamates. *Br. J. Nutr.*, **47**, 183–9.

Pippen, E.L. and Potter, A.L. (1975) Quantitating the recovery of thiamine (vitamin B_1) from Decalso in the thiochrome method for the determination of thiamine. *J. Agric. Fd Chem.*, **23**, 523–6.

Polansky, M.M. (1981) Microbiological assay of vitamin B-6 in foods. In *Methods in Vitamin B-6 Nutrition. Analysis and Status Assessment* (eds J.E. Leklem and R.D. Reynolds), Plenum Press, New York, pp. 21–44.

Rees, D.I. (1989) Determination of nicotinamide and pyridoxine in fortified food products by HPLC. *J. Micronutr. Anal.*, **5**, 53–61.

Reingold, R.N. and Picciano, M.F. (1982) Two improved high-performance liquid chromatographic separations of biologically significant forms of folate. *J. Chromat.*, **234**, 171–9.

Reyes, E.S.P. and Subryan, L. (1989) An improved method of simultaneous HPLC assay of riboflavin and thiamin in selected cereal products. *J. Fd Comp. Anal.*, **2**, 41–7.

Reyes, E.S.P., Norris, K.M., Taylor, C. and Potts, D. (1988) Comparison of paired-ion liquid chromatographic method with AOAC fluorometric and microbiological methods for riboflavin determination in selected foods. *J. Ass. Off. Analyt. Chem.*, **71**, 16–19.

Ruddick, J.E., Vanderstoep, J. and Richards, J.F. (1978) Folate levels in food – a comparison of microbiological assay and radioassay methods for measuring folate. *J. Fd Sci.*, **43**, 1238–41.

Russell, L.F. and Vanderslice, J.T. (1990) A comprehensive review of vitamin B_2 analytical methodology. *J. Micronutr. Anal.*, **8**, 257–310.

Russell, L.F. and Vanderslice, J.T. (1992) Comments on the standard fluorometric determination of riboflavin in foods and biological tissues. *Fd Chem.*, **43**, 79–82.

Shane, B., Tamura, T. and Stokstad, E.L.R. (1980) Folate assay: a comparison of radioassay and microbiological methods. *Clin. Chim. Acta*, **100**, 13–19.

Thompson, J.N. (1982) Trace analysis of vitamins by liquid chromatography. In *Trace Analysis*, Vol. 2 (ed. J.F. Lawrence), Academic Press, New York, pp. 1–67.

Toma, R.B. and Tabekhia, M.M. (1979) High performance liquid chromatographic analysis of B-vitamins in rice and rice products. *J. Fd Sci.*, **44**, 263–5, 268.

Tsunoda, K., Inoue, N., Iwasaki, H., Akiya, M. and Hasebe, A. (1988) Rapid simultaneous analysis of nicotinic acid and nicotinamide in foods, and their behaviour during storage. *J. Fd Hyg. Soc. Japan*, **29**, 262–6 (in Japanese).

Tyler, T.A. and Genzale, J.A. (1990) Liquid chromatographic determination of total niacin in beef, semolina, and cottage cheese. *J. Ass. Off. Analyt. Chem.*, **73**, 467–9.

Walsh, J.H., Wyse, B.W. and Hansen, R.G. (1979) A comparison of microbiological and radioimmunoassay methods for the determination of pantothenic acid in foods. *J. Fd Biochem.*, **3**, 175–89.

Wehling, R.L. and Wetzel, D.L. (1984) Simultaneous determination of pyridoxine, riboflavin, and thiamin in fortified cereal products by high-performance liquid chromatography. *J. Agric. Fd Chem.*, **32**, 1326–31.

White, D.R. Jr (1990) Determination of 5-methyltetrahydrofolate in citrus juice by reversed-phase high-performance liquid chromatography with electrochemical detection. *J. Agric. Fd Chem.*, **38**, 1515–18.

White, D.R. Jr, Lee, H.S. and Krüger, R.E. (1991) Reversed-phase HPLC/EC determination of folate in citrus juice by direct injection with column switching. *J. Agric. Fd Chem.*, **39**, 714–17.

Wills, R.B.H., Wimalasiri, P. and Greenfield, H. (1983) Liquid chromatography, microfluorometry, and dye-titration determination of vitamin C in fresh fruit and vegetables. *J. Ass. Off. Analyt. Chem.*, **66**, 1377–9.

Wills, R.B.H., Wimalasiri, P. and Greenfield, H. (1985) Comparative determination of thiamin and riboflavin in foods by high-performance liquid chromatography and fluorometric methods. *J. Micronutr. Anal.*, **1**, 23–9.

Wilson, D.S., Clifford, C.K. and Clifford, A.J. (1987) Microbiological assay for folic acid – effects of growth medium modification. *J. Micronutr. Anal.*, **3**, 55–67.

Wilson, S.D. and Horne, D.W. (1984) High-performance liquid chromatographic determination of the distribution of naturally occurring folic acid derivatives in rat liver. *Analyt. Biochem.*, **142**, 529–35.

Ziegler, S.J., Meier, B. and Sticher, O. (1987) Rapid and sensitive determination of dehydroascorbic acid in addition to ascorbic acid by reversed-phase high performance liquid chromatography using a post-column reduction system. *J. Chromat.*, **391**, 419–26.

Index

Page numbers in **bold** type refer to figures and those in *italics* refer to tables.

GPSR Compliance

The European Union's (EU) General Product Safety Regulation (GPSR) is a set of rules that requires consumer products to be safe and our obligations to ensure this.

If you have any concerns about our products, you can contact us on ProductSafety@springernature.com

In case Publisher is established outside the EU, the EU authorized representative is:

Springer Nature Customer Service Center GmbH
Europaplatz 3
69115 Heidelberg, Germany

Batch number: 10682207

Printed by Printforce, the Netherlands